INTEGRATED RESEARCH METHODS IN PUBLIC HEALTH

INTEGRATED RESEARCH METHODS IN PUBLIC HEALTH

MURIEL JEAN HARRIS
BARAKA MUVUKA

JB JOSSEY-BASS
A Wiley Brand

© 2023 John Wiley & Sons, Inc.

All rights reserved. No part of this publication may be reproduced, stored in a retrieval system, or transmitted, in any form or by any means, electronic, mechanical, photocopying, recording or otherwise, except as permitted by law. Advice on how to obtain permission to reuse material from this title is available at http://www.wiley.com/go/permissions.

The right of Muriel Jean Harris and Baraka Muvuka to be identified as the author of this work has been asserted in accordance with law.

Registered Office
John Wiley & Sons, Inc., 111 River Street, Hoboken, NJ 07030, USA

Editorial Office
111 River Street, Hoboken, NJ 07030, USA

For details of our global editorial offices, customer services, and more information about Wiley products visit us at www.wiley.com.

Wiley also publishes its books in a variety of electronic formats and by print-on-demand. Some content that appears in standard print versions of this book may not be available in other formats.

Limit of Liability/Disclaimer of Warranty

The contents of this work are intended to further general scientific research, understanding, and discussion only and are not intended and should not be relied upon as recommending or promoting scientific method, diagnosis, or treatment by physicians for any particular patient. In view of ongoing research, equipment modifications, changes in governmental regulations, and the constant flow of information relating to the use of medicines, equipment, and devices, the reader is urged to review and evaluate the information provided in the package insert or instructions for each medicine, equipment, or device for, among other things, any changes in the instructions or indication of usage and for added warnings and precautions. While the publisher and authors have used their best efforts in preparing this work, they make no representations or warranties with respect to the accuracy or completeness of the contents of this work and specifically disclaim all warranties, including without limitation any implied warranties of merchantability or fitness for a particular purpose. No warranty may be created or extended by sales representatives, written sales materials or promotional statements for this work. The fact that an organization, website, or product is referred to in this work as a citation and/or potential source of further information does not mean that the publisher and authors endorse the information or services the organization, website, or product may provide or recommendations it may make. This work is sold with the understanding that the publisher is not engaged in rendering professional services. The advice and strategies contained herein may not be suitable for your situation. You should consult with a specialist where appropriate. Further, readers should be aware that websites listed in this work may have changed or disappeared between when this work was written and when it is read. Neither the publisher nor authors shall be liable for any loss of profit or any other commercial damages, including but not limited to special, incidental, consequential, or other damages.

Library of Congress Cataloging-in-Publication Data

Names: Harris, Muriel, 1989– author. | Muvuka, Baraka, author.
Title: Integrated research methods in public health / Muriel Harris, Baraka Muvuka.
Description: First edition. | Hoboken, NJ : Jossey-Bass, [2023] | Includes bibliographical references and index.
Identifiers: LCCN 2022026758 (print) | LCCN 2022026759 (ebook) | ISBN 9781119619888 (paperback) | ISBN 9781119619901 (adobe pdf) | ISBN 9781119619895 (epub)
Subjects: LCSH: Public health—Research—Methodology.
Classification: LCC RA440.85 .H38 2023 (print) | LCC RA440.85 (ebook) | DDC 362.1072—dc23/eng/20220715
LC record available at https://lccn.loc.gov/2022026758
LC ebook record available at https://lccn.loc.gov/2022026759

Cover Design: Wiley
Cover Image: © Jorg Greuel/DigitalVision/Getty Images

Set in 12/14 pts and Times New Roman MT Std by Straive

DEDICATION

Muriel Jean Harris' Dedication
To the memory of my twin brother, Howard Evelyn Cummings, of blessed memory.

Baraka Muvuka's Dedication
To my husband, Steven O. Nwaokolo, and parents, Dr. Muteho Kasongo and Dr. Kambale Karafuli, for their unconditional love and support.

CONTENTS

Preface	xi
Acknowledgments	xiii
About the Companion Website	xv

1 MODULE 1: SETTING THE STAGE FOR PUBLIC HEALTH RESEARCH — 1

Section 1: Fundamental Concepts in Research	2
Introduction	2
Philosophical Underpinnings	7
Theoretical and Conceptual Frameworks	11
Human Subjects Protection	13
Section 2: Research Study Design Framework	20
The Research Study Design Framework	20
Funding Research	31
Section 3: Conducting The Literature Review	34
Types of Literature Reviews	34
The Literature Review Process	38
References	52

2 MODULE 2: QUANTITATIVE RESEARCH — 55

Section 1: Basic Principles of Quantitative Research	56
Introduction	56
Philosophical Underpinning	56
Ethical Responsibilities	57
Cultural Responsiveness	58
Research Designs	58
Threats to Validity	63
Step 2A: Designing and Implementing the Research Study	66
Introduction	66
Planning for Research	66
Designing the Study	74
Survey Research Design	78
Sampling	83
Sample Size Calculations	87
Step 2B: Designing and Implementing the Research Study	89
Designing a Survey Instrument	89
Translating Survey Instruments	99

Step 2C: Designing and Implementing the Research Study	102
Collecting Survey Data	103
Distributing and Delivering Surveys	104
Step 2D: Designing and Implementing the Research Study	108
Analyzing and Interpreting the Survey Data	109
Step 3: Pulling It All Together: An Overview of Grant Writing	121
Introduction	121
Application and Review	130
References	133

3 MODULE 3: QUALITATIVE RESEARCH METHODS — 149

Section 1: Introduction to Qualitative Research	150
Introduction	150
Philosophical Underpinnings	151
Attributes of Qualitative Research	151
When to Use Qualitative Research	153
Qualitative Research Designs	154
The Qualitative Research Process	161
Section 2: Conceptualizing A Qualitative Research Study	163
Introduction	163
Selecting a Broad Research Area	164
Defining the Research Topic	165
Conducting a Literature Review For a Qualitative Research Study	170
Defining the Research Problem	171
Defining The Purpose of The Study	174
Formulating the Research Questions	175
Using Theoretical and Conceptual Frameworks in Qualitative Research	178
Section 3: Designing and Implementing a Qualitative Research Study	180
Introduction	181
Writing a Qualitative Research Proposal	181
Ethical Considerations	183
Selecting the Study Sites and Participants	187
Collecting Qualitative Data	192
Ensuring the Trustworthiness of the Findings	205
Managing Qualitative Data	206
Analyzing and Interpreting Qualitative Data	208
Reporting and Disseminating the Research Findings	212
References	218

4 MODULE 4: RESEARCH METHODOLOGY—MIXED METHODS APPROACHES — 223

Introduction	223
Section 1: Mixed Methods Design	224
Introduction	224

Philosophical Underpinning	225
Theoretical Frameworks in Mixed Methods Research	226
Convergent/Concurrent Designs	229
Sequential Designs	231
Complex Designs	233
Ethical Responsibilities	241
Informed Consent	241
Cultural Responsiveness	241
Section 2: The Two Paradigms—Mixed Methods Research Designing the Research Study	243
Planning for Research	243
Quantitative Data	253
GIS Mapping	255
Qualitative Research	255
Individual Interviews	255
Report the Findings	260
Data Transformation	261
Ethical Considerations	262
Section 3: Case Study—Embedded Mixed Methods Design	264
Introduction	264
Literature Review And Problem Statement	265
Individual Factors	266
Interpersonal Factors	266
Community Factors	267
Organizational Factors	267
Policy Factors	267
Best Practices in Prenatal Care	268
Evaluation Design	268
The Study Setting	269
Methodology	270
Review of Existing Databases	270
Patients, Providers, and Staff Surveys (Quant)	270
Observations (Qual)	271
Document Review (Qual)	271
GIS Mapping (Qual)	271
Data Analysis	271
Results	271
A Review of Family Health Centers' Prenatal Care Materials and Website	275
Provider and Staff Recommendations to Increase Early Entry into PNC	278
Discussion	279
Recommendations	280
The Literature Review and Problem Statement	280
Conclusions	291

Study Limitations	291
Acknowledgment	291
References	292

5 MODULE 5: WRITING AND DISSEMINATING THE RESEARCH FINDINGS — 295

Section 1: Writing the Research Report	296
Introduction	296
The Structure and Content of the Report	297
Reporting Guidelines and Tools	302
Ethical, Legal, and Cultural Considerations in Writing a Research Report	304
Section 2: Disseminating the Report to Academic Audiences	309
Introduction	309
The Peer-Review Process of a Journal Article	320
Scientific Conference Presentations	322
Ethical Considerations in Publishing The Findings	325
Section 3: Disseminating The Report To Nonacademic Audiences	326
Introduction	326
Disseminating the Findings to Practitioners	327
Disseminating the Findings to Communities or The General Public	327
Disseminating the Findings to Policymakers	332
Disseminating the Findings to the Media	335
References	339

INDEX — 343

PREFACE

Integrated Research Methods in Public Health is inspired by our collective research, teaching, and service experiences in diverse sociocultural contexts. It is also informed by theoretical and empirical evidence on effective research and pedagogical approaches. Its pedagogical underpinning rests on the co-construction of learning, which requires the active participation of both students and instructors in the learning process within an interactive, inclusive, and learner-centered environment. Since we perceive learners as active participants in their own learning, our specific objectives are to (a) empower learners to become critically engaged, analytical, reflective, and independent researchers; (b) facilitate mastery and integration of fundamental research concepts and frameworks; and (c) enable the development and application of core research competencies. This book therefore incorporates real-world examples, practical mini case studies, and interactive individual and small group exercises or assessments (stop, think, and apply) to prompt learners' active participation, critical thinking, problem-solving, and knowledge application (Figure P.1).

This book's design centers integrative learning. Traditional approaches to teaching are siloed and organized into fragmented or stand-alone chapters, with minimal integration of concepts across chapters. Learning should not be a siloed process; integrative teaching and learning approaches connecting core concepts enable students to develop a holistic mental model that facilitates knowledge application and translation. This book incorporates strategies to help learners develop mental models and connect new information to prior knowledge. For instance, we encourage concept mapping to visually display and explain relationships between concepts. More specifically, this book presents fundamental research concepts and frameworks while integrating the following overarching concepts across the five modules: literature review, philosophical underpinnings, stakeholder engagement, ethics, and cultural considerations.

FIGURE P.1. *The conceptual model for teaching and learning integrated research methods in public health.*

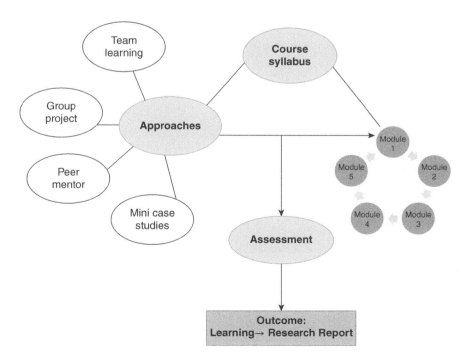

FIGURE P.2. *The iterative research model of the integrated research methods in public health book.*

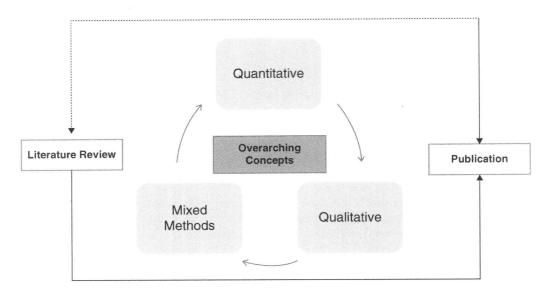

The iterative research model of the integrated research methods in public health book provides co-constructive and integrative approaches intended to enable transformational learning (Figure P.2). Learning is a lifelong process of transforming one's knowledge, beliefs, attitudes, skills, and behaviors. It is influenced by a combination of learner, educator, and contextual factors including the learner's background, learner's level of engagement, learner's self-efficacy, instructional design and delivery, educator's teaching philosophy, educator's background, and the learning environment. This book's readings, examples, and exercises are designed to build learners' skills in key research areas such as conducting a literature review, designing a research study, grant writing, and writing for publication. They also provide learners with the opportunity to reflect and think critically about core research components including the researcher's theoretical and philosophical orientations, social justice, ethics, and community-centered research. The book incorporates cultural references and examples from diverse settings to transform the learner's perspectives on these issues.

Overall, this book presents an iterative research model in the following five modules:

Module 1: Setting the Stage for Public Health Research
Module 2: Quantitative Research Methods
Module 3: Qualitative Research Methods
Module 4: Mixed Methods Approaches
Module 5: Writing and Disseminating the Research Findings

This book is designed to serve as a primary textbook for academics and researchers in the fields of public health, allied health professions, and social sciences. The following are the intended primary users:

- Senior undergraduates and graduate students in public health required to write a thesis or dissertation as a culminating product

- Students and academics in public health, allied health, and social sciences research oriented toward social justice and cultural competency

- Public health practitioners and other staff in public health-oriented organizations who conduct research, needs assessments, or program evaluation

ACKNOWLEDGMENTS

We would like to acknowledge our students, mentors, colleagues, and community partners with whom we engaged in the critical and challenging research conversations that inspired this work.

ABOUT THE COMPANION WEBSITE

This book is accompanied by an instructor's companion website found here: www.wiley.com/go/harris/integratedresearchmethods.

It contains the following components:

- Instructor's manual
- Test banks
- PowerPoint lecture slides

CHAPTER 1

MODULE 1: SETTING THE STAGE FOR PUBLIC HEALTH RESEARCH

Module 1 sets the stage for research in public health and provides an overview of the research study design and approach. Concepts in this chapter will be developed further in module 2 (Quantitative Research), module 3 (Qualitative Research), module 4 (Mixed Methods Research), and module 5 (Writing and Disseminating the Research Findings). This module is divided into three sections. The first section provides an overview of the research and describes its philosophical underpinnings, specifically in its application to public health. The second section describes stakeholder engagement and culturally appropriate research approaches and considerations. The final section considers ethical concerns before and during the conduct of research and provides the reader with a systematic approach to conducting a literature review. Each section focuses on one module learning objective.

By the end of Module 1, learners will be able to:

1. Explain the fundamental concepts in research.

2. Outline a study using the research study design framework.

3. Conduct a literature review as the first step to conducting the research study.

Integrated Research Methods In Public Health, First Edition. Muriel Jean Harris and Baraka Muvuka.
© 2023 John Wiley & Sons, Inc. Published 2023 by John Wiley & Sons, Inc.
Companion website: www.wiley.com/go/harris/integratedresearchmethods

Module 1: Setting the Stage for Public Health Research

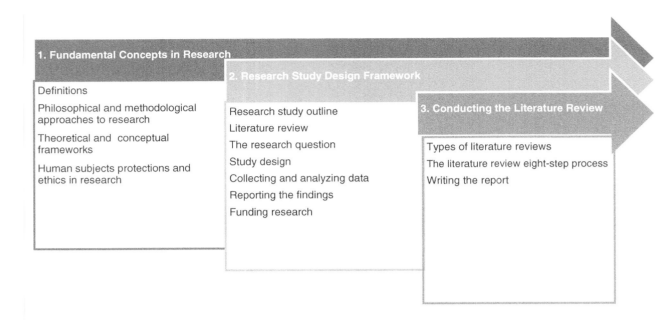

SECTION 1: FUNDAMENTAL CONCEPTS IN RESEARCH

By the end of this section, learners will be able to:

- Explain the fundamentals of the research enterprise.
- Compare the different philosophical and methodological approaches to research.
- Apply ethical standards to research.

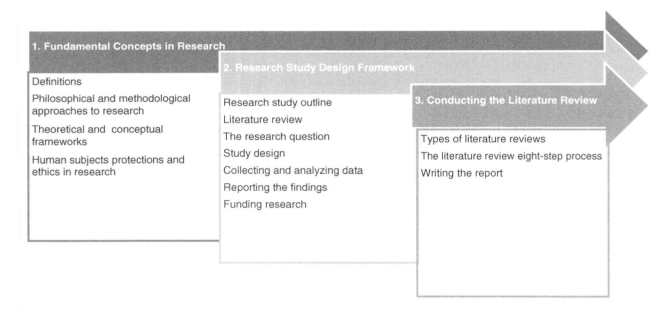

INTRODUCTION

Research is a detailed study of a subject to discover information or achieve a new understanding. It may be described as a careful search, a studious inquiry, or an examination of a particular subject. It is also defined as a systematic investigation designed to develop or contribute to generalizable knowledge. The National Academy of Sciences states that the intent of research is to "extend human knowledge of the physical, biological, social world beyond what is already known" (US Department of Health and Human Services, www.ori.hhs.gov). Traditionally, research is undertaken to gather evidence for practice; for understanding a phenomenon; or for the purposes of developing programs or policy. Yet others have come to define research in more transformative terms (Chilisa, 2012; Lapan et al., 2012) in indigenous approaches that are rooted in relationships and foster authentic partnerships with local communities to challenge deficit thinking and empower people to change society through their empowerment. This research is informed by critical theory, postcolonial discourse, feminist, and race-specific theories.

The systematic method that encapsulates positivist and postpositivist thought depends on quantifiable observations, which create and test hypotheses specifying factors important to study and how they are interrelated. The initial factors are discoverable through a systematic review of the literature. The observations are usually obtained from surveys and lead to statistical analyses that clarify hypothesized relationships. Postpositivist research emphasizes statistical, mathematical, and numerical data to quantify attitudes and opinions of individuals about a range of characteristics, situations, and phenomena. The data are presented in graphs, tables, and charts.

However, qualitative research encapsulates an inductive approach, in a process of naturalistic inquiry that seeks to understand social phenomena. It focuses on the reasoning behind behaviors, actions, or situations. It uses data primarily from open-ended questions in focus group and individual interviews as well as pictorial, video, and observational approaches that are analyzed through content and thematic analysis or grounded theory approaches. Qualitative research is generally described as dealing with words and meanings.

What Is Research?

It is important to strive for a full and complete understanding of a phenomenon through valid research before drawing conclusions, recognizing that our actions are based in assumptions and research opens doors to our understanding. A poem by John Godfrey Saxe (1816–1887) describes very vividly how six blind men of Indostan went to see an elephant, and each came back with a very different perception of the elephant based on their assumptions and what they observed. As they encountered different parts of the elephant's body, they thought it felt like a wall, spear, snake, tree, fan, and rope. Each thought he was right. The writer closes the poem by saying, "Though each was partly in the right, all were in the wrong" (Saxe, 1873).

In many ways, researchers are like those six blind men as they investigate a question and try to get to the right answer. It is only over time, with each of us conducting valid studies, that we arrive collectively at somewhat of the right answer. Research approaches require applying a framework based on standard philosophical foundations, appropriate methods, skills, and procedures to produce valid and unbiased and repeatable results. Valid research therefore is based not on a particular philosophical approach but instead on "well-grounded or justifiable: being at once relevant and meaningful."

Basic research, which is the most familiar, often characterizes positivism and postpositivism inquiry as associated with the development of methods and expanding existing scientific knowledge. In contrast, applied research primarily assesses situations for the purposes of furthering knowledge or evaluating programs, policies, or persons. It differs from basic research by being related to understanding why and how well an intervention or policy worked and whether it worked for particular stakeholders in an analysis that has a health equity lens. Research questions in basic research are usually dictated by the researcher's agenda, whereas applied research is dictated by the needs of the stakeholder (Harris, 2017). Ultimately, research is a process of solving problems and finding facts in an organized and systematic way. It is undertaken by applying what is known and building on it. Knowledge is gained, new theories are built, or old theories are tested by trying to better understand and explain observations or phenomena of interest around us. To think critically is to consider that theories explain how the world is supposed to work and to recognize that theories change as the variables that make up that theory also change (Brookfield, 2012). Many theories were developed many years ago yet today must be applied to a very different population. To do this, we must reconceptualize theory and consider constructs through a cultural lens. This may well require incorporating constructs from other theories and through other lenses such as feminism or critical race theory.

Formal research occurs in a range of environments, but it happens all the time in our daily lives without us realizing it. Consider for a minute the decisions surrounding what outfit you'll wear on a particular day. You might:

- Check the weather on your weather app.
- Look up the day's agenda—meetings or not, dress up or down (formal, business casual, informal).
- Assess the options depending on the activities of the day.

In some ways, this is how traditional research steps work, but it gets a little more involved with public health.

What Is Public Health Research?

The art and science of preventing disease and prolonging life, public health is a component of the health sciences that:

- Detects and tracks disease including outbreaks
- Prevents injury
- Works to ensure that all people are given the chance to be healthy through
  - Promoting healthy lifestyles
  - Clean, healthy, and safe environments for individuals to be born, live, work, play, and be fulfilled
- Addresses the causes of illness and disease

It is undergirded by the social justice principle that health is a right and that everyone has the right to live in a community that supports their health. The National Education Association defines it as "a concept in which equity or justice is achieved in every aspect of society rather than in only some aspects or for some people" (http://www.nea.org/tools/30414.htm).

Research is "a detailed study of a subject, especially to (new) information or reach a (new) understanding (Cambridge Dictionary, n.d). In public health the topics span the gamut from identifying risk factors resulting in disease and disability to pinpointing individuals' behaviors influencing the environment and the environment's influence on individuals and their behavior. Public health recognizes that individuals are healthy only when their environments are safe and healthy, and it challenges us to provide an equitable society where all people can be healthy. The environment is defined as being at multiple spheres of influence: the interpersonal, community, institutional and policy levels. It includes the social, physical, and political environment. Topics that have been researched include communicable (e.g., sexually transmitted infections like HIV/AIDS, Ebola, and COVID) and noncommunicable diseases (e.g., diabetes, heart disease), access and opportunities for healthy living (e.g., healthy foods, exercise, safety), mental and emotional health, violence (e.g., intimate partner, guns), and maternal and child health. In addition, the focus of the research question could be on the geographic area, a particular time frame, a population group, or a particular area of the health care sector. It can also embrace the social or physical environment.

Who Conducts Research?

Research is conducted by a range of persons in any profession. It is conducted in medicine to answer critical questions regarding patient health, in education to answer questions related to education at elementary, secondary, tertiary or community levels, in history, or engineering as well as in public health. While a range of persons in any profession can carry out an investigation to answer a question or solve a problem, this book will focus on individuals at various stages of their careers as students or as fully trained professionals who are attempting to address population-level influences that impact health outcomes at the individual and environmental level. Most importantly, systematic research requires skills in areas that range across the spectrum from designing a research study to reporting on the findings from the study. Research may take place in a laboratory, classroom, or field setting. The field or natural setting may be in the community, the hospital, or any other site where individuals who might be participants in the research may be found. The individual who has overall responsibility for the research study is generally referred to as the principal investigator (PI), and others on the research team may include staff scientists, clinical fellows, postdoctoral fellows, and medical and graduate students. Each person on the team bears responsibility for ensuring the research study is conducted in such a way as to ensure the results are valid and replicable.

Cross-Cultural Research

Culture plays an important role in determining the validity of research requiring researchers to be culturally competent. Perez and Luquis (2008) identify three characteristics in working cross culturally as, cultural desire, cultural awareness and cultural sensitivity. The ability to be a culturally responsive public health researcher requires awareness, knowledge, skill, and cultural dexterity (Figure 1.1). Additional skills include having the capacity to listen, communicate, understand, and respond genuinely to a given situation. Valid research requires the researcher is authentic and possesses the ability to work effectively and develop meaningful relationships with people of various cultural backgrounds. It requires that in the absence of these traits, researchers surround themselves with stakeholders who have the dexterity and the ability to conduct culturally relevant and culturally appropriate research.

FIGURE 1.1. *Components of culturally responsive research.*

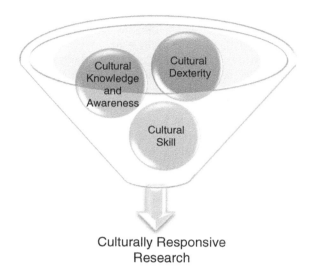

In collective cultures, custom requires that permission is sought from the chief or other leaders to enter the community to conduct research. However, this permission is not a substitute for individual permissions and informed consent (CIOMS, 2002, 2016). Communication must be in the local language. The onus is on the researcher to ensure that the potential research participants understand the contents of the consent form, especially if there are unfamiliar concepts like clinical trials or investigative therapies (CIOMS, 2002, 2016).

Differences in backgrounds that result in cross-cultural missteps include race, age, gender, beliefs, customs, language, or behaviors. The difference may emanate from researchers being from different regions of the world or country or different sides of town or from varied educational levels and academic disciplines. These differences influence how we interact as well as the appropriate methodology for answering the research question. As we engage in new spaces, we must also be aware that what might be acceptable in one culture is not necessarily acceptable in another, and a gesture in one group might be offensive in another. We must take the time to learn about the groups we intend to work with before we engage in our research. It shows respect and a cultural sensitivity that will invariably lead to our success. It also means that every stage of the research process must be recognized as being a cultural encounter, and the more authentic the encounter, the more likely it is that the data collected will be valid (Casado et al., 2012).

Stakeholder Engagement

One way to build cross-cultural understanding is to engage stakeholders. This includes anyone interested in the research, whether it be positive or negative. While negative stakeholders may provide a more challenging environment to work in, our engagement with that group may be the difference between our success and our failure. There are multiple opportunities for engaging citizens during the process. However, it is important to pay attention to issues of power and difference, particularly when engaging disadvantaged and marginalized groups (Pratt, 2019). They are most likely to be involved in participatory research approaches when the goals of sharing power, shaping the research questions, and creating change that is beneficial to the community require that marginalized and disadvantaged groups have a voice at the table (Pratt, 2019).

In addition to the expected team of researchers, the success and validity of the work depends on the engagement of stakeholders. In this instance, stakeholders are defined as community members who provide insights that help ensure the data collected are both reliable and valid. They provide input into the culture and community norms of the community. They facilitate the process and provide legitimacy for the research. Their participation can be symbolic (i.e., cooperation and involvement in Hwang ecoordination) or active, meaning they are fully engaged in decision-making as evidenced in community-based participatory research (Goodman and Thompson, 2017). In a study of clinical trials recruitment planning, Huang et al. (2018) identified a role of stakeholders as being actively engaged in the protocol design. Research that relies less on stakeholders for input may engage members of the community only in the data collection aspects of the study.

Irrespective of what role they play researchers are an important constituency. Some stakeholders are engaged in the design stage of the research, in the conceptualization of the research question, in conducting the literature review, in providing a keen eye in the methodological aspects of the study, or in ensuring that the study is ethical (Harris, 2017). Others may assist in identifying a study population and helping collect the data. Stakeholder participation is critical in ensuring that the study population is knowledgeable about the work and is willing to participate. Of course, there are those who, when it is all said and done, will be most critical in ensuring the research findings from the study are made actionable. These are the practitioners. The new normal in health research is that findings must have some value for changing lives, hence the increasing importance more recently in translational research. In his commentary, Woolf (2008) highlights the importance of translational research, emphasizing its focus by the National Institutes of Health in the United States and the European Commission. In both cases, he says, translational research centers have been established to further this field of research. In an application of the translational research process, Love et al. (2019) were able to scale their infant program within the health care delivery system.

Strekalova (2018) identified two important factors in the recruitment of participants for research: communication and the perceptions that potential participants have given certain terms. *Clinical trial* was the least popular term in their study, whereas the *health-related research* was associated with the highest intention to participate (Strekalova, 2018). Organization, values, and practices are identified as three principles related to stakeholder engagement for effective practice in a systematic review by Boaz et al. (2018). At the organizational level, engagement requires a clarification of objectives and roles, while the values of engagement are expectations of the relationship and factors that are important to foster such as shared commitment for the present and future. The value, however, of stakeholders is enhanced when there is a plan for how stakeholders are engaged in the work as well as a flexibility that allows the stakeholder who may be a volunteer to enter and leave the relationship in ways that enhance their value to the team and to the volunteer (Table 1.1).

Indigenous research reaffirms the importance of roles and responsibilities of researchers and stakeholder partners in the community and considers multiple expectations that include incorporating the new and different worldviews, values and cultures of indigenous peoples, assuming roles of transformative healers, and promoting a relational approach to research. In promoting a relational approach, consent is both individual and collective, incorporating researcher reflectivity informed by an I–we relationship (Chilisa, 2012). Euro-Western research includes attention in language to issues of gender, race, ethnicity, ableness, health, socioeconomic status, sexual orientation, and age, which often seeks to highlight their *otherness* and identify it as different from indigenous and ethnic research, which seeks to be inclusive in its methodologies. Ways of knowing in indigenous and ethnic knowledge systems are shaped by an

TABLE 1.1. Principles Associated with Stakeholder Engagement in Research

Principle	Characteristics
Organization	▪ Clarify objectives ▪ Embed stakeholder engagement in the research framework ▪ Identify resources ▪ Ensure organizational learning ▪ Rewards ▪ Allow stakeholders to play key roles
Values	▪ Foster a shared commitment of stakeholder engagement ▪ Encourage the engagement of stakeholders across organizations ▪ Recognize potential tension between productivity and inclusion ▪ Generate a shared commitment for continued stakeholder engagement
Practices	▪ Plan for stakeholder engagement as part of the work ▪ Build in flexibility to ensure meaningful engagement ▪ Incorporate systematic data collection to allow for full participation of stakeholders ▪ Recognize the iterative and ongoing involvement of stakeholders

ongoing struggle to resist a continual assault on their culture by those from the outside whose research paradigms are different from their own. Indigenous and ethic research operates within four dimensions that (a) identify local issues and concerns to define the research question, (b) ensure context sensitivity that create locally relevant approaches, (c) integrate all cultural perspectives and what counts as reality, and (d) embeds its research approaches in knowledge and values that are informed by local culture (Chilisa, 2012). Therefore, centering indigenous and ethnic people and their approaches in research is both a research and ethical responsibility (Chilisa, 2012; Lahman, 2018) and one that, if embraced, increases the credibility of the research.

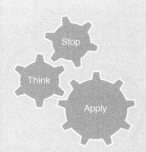

Identifying our Assumptions about Research!

Discuss the following questions in groups of two to three.

- How do you see the world?
- How would you define your approach to research?
- What makes you define it this way?
- What assumptions do you bring into your research?
- What experiences do you have that have helped you develop this worldview? (f) How is your present worldview likely to influence your research agenda and practice?

Remember: there is no right or wrong answer. We all see the world differently based on our myriad experiences growing up and as we learn about the world around us.

Write down your philosophy of research in a short paragraph of about 150 words. Keep it in a safe place and revisit it after your first research project. Reflect on it. Do you need to make any changes to it?

PHILOSOPHICAL UNDERPINNINGS

Philosophical underpinnings include the most basic beliefs, concepts, and attitudes of individuals or groups. In science and in public health science, research is based on a variety of assumptions that are defined by the research approach and made explicit by the researcher. Underlying the assumptions is a series of philosophical positions such as positivism and postpositivism, adopted in qualitative research and constructivism and transformativism, which are related to qualitative research.

Positivism and Postpositivism

Positivism is associated with quantitative research and is the more traditional form of research and most often referred to as "scientific" research. This approach is usually associated with conducting surveys with closed-ended questions often created as a result of extensive research to understand the factors being included in the research. This approach is challenged by researchers in favor of what is referred to the postpositivist approach. Postpositivist research challenges the notion that scientific research gets at the truth and holds that there is a relationship between the cause and the effect or outcome. In spite of the challenge, however, it retains the basic assumptions of positivism, the possibility and desirability of an objective truth, and the use of experimental design methodologies. It is controlled, rigorous, systematic, verifiable, empirical research with the ability to withstand critical scrutiny (Kumar, 2014). In real life and with human behavior it is almost impossible to control the process and the outcome,

TABLE 1.2. An Overview of Epidemiology Study Designs

Study name	Description
Case–control	Individuals are selected on the basis of the outcome after the exposure had already been determined where those with the outcome are considered cases, while those without are controls
Cohort	Compares exposure before cases are detected and measures incidence over time within the same group of individuals
Cross-sectional	Compares the prevalence of the outcome or the phenomenon and the exposure simultaneously taking a cross section of the population
Ecological	Population level observational studies that assess prevalence or incidence of cases using cross-sectional or cohort methods
Intervention	Compares intervention and control groups in experimental or quasi-experimental research designs

although laboratory science and experimental research may achieve this. One example of a research approach that achieves control involves mice or plants in a controlled environment. Public health researchers—specifically epidemiologists—who have a positivist or postpositivist approach to research use five primary methodologies involving quantitative data (Table 1.2).

Constructivism

Constructivist researchers on the other hand believe that individuals develop meanings from their lived experience and as such they rely on the perspectives of the research participants. Unlike postpositivists, they do not believe that theory and practice can be separated, but that theory drives practice and vice versa and practice exists both before and after theory (Mir and Watson, 2000). Constructivists challenge the notion that research is impartial, detached and value neutral and argue that theory drives empirical research, including what gets researched and what measurement techniques are used (Mir and Watson, 2000). Qualitative data forms the basis for this type of research and may involve individual and group interviews, documents, photographs, song, drama, or various forms of art (Table 1.3). I was fascinated a few years ago when I listened to a lecture of the analysis of form, colors, and content of graffiti by a qualitative researcher. In this philosophical approach, the researcher tries to understand the social, cultural, and historical context of the material through iterative questioning and relies on continual construction of the narrative. Rather than starting with the theory as the positivist and the post positivist, the constructivist develops patterns from within the data as the narrative unfolds to develop a theory or identify common patterns.

> Critical research asks about the sources of inequality and oppression in society, how language and communication patterns oppress and how individuals achieve autonomy

Within this paradigm there are two perspectives, *interpretivist and the critical research*. Interpretivist research includes interviews, narrative inquiry, ethnography, case study, photovoice, arts-based and program evaluation (Bartlett and Vavrus, 2017). The interpretivist approach is rooted in the social constructivist approach emphasizing the importance of the experience of the respondent and exploring the meanings associated with their actions with a strong focus on qualitative research. While critical research focuses on issues of power embedded in the structure of society and how individuals become empowered through principles of social justice to eventually change society (Lapan et al., 2012; Mertens and Wilson, 2019; Oparah et al., 2015).

TABLE 1.3. An Overview of Common Qualitative Research Approaches

Study name	Description
Arts-based	Research approach that employs any form of art to raise questions about social issues, social practices and cultural artifacts.
Case study	Research approach to describe complex phenomena of a case that sets out to answer questions about the entity or to support the development of theory or the explanation of a phenomena
Ethnography	Primarily used by anthropologists to interpret culture from an emic(internal) or etic (outside) perspective and capture the very essence of the society using observation, individual, and group interviews
Interview	Used to gather information either at the individual (in-depth or key informant) or group level (focus group)
Narrative Inquiry	Includes biography, autobiography, life story research and oral history as they allow the participant to be reflective as they describe their surroundings, note actions and participate in a dialogue with the researcher
Phenomenology	Describes the lived experience from the perspective of the respondent through a series of individual interviews
Photovoice	Involves study participants taking photographs on a given theme, describing the photograph(s) and discussing them in group sessions with the goal of building consciousness and subsequent action

Participatory Research

The fundamental difference between basic research and applied research is in their purpose. Basic research is conducted for the purpose of exploring issues and the relationships between them based on the researcher's initiative while applied research is undertaken for the purpose of addressing and exploring issues in close association with identifying solutions for action. It is driven by the community's needs. Action research is one of many participatory research approaches that fall into the category of applied research. Research on social actions that could lead to changes in the community and further action is referred to as action research. Action research and other participatory action research emphasize empowerment and critical consciousness of participants in collaborative relationships with academic partners. They draw from the philosophical foundations of critical theory and use qualitative and quantitative methodologies with the intentional integration of data in mixed model designs (Creswell and Creswell, 2018). Participatory approaches strive for a true partnership with the community, utilize an ecological framework and adopt a worldview that recognizes the individual is within and influenced by the social determinants of health and equity.

In community-based participatory action research, a social justice-based approach gives voice to those who are the subjects of the research and is intended to reinforce practices that are action oriented and have the potential to sustain those who are researched. Participatory research is a philosophy that focuses on multiple ways of knowing based on reciprocity with community members, collaborative decision-making, and power sharing. These methodologies require full participation of community members in putting the plans that are described in the final report, into action followed by their evaluation. The most important feature however of participatory research is in building trust, reciprocity, and a shared vision (Christopher et al., 2008). Reflecting on the process and ensuring that there is a significant element of knowledge sharing and skills building are important components.

Transformative Research

Transformative research holds that the inquiry is intertwined with a political change agenda to confront social oppression in an act of self-determination and community transformation focusing on issues of power and addressing inequities (Mertens and Wilson, 2019; Oparah et al., 2015). This type of research emerged from the work of Paulo Freire who through conscientization helped poor women in South America to move toward the awareness of power and oppression and learn how to act on their own behalf (Frier, 2018). It includes and results in change to the lives and the institutions where people live. The social justice approach to research is achieved when research gives voice to those who are the subjects of the research and ensures that marginalized peoples are at the center of the research. Marginalized and "othered" groups are identified based on age, race, socioeconomic status, sexual orientation, migration, geographic residence and physical or emotional ability.

Indigenous research refers to the non-Euro western cultural ways of knowing and focuses on the reality of diverse cultural groups (Chilisa, 2012). Like indigenous research, social justice moves the research from a deficit to an empowerment-based approach in a participatory research methodology that has multiple advantages. Indigenous research helps to (a) increase the likelihood that the researcher will complete the research, (b) provide support for the recruitment and retention of study participants, (c) facilitate the investments and commitments from the participants, and (d) ensure that interventions developed as a result of the research are culturally relevant and effective.

Participatory rural appraisal is also classified as a people centered approach that allows researchers to learn from those being researched in a process that facilitates the community's ownership of the research process and outcomes. The three principles emphasized in this participatory research approach are as follows (Chilisa, 2012):

a. Be flexible, creative, patient, respectful, and willing to listen.

b. Present information and ideas visually so that nonreaders, persons with disabilities, the elderly, and children are able to participate.

c. Use multiple methods such as local history, narratives and folklore, songs, poetry, and dance in mixed methods designs to increase precision in measurement.

Like Oparah et al, (2015), Chilisa (2012) argues for a relationship between the researchers and the researched based on an ethically responsible partnership where the researched are involved in decision-making and what is being written and disseminated about them (Oparah et al., 2015).

> *"Those of us whose bodies are metaphorically placed under a scalpel are seldom consulted about the research agendas, design, findings, or recommendations"* (p. 117).

Author and advocate Chimamanda Ngozi Adichie (n.d) describes "The Danger of a Single Story" and defines our lives as composed of many overlapping stories. A useful analogy in research is the danger of a single approach relying on one methodology to tell the whole story and answer the research question completely. It is true that research benefits from overlapping philosophies. The researcher's perceptions of reality, what counts as knowledge, and what is valued determines the research questions, the data collection approaches, how the results are interpreted, and how and to whom they are disseminated. Distributing research only among other researchers in peer-reviewed publications denies the community of knowing what was discovered about them and the opportunity to defend themselves when they are misrepresented. Research should and must be viewed from multiple perspectives and paradigms if it is to fully understand the phenomenon being observed. Cross-cultural or multicultural research involves conducting research across cultures, countries, and populations. It primarily involves ethnographic research and focuses on systematic comparisons that answer questions about incidence, distribution, causes of disease, and associations of cultural variation in unbiased, reliable, and replicable designs (Ember and Ember, 2009). However, cross-cultural research may also be conducted across populations considering aspects of public health other than a focus on disease.

Pragmatism

Pragmatism as a worldview describes an approach to research that considers an action's consequences, is centered on problem, is pluralistic, and is oriented in the real world in contrast to the postpositivist view, which focuses on the antecedents of actions or conditions. Pragmatism adopts a mixed methods approach to research (Creswell and Creswell, 2018). Summarizing the work of multiple researchers, Creswell and Creswell (2018) provide the components of what they consider to be the basis for this approach to research (pp. 10–11):

- Not committing to any one system of philosophy and reality

- Determining what and how to research and adopting a systematic approach to mixing the methods
- Occurring in a social, historical, political, or other context that may include social justice study aims and lens
- Having the freedom to choose methods, techniques, and procedures across data collection and data analysis approaches

Mixed Methods

Mixed methods research integrates qualitative and quantitative data on multiple levels. It combines paradigms, methodologies, or data in myriad formats, postpositivism, constructivism, and transformative and pragmatic philosophical views (Creswell and Creswell, 2018). Kumar (2014) defines mixed methods as the use of two or more methods, either quantitative or qualitative or both, for the whole or part of a research process that contributes to the mixed or multiple methods approach (p. 23). Factors important in choosing a mixed methods design include the research questions, expected outcomes of the study, and the approach to mixing qualitative and quantitative data. There are three common approaches for conducting a mixed methods research:—convergent, explanatory, and exploratory sequential designs—and the less common complex design (Creswell and Creswell, 2018). These are described more fully in Module 4 of this book.

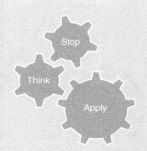

Differentiating Between the Different Philosophical Approaches

What is your research philosophy? Write a one- to two-page essay discussing your research philosophy or philosophical position. Explain why you selected this approach and how the philosophy you select guides your approach to research and its data collection methods. Make sure to use the literature to support your explanation. Cite your sources both within and at the end of the paper.

THEORETICAL AND CONCEPTUAL FRAMEWORKS

The theoretical and conceptual frameworks are situated within the philosophical paradigm (Figure 1.2) and serve as critical foundations for the research study. While the terms *theoretical* and *conceptual* are often used interchangeably, they are distinct in that the theoretical framework is developed prior to the conceptual framework. The empirical and theoretical findings derived from the literature review form the basis for developing the theoretical and conceptual frameworks guiding the study, and together they shape the researcher's perspectives and methodological decisions.

The theoretical framework is the broad theoretical lens through which the study or knowledge is processed (Merriam, 2009). It is a road map that guides the formulation of research questions and informs decisions on study design, methods, and analysis (Calba et al., 2015) formed from the literature. The theoretical framework may be based on myriad theories and their constructs across multiple disciplines, forming a theoretical lens through which knowledge related to the phenomenon is processed. The conceptual framework is the culmination of that work, with the researcher developing a conceptualization for their study grounded in the philosophical paradigm and the theoretical framework.

Quantitative studies incorporate theories from the beginning of the study and primarily test and verify these theories in the research process. While qualitative research is primarily designed to build or modify theory from the data that was collected during the study (Merriam, 2009) to offer a new or revised conceptualization of the topic. Unlike quantitative studies that start with a theoretical framework developed from the literature review, the use of a theoretical

FIGURE 1.2. *Conceptual frameworks and the research study.*

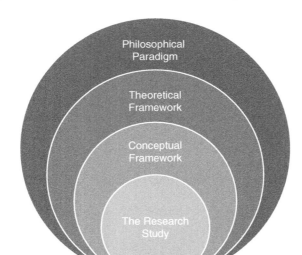

framework in qualitative research is highly variable. Some qualitative designs such as grounded theory discourage the development or utilization of a theoretical framework at the beginning of the study and aim to construct a theory that is grounded in the data. The theoretical framework informs all decisions made throughout the research process. It shapes the conceptual framework.

The conceptual framework is more specific and more concrete than a theoretical framework. It is a logical narrative or visual representation of the main ideas, concepts, and relationships that the study plans to explore (Miles and Huberman, 1994; Reichel and Ramey, 1987). It can be viewed as a concept map that displays the main concepts of the study and their interrelationships, some grounded in the literature and others based on experience and pilot or exploratory studies that might have been conducted by the researcher. Since the conceptual framework offers a tentative theory of the relationships between the main concepts of the study, the conceptual framework can be revised in light of new findings during the study for qualitative research and at the end of the data analysis for quantitative research.

Theory in Quantitative Research

In quantitative research, the researcher aims to advance theory by undertaking a study to determine if a predefined relationship between concepts is supported to explain and predict a specified outcome. The theory or combination of concepts that is identified in the literature becomes the framework or the conceptual model for the study. When concepts are specifically defined within a theory they are known as constructs that for measurement purposes are operationalized as variables (Glanz et al., 2015). Theories in research can be proposed in a number of different ways to define these relationships in (a) hypotheses, (b) "if this then that" logic statements, and (c) diagrams that depict the relationships between the constructs. Theory in research helps explain how the independent variables predict the dependent variable. Theories emerge when researchers test the relationship between variables over and over and establish the authenticity of the effect of the predictor variables on the outcome variable. The resulting theory is tested among different populations and settings. These relationships have been tested by multiple researchers using a variety of populations and settings to produce well-established theories that are in use today.

Theory in Qualitative Research

Qualitative research recognizes two primary approaches in the use of theory: (a) theory as the foundation for the study; and (b) theory as the product of research although there remains some controversy across qualitative researchers. When theory is used as the foundation of the research study, to frame the research, it may be somewhat similar to its use in quantitative research. As in quantitative research the literature is used to identify the theoretical framework upon which the conceptual framework is built. Known as the *grounded theory method*, this approach endorses the notion of multiple socially constructed realities and views the researcher and participants as active co-constructors of the knowledge that is interpreted to generate the grounded theory or conceptual framework. This approach encourages the use of the literature and formulation of research questions prior to conducting the study (Charmaz, 2014). The alternative grounded theory does not start with a literature review or a conceptual framework but intends the outcome of the study to be a theory—and in some versions a conceptual framework, model, or schema—that describes, explains, predicts, and interprets structures and processes related to the phenomenon being investigated (Sbaraini et al., 2011). Grounded theory is a constant comparative process that involves data collection, formulation and testing the theory in an iterative process. Qualitative research may be the precursor to quantitative research once the pathways between the independent variables and the dependent variable are fairly well understood or a component of mixed methods research when it may be adopted in convergent, explanatory, or complex designs.

HUMAN SUBJECTS PROTECTION

Biomedical ethics is influenced by a long history of ethics in medical practice as well as by post–World War II ethical lapses in medical research, when doctors carried out experiments in concentration camps in Nazi Germany. The violation of human rights was exposed during the Nuremburg Trials in 1947 that resulted in ethical standards being set for research with human subjects (Carlson, Boyd, and Webb, 2004; Carlson and Webb, 2004). More recently, lapses in ethical practice include the Tuskegee Study of Untreated Syphilis in the Negro Male from 1932 to 1972, that observed Black men who had syphilis and withheld treatment from them even after Penicillin became available in 1947 to research the natural course of syphilis. This study ultimately led to the US National Commission for the Protection of Human Subjects in Biomedical and Behavioral Research in 1974 with the responsibility to ensure ethical research. The Belmont Report identifies basic ethical principles and guidelines (U.S. Department of Health and Human Services, n.d.b) for use by researchers and ethics or institutional review boards. In addition, the World Medical Association adopted the Declaration of Helsinki in 1964 to guide members of the medical profession in their conduct of research. One of its provisions was the review of medical research protocols by specifically appointed ethics review committees, which are known by various names including ethics committee, institutional review board (IRB), ethical review board (ERB), research ethics committee (REC), or research ethics board (REB). They are established within a university or a government entity such as a hospital, a prevention center, or a research institute. They are made up of an independent panel of researchers and community members with primary responsibility to review and provide guidance for biomedical and sociobehavioral research.

Ethics Review Boards

Ethics boards or IRBs oversee the ethical conduct of scientific research in institutions all over the world. They are responsible for reviewing research proposals and monitoring research studies to ensure their compliance with international and local ethical codes for conducting research with human participants. IRB clearance is required for any study that is considered to be research and can be characterized as being a systematic investigation that is intended to be generalizable. Ethics or IRBs are established on federal guidelines with specific provisions that must be followed. Ongoing monitoring of the research project is dependent on the risk associated with the study, but all researchers must seek approval for any changes to an approved protocol.

Ethics review boards in the United States must comply with regulations that govern ethical human subjects research such as the U.S. Department of Health and Human Services policy for the Protection of Human Subjects (US), as outlined in 45 Code of Federal Regulations (CFR), Part 46. The regulations contain four parts: (a) the Common Rule—subpart A; (b) the protections of pregnant women, human fetuses, and neonates—subpart B; (c) protections for prisoners; and (d) protections for children. The Common Rule outlines the basic provisions for review boards, informed consent, and assurances of compliance. These same principles have been adopted worldwide. The Declaration of Helsinki reminds us that, while the primary purpose of medical research is to generate new knowledge, this goal can never take precedence over the rights and interests of individual research subjects.

The Council for International Organizations of Medical Sciences (CIOMS) in collaboration with the World Health Organization (WHO) published two sets of guidelines governing biomedical research following the Declaration of Helsinki in 1964 but that has undergone some revision. The International Guidelines for Ethical Review of Epidemiological Studies (published in 1991) and the International Ethical Guidelines for Biomedical Research involving Human Subjects (1993) left many unanswered questions, and an update of the 1993 guidelines was published in 2002. This publication and a more recent version provide guidelines for low-resource countries in establishing mechanisms for ethical review of human subjects' research (CIOMS, 2002, 2016).

The foundational bioethics in research outlined in the Belmont Report and other ethics documents highlights three principles that are described as prima facie and must be considered together unless specifics of the situation require that one principle takes precedence: *Respect for persons*, *Beneficence* and *Justice* (a complete discussion of these concepts can be found in Chapter 2 of this book). In many cases the poor are more likely to be recruited for research, yet they are often the least likely to benefit from the research. There are multiple examples such as the Tuskegee study referred to earlier that recruited disadvantaged, rural Black men to study the natural course of an untreated disease. An earlier violation of human rights than was described in the Tuskegee study of the 1950s was one in which researchers performed experiments on vulnerable people in Guatemala to test treatments for sexually transmitted infections after being deliberately exposed to syphilis or gonorrhea. These and other violations have resulted in a greater awareness of the need to be vigilant in research to ensure high ethical standards. Hlongwa (2016) concludes that a discussion of ethical issues regarding HIV-preventive vaccine trials should be highlighted in developing research in resource-poor countries. In addition, the author suggests that mechanisms to monitor participants and address grievances should be put in place.

Research that is conducted with individuals or from identifiable private information is subject to IRB approval and clearance. Research may involve the individual in intervention research such as a clinical trial or testing a technology or research that does not require an intervention such as a survey that is only asking questions or accessing an individual's clinical records. The researcher must be able to specify the likelihood of any negative consequence or harm to the individual participating in the study. A negative consequence or harm could take the form of physical or psychological harm or a breach of privacy or confidentiality of the individuals' private information or information gathered as a result of the study. The risk associated with a study is generally assessed by the IRB as minimal or harmful. On this basis studies are categorized as exempt, expedited, or full review. Exempt and expedited studies generally pose the least amount of risk to their study participants, while studies classified as requiring full review are considered to be somewhat of higher risk either to the individual's physical or psychological well-being. These studies are reviewed by the full IRB and are also carefully monitored during study implementation.

BOX 1.1 Justifications for Ensuring Ethically Responsible Research (Resnick, 2015)

- Support values of respect and fairness in collaboration
- Accountability to the colleagues, public, and funders
- Support of research
- Support of the principle Do No Harm
- Promote the aims of research through publications to expand knowledge

---

A set of ethical principles adopted by community-based participatory practice (Center for Social Justice and Community Action, 2012) addresses more than the informed consent process but expands the narrowly interpreted principles of respect for persons, beneficence and justice that primarily focuses on those being researched to include the wider research enterprise (Table 1.4).

TABLE 1.4 Ethical Principles and Their Applications in Community-Based Participatory Research

Principle	Application of the Principle
Mutual respect	Developing research relationships based on mutual respect, including a commitment to: • agreeing on what counts as mutual respect in particular contexts • everybody involved being prepared to listen to the voice of others • accepting that there are diverse perspectives

TABLE 1.4 (Continued)

Principle	Application of the Principle
Equality and inclusion	Encouraging and enabling people from a range of backgrounds and identities (e.g., ethnicity, faith, class, education, gender, sexual orientation, (dis)ability, age) to lead, design, and take part in the research, including a commitment to: - seeking actively to include people whose voices are often ignored - challenging discriminatory and oppressive attitudes and behaviors - ensuring information, venues and formats for meetings are accessible to all
Democratic participation	Encouraging and enabling all participants to contribute meaningfully to decision-making and other aspects of the research process according to skill, interest, and collective need, including a commitment to: - acknowledging and discussing differences in the status and power of research participants, and working toward sharing power more equally - communicating clearly using language everyone can understand - using participatory research methods that build on, share and develop different skills and expertise
Active learning	Viewing research collaboration and the process of research as an opportunity to learn from each other, including a commitment to: - ensuring there is time to identify and reflect on learning during the research, and on the ways, people learn, both together and individually - offering all participants, the chance to learn from each other and share their learning with wider audiences - sharing responsibility for interpreting the research finding and their implications for practice
Making a difference	Promoting research that creates positive change for communities of place, interest, or identity, including: - engaging in debates about what counts as positive change, such as broader environment sustainability and human needs or spiritual development and being open to the possible of not knowing in advance what making a positive difference might mean - valuing the learning and other benefits for individual and groups from the research process as well as the outputs and outcomes of the research - building the goal of positive change into every stage of the research
Collective action	Individuals and groups working together to achieve change, including a commitment to: - identifying common and complementary goals that meet partners' differing need for the research - working for agreed visions of how to share knowledge and power more equitably and promote social change and social justice - recognizing and working with conflicting rights and interests expressed by different sections and communities or by different communities
Personal integrity	Participants behaving reliably, honestly, and in a trustworthy fashion, including a commitment to: - working within the principles of community based participatory research - ensuring accurate and honest analysis and reporting of research - being open to challenge and change and prepared to work with conflict

In research, autonomy has become the central ethical principle requiring researchers to document the study participants' voluntary participation in the research following full disclosure of the research study, its risks and benefits to the participant. This principle requires that potential subjects are given the opportunity to choose whether they will or will not participate in the study and recognition of the cultural factors that influence their participation in research must be a consideration. Maria Lahman (2018) describes culturally responsive relational reflexive ethics as an ethical stance in which the researcher will not always understand the perspective of the various cultures; they work with but will be flexible and open to examining ethical issues that arise. A culturally responsive researcher is able to accommodate their participants in ways that make it easier for them to collect trustworthy information.

Informed Consent

Obtaining voluntary informed consent is considered one of the most important aspects of a research study that requires the researcher to consider risk and benefits not only to the individual exposed to the research but also to the larger community that may be affected a negative outcome. Research studies recognize the autonomous status of their respondents throughout the research process, and due consideration is given to individuals who are invited to participate in a research study. The *informed consent* document must be written so that a member of general public who is literate in the language can understand what the research study is about and the individual is able to make a judicious decision. Each study will have very explicit guidelines for how the informed consent process is implemented. The information must be complete and provide the potential participant with a clear understanding of benefits associated with the study to them personally and to the larger population, but more importantly researchers must be clear about their risk. Imagine being asked to participate in a study and not being told the risk inherent in participation. Lahman (2018, pp. 19–20) proposed several questions that can be used to assess a person's capacity to understand the risk associated with the research and be able to provide truly informed consent (Box 1.2).

BOX 1.2 Questions Regarding a Person's Capacity to Give Informed Consent

- Does the participant have the capacity to deliberate about whether to participate?
- Is the participant liable to the authority of others who may have an independent interest in that participation?
- Is the participant given to patterns of deferential behavior that may mask an underlying unwillingness to participate?
- Has the participant been selected, in part because they have a serious health-related condition for which there are no satisfactory remedies?
- Is the participant seriously lacking in important social goods that will be provided as a consequence of their participation in the research?
- Does the political, organizational, economic, and social context of the research setting possess the integrity and resources needed to manage the study?

All research is required to be reviewed by an ethics review board in the country in which the research is being conducted. While ethical review of research is well developed in the US and in Europe, programs in Sub-Saharan Africa countries have only relatively recently initiated research ethics capacity development in health sciences (Ndebele, 2019). In South Africa, a local ethics committee reviews all biomedical research and researchers. Silaigwana and Wassenaar (2019) in their review of ethical issues raised, found that most queries involved informed consent, respect for participants, and scientific validity, providing additional evidence of the importance of the educational role of research ethics review boards. Without sufficient training, ethics boards run the risk of inadequate oversight of ethical rules and regulations.

The Ethics Review and Approval Process

The ethics review and approval process and guidelines vary across institutions and settings, but they include some basic components: preparation and submission of the application to the local or international board as necessary, followed by monitoring of the approved study ethics guidelines, and finally a request to close the study once all aspects of the research study are completed (Figure 1.3).

FIGURE 1.3. *Ethics review and approval of a research study with human participants.*

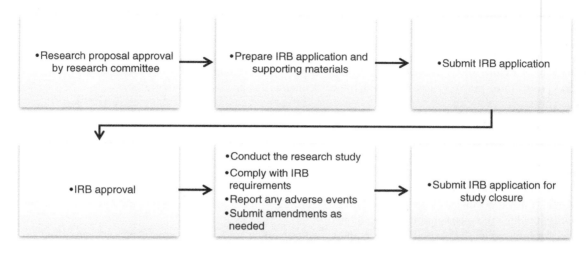

The following materials make up the submission packet that is commonly required for an ethics review, most of which are developed as part of the research proposal:

- An approved research proposal or protocol (usually a condensed version)
- Recruitment and screening materials
- Consent documents
- Authorization/permission letters and memorandums of understanding (if applicable)
- Data collection tools
- Completed ethics review application form (in print or electronic)
- Certificate or proof of human subject's protection training for all research personnel involved in the research study

Many ethics committees require the completion of a human subject's protection training to engage in any research with human participants. The Collaborative Institutional Training Initiatives (CITI) program is a standard online research ethics training that has been widely adopted by several ethics committees and universities within and outside the United States (CITI, n.d.). It is designed to educate researchers on the protection of human participants in research within two disciplinary categories: biomedical research and social behavioral educational research.

Since ethical codes and principles may vary across sociocultural contexts, there are special ethics review guidelines for international research studies to ensure their compliance with ethical standards within the local and sociocultural context of the study. International studies typically undergo at least two ethics reviews and approvals: one in the country sponsoring the study and another in the host country in which the research will be conducted. These ethics reviews can be done concurrently or sequentially depending on the institution's guidelines. Ethics review boards in host countries often require the study's approval by the ethics review board in the sponsoring country prior to being reviewed in the host country. For international or cross-cultural research, both original and translated versions of the recruitment, consent, and data collection materials must be submitted to the Ethics Review Board. In the event of conflicting reviews between two ethics review boards, any proposed changes by the host ethics committee may need to be submitted as an amendment to the review board in the sponsoring country. Alternatively, some review boards require that the researcher meet the higher ethical standards in the event of conflicting reviews. The research can be conducted only once both approvals have been secured. It is important to involve local stakeholders because they can provide assistance in navigating and following up on local ethics review procedures.

Once the approval has been secured and communicated by the ethics review board, the research activities can begin. The approval letter by a local review board is often required when requesting for authorization to access the study sites for recruitment and data collection purposes. When conducting the study, the researchers must comply with the ethical guidelines established by the review board, as specified in the approval packet. This includes administering informed consent prior to collecting data, immediately reporting any adverse events related to the study, and submitting amendments for review by the ethics review board when making changes to the originally approved research protocol or research forms. Upon completion of the study, when the data have been analyzed, deidentified, and reported, the ethics review board may require the researcher to submit an application for a formal study closure. This application contains additional questions eliciting information pertaining to the reason for the study closure, the occurrence of any adverse events over the course of the study, and the status of the research data at the time of the study closure (e.g., identifiable or deidentified). The researcher is required to keep the research materials in a secure storage for a specified time period (e.g., three to five years), after which the documents can be destroyed or erased.

Ethical Review in Emergencies

Emergencies have arisen around the world, and researchers engage in research often in very difficult conditions. However, informed consent to conduct research with human subjects' remains a critical element. A necessary review of the role of ethics committees resulted in a set of Council for International Organizations of Medical Sciences guidelines (2002) that include a section on ethical review of emergency compassionate use of investigational therapy. They specify that "informed consent should be obtained according to the legal requirement and cultural standards of the community in which the intervention is carried out."

A research-based model for collaboration and expediting ethics review in an emergency was proposed by Aarons (2018) for countries in the Caribbean region although cross country ethics review would occur through the Caribbean Public Health Agency (CARPHA). Components of the local model would include formation of an ad hoc research ethics committee made up of six to seven chairs of ethics committees, the local ministry of health and members of the community. Communication must go through the chairs of the committees back to their committees and institutions electronically and secretarial and trained administrative support. This could form the basis for other community collaboration for the development of ethical guidelines during emergencies.

Misconduct in Research

42 CRF 93.103 of the US CFR defines misconduct in research under three categories but does not include honest error or difference of opinion. The three areas are:

1. Fabrication of data or results and recording or reporting them
2. Falsification (manipulation) of research methods, equipment, or processes or changing or omitting data or results
3. Plagiarism as the appropriation of another person's ideas, processes, results, or words without giving appropriate credit

Misconduct in research can lead to wasteful squandering of resources and a negative perception of science, which in turn can have negative consequences for funding (Coughlin, 2009) (Box 1.3).

BOX 1.3 Misconduct in Research

- Selectively reporting findings
- Phishing or milking the data in the analysis using several methods to find a significant result that is unrelated to the original research hypothesis
- Inappropriate reporting of research findings to look like the study yielded publishable results given the bias by publishers against reporting negative findings
- Misleading discussion and conclusion
- Inadequate and biased reporting of study limitations to deny the reader the opportunity to judge the validity of the study independently

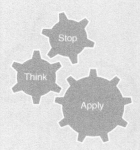

Thinking Through an Ethical Dilemma

In groups of three or four, discuss the following scenario. It is important to conduct research among homeless individuals for purposes of providing appropriate public health interventions, yet there are many reasons such research could be considered unethical. Consider the implications for conducting a public health–related intervention research study with this potentially vulnerable population.

- What issues surround research involving homeless individuals?
- What does it mean to ask a homeless individual to give informed consent? Discuss the risks and benefits for the individual.
- Should individuals who are homeless be compensated for their participation? Why or why not?

 SUMMARY

Research is a detailed study of a subject or phenomena to get a deeper and often new understanding. It is important to get a full and complete understanding of a phenomenon through valid research before drawing conclusions.

Perez and Luquis (2008) identify three characteristics in working cross culturally: cultural desire, cultural awareness, and cultural sensitivity. Being a culturally responsive researcher requires cultural awareness, cultural knowledge, and cultural skill as well as cultural dexterity.

Underlying the assumptions in public health research is a series of philosophical positions such as positivism/postpositivism, constructivism, and transformativism.

The theoretical framework and conceptual framework are situated within the philosophical paradigm and serve as important foundations for research. Although the terms are often used interchangeably, the theoretical framework is developed before the conceptual framework. The conceptual framework forms the basis for the research study that is being conducted.

Ethics boards or IRBs oversee scientific research in institutions all over the world. *Clearance from these boards is required for any study that is research and can be characterized as being a systematic investigation that is intended to be generalizable.*

The Belmont Report and other ethics documents highlight three principles that are critical to be considered in research. They are respect for persons, beneficence, and justice.

Obtaining informed voluntary consent is considered one of the most important aspects of a research study. It requires the researcher to consider risk and benefits not only to the individual who participates in the research but also to the larger community that may be affected by a negative outcome.

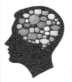

Now that I have reached the end this section, I am able to:

Course Objective	Strongly Agree	Somewhat Agree	Neutral	Somewhat Disagree	Strongly Agree
Explain the fundamentals of the research enterprise					
Compare the different philosophical and methodological approaches to research					
Apply ethical standards to research					

SECTION 2: RESEARCH STUDY DESIGN FRAMEWORK

By the end of this section, learners will be able to:

- Outline a research study using the research study design framework
- Discuss validity and reliability
- Describe how research is funded

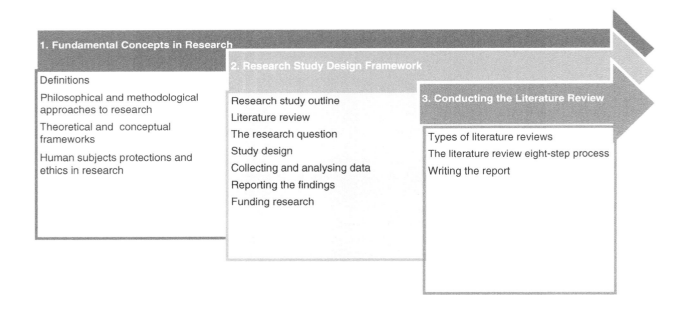

THE RESEARCH STUDY DESIGN FRAMEWORK

The basis for the research study is the review of the literature, the philosophical grounding and interest of the researcher, and funding of the research team. The research plan is the backbone of good research and is at the intersection of philosophy, research design, and the specific methods identified by the researcher. The research study design framework provides the overall conceptual structure for the study to provide insights into the research problem and answer the research question from the data collection and data analysis. The research study plan components include conducting the literature review, specifying the research question, the methodology for conducting the research, the data analysis, and reporting the findings (Figure 1.4). These components must each be developed with fidelity to ensure the

FIGURE 1.4. *Research study design framework.*

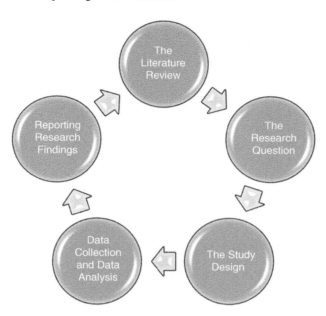

soundness of the research study. This section provides an overview of the research process. Modules 2–4 will describe the components in more detail in quantitative, qualitative, and mixed methods research.

Developing the research study plan is probably the most important component in conducting a research study as it requires the researcher to take the time to organize their thoughts and consider the core question of the research study and the research approach that will provide the most reliable results that avoid the risk of misleading and false conclusions. Research benefits from having input from fellow researchers and the stakeholders about who the research is intended for.

The Literature Review

Conducting a literature review is a crucial and preliminary step of the research process as it establishes what is known and not known about a given topic, pointing the researcher to future research directions. Its utility spans the entire research process from the topic development to the interpretation of the research findings (Figure 1.5). A literature review can be conducted (a) as a section or chapter of a research study (e.g., thesis or dissertation), grant, or project proposal/report—also known as an "embedded review" (Efron and Ravid, 2019, p. 173); or (b) as a stand-alone research project. Common struggles in conducting a literature review include formulating focused searches and critically synthesizing large volumes of information retrieved from the literature. Conducting a literature review is therefore an essential competency for scholars as it builds the foundation and justification for the research study (Shah et al., 2018).

The literature review is a structured and objective *search*, *critical analysis*, and *synthesis* of the evidence (i.e., research, theories, practices, and methodologies) produced on a given topic by scholars, researchers, and practitioners (Fink, 2019). It retrieves and critically synthesizes information from a variety of scholarly and professional sources including peer-reviewed journals, books, government/organizational reports, and web-based sources. A literature review should be distinguished from other types of reviews and reports of the literature such as an annotated bibliography, a literary review, or an account of the researcher's opinion in the following ways:

- It is a critical evaluation and synthesis that captures interrelationships, areas of agreement and contradiction, controversies or debates, strengths, and limitations of existing evidence from a variety of sources. It also identifies critical knowledge gaps on a topic and proposes areas for future research. It is not an annotated bibliography that provides a concise summary of the findings, quality, and relevance or utility of each source (Efron and Ravid, 2019).

- It is a critical integration and synthesis of findings, theories, and methodological approaches from a variety of sources. It is not a literary review (e.g., book review) that critiques the style, content, and merits of a specific literary work (e.g., novel, play).

- It critically interprets, compares, and contrasts the findings, arguments, or ideas of other scholars in the field. The researcher's synthesis of the existing literature can reveal new patterns or themes that trigger new perspectives and debates on the topic. It is not an account of the researcher's own opinion (Efron and Ravid, 2019). The researcher's position or assertions should be stated explicitly and supported by the literature or appropriate citations (Ridley, 2012, p. 158).

A full discussion of how to conduct a literature review is in Section 3 of this Module.

FIGURE 1.5. *The utility of a literature review throughout the research process.*

Identifying and defining the research problem
- Gives background information on the problem, highlights its significance, provides justification for the study
- Identifies prior research and offers new perspectives for understanding the topic
- Reveals research gaps, biases, contradictory findings, and inconclusive results, thus establishing future research directions and priorities

Formulating research questions and hypotheses
- Reveals research gaps, contradictory findings, and inconclusive results that form the basis for formulating, refining, and focusing research questions
- Reveals relationships between constructs that can be used to formulate hypotheses

Developing a theoretical and conceptual framework
- Identifies relevant concepts (including their interrelationships), theories, and their applications to the topic of interest, which informs the development of theoretical and conceptual frameworks for a study

Selecting a study design and methodology
- Examines the strengths and limitations of research methodologies and study designs employed in prior studies
- Identifies how others have defined and measured key concepts (i.e., variables), including the existing data collection and analysis tools and procedures. This guides the development of data collection tools and analysis strategies
- Provides an overview of samples and sampling methods in previous research to inform sampling decisions

Analyzing and interpreting data
- Generates theoretical, conceptual, and methodological evidence that informs the interpretation of study findings
- Compares and contrasts current findings to previous findings, highlighting a study's unique contribution (revise, refine, advance) to the body of knowledge on a given topic

Disseminating Findings
- Presents a structured and concise synthesis of existing literature on a given topic and highlights a study's contribution (revise, refine, advance) to the body of knowledge

The Research Question

Selecting a topic for public health research is also both a science and an art. The science is selecting a topic that is of value and significance to public health and society. Therefore, it covers an aspect of health, which can be investigated using formulae and traditions found in science and art, that is required to collect and analyze the data to answer the research question. Here are a few ideas for how to select a topic:

- Brainstorm ideas of public health–related topics
- Identify topics that are well covered in the literature or are of particular interest
- Define the topic by using a focused question
- Make a list of key words and combinations of key words that will help the search
- Scan at least 10 articles on the topic looking particularly at the results sections
- Formulate a research question to answer

A good research question is focused, researchable, and feasible to answer given the technical, practical, and financial resources available. It should be complex enough to be able to develop a reasonable answer and must be relevant to the field of study: in this case public health. The research question may serve one of two purposes: (1) to ask a basic scientific question to generate new knowledge; or (2) to solve a problem. The basic scientific question is generally asked by the researcher and expands on previous research. The question that relates to solving a real-world problem may also be asked by clients and non-scientific researchers. The type of question also depends on the training and interest of the researcher or the research team. A team with a wide range of data collection and analysis skills may be less limited in the number or range of questions. A large team may ask questions that bring together expertise from both quantitative and qualitative approaches and based on both postpositivist and constructivist philosophies.

Qualitative research questions will typically be asked when the goal is to understand respondents' concepts, thoughts, and experiences to provide in-depth insights into a topic that may not be well understood. Sample sizes for qualitative data are usually small, and the results are not generalizable to the larger population. The questions may apply to only that study, and data may be collected to get a deeper understanding of the phenomena, to develop a questionnaire, or to develop a theory for grounded theory approaches. Qualitative approaches may also be used in applied research approaches.

Quantitative data are collected when the focus of the study is to generate findings that are generalizable to the larger population, in which case the research will focus on collecting data using surveys and large sample sizes. Not all quantitative data are generalizable, such as with research studies done with a small sample homogenous population or data collected in the context of program evaluation. Quantitative research is used to test or confirm theories or assumptions. It is used in a range of research design studies in surveys to classify subjects, provide the characteristics of a study population and to describe a phenomenon on numerical terms.

The Hypothesis

Once the research questions are written, researchers will often also develop hypotheses following a literature review. Like the research questions, it is involved in the process of determining how to proceed with the research study. It is based on an expectation of a particular relationship between the variables. A hypothesis has to be simple, specific, clear, and measurable and should test only one relationship at a time. There are two types of hypothesis: null and alternative. The null hypothesis (H_0) is essentially the test of the assumed relationship between variables. The alternative hypothesis (H_A) is the opposite of the null hypothesis. The alternative hypothesis may also be referred to as H_1.

Research Question—Does competency-based teaching have an effect on perceived competence of new graduates of public health programs?

H_0 Competency-based teaching has no effect on the perceived competence of new graduates.

H_A Competency-based teaching has a positive effect on the perceived competence of new graduates.

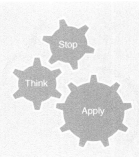

Formulating Research Questions

In groups of three to four, think about and brainstorm ideas for a public health–related topic. Make a list of key words and take about 20–30 minutes to do a literature search using accessible internet tools (e.g., Google Scholar).

- Write down ideas that emerged from the scan of the literature.
- Write down a research question that came to mind about the topic as you scanned the literature.
- Discuss each of your research questions.
- Decide which research question the group would like to answer as a research project.

Individually, write a half-page summary of how multiple voices helped frame the final research question. At the end of the process, what word or phrase best describes your experience?

Study Design

At this point of the research study design framework (Figure 1.3), the researchers have declared their philosophical approach to the research study, completed the literature review that reflects the theoretical framework for the study and have determined the research question (or questions) for the study. The next step is to develop the concept map/conceptual framework that will guide the development of the plan for data collection and data analysis. The conceptual framework reflects the variables of interest and when appropriate it shows the assumed relationship between the constructs that formed the basis for the research question. It forms the basis for the hypothetical relationship between the variables that will be the focus of the study in the case of a quantitative research and for a qualitative study when it is appropriate.

Designing the Methodology

The design of the methodology allows the researcher to find valid answers to the selected research question. It sets out the specific details of the research study. A faulty design leads to misleading and mislabeled findings. In the absence of a valid study design, results from the study will be dismissed. A literature review is important to show how similar research questions have been tackled in the past. It highlights what study population may be the most appropriate, what methods have been used, and the limitations of the methods. It provides insights into what approach would be most likely to be a helpful addition to the field. For example, previous research may be primarily focused on exploratory studies with small sample sizes, and there may be sufficient information to consider conducting a large quantitative study to measure the prevalence of the trait within a given community.

The data collection method is dependent on the type of study as well as the specific research question. Quantitative research will most likely collect data using a survey, whereas a qualitative research study will have a wide range of options. Specifically, for the question "What factors influenced the relationship between a foundation and a not-for-profit child health organization?" could be answered using quantitative or qualitative data (Table 1.5), and the choice will largely depend on the number of entities, what opportunities there are to use existing surveys, and a collection of individual interview data to understand the nuances a survey may not be able to provide for purposes of expanding the understanding of this phenomena. Another consideration during this phase of the study is the research design that influences the research question and is also influenced by the research question. For example, in Table 1.6 when the underlying purpose of the question, "Does competency based teaching have an effect on perceived competence of new graduates of public health programs?" is to *assess the cause and effect* of an

TABLE 1.5. The Relationship Between the Question, the Underlying Purpose, and the Type of Study

The question	Purpose of the question	Type of research
Do individuals who are exposed to a certain risk have higher levels of disease?	To test a hypothesis	Quantitative
What factors influenced the relationship between a foundation and a nonprofit child health organization?	To explore a new idea	Mixed methods
What is the distribution of risk factor X across population Y?	To determine the extent of a situation/phenomenon across the population	Quantitative
How does population Z describe their experience of acculturation after living in a refugee camp?	To explore an underresearched population?	Qualitative
Does competency-based teaching have an effect on perceived competence of new graduates of public health programs?	To assess cause and effect	Quantitative
What are the characteristics of the study population participating in the case–control study?	To determine the characteristics of study subjects	Quantitative

TABLE 1.6. A Comparison of Features That Distinguish Different Research Designs

	Research Designs	Characteristics
1	Basic	Develops knowledge, theories, and predictions and tests relationships
	Applied	Develops and evaluates techniques, products and procedures and answers real-world problems
2	Exploratory	Explains the main aspects of an underresearched problem
	Explanatory	Explains the causes and consequences of a well-defined problem
3	Inductive	Traditional research to develop or test a theory
	Deductive	Explores the underling factors that are not well understood
4	Qualitative	Emphasis is on words or text and understanding
	Quantitative	Emphasis is on numbers and statistics
5	Descriptive	Gathers and interprets data on the characteristic of a phenomenon without controlling for any variable
	Experimental/Quasi-experimental	Manipulates outputs and variables to detect cause and effect

intervention a corresponding study design would be an *experimental/quasi-experimental design* (Table 1.7). The experimental/quasi-experimental design requires the researcher to compare the treatment group with a control group that has not received the treatment in a pre/post intervention design.

Without using a control group in the study, the researcher cannot conclude that the treatment caused the outcome (effect) and it was not caused by something other than the treatment. In this design, the researcher will collect quantitative data to answer the research question. In addition, the researcher will also collect descriptive data to understand the characteristics of the study populations. However, none of this prevents the researchers from asking a third question about the experience of the individuals who participated in the study in individual interviews; therefore, collecting qualitative data in a pre-planned mixed methods design.

Mixed methods approaches may be used to increase the validity of a study through a mechanism known as triangulation (Silverman, 2001). The objective of triangulation is to use a combination of methodological or theoretical approaches to answer a research question, so as to increase confidence in the conclusions from two or more independent measures (Graham, 2005). Using different methods allows a different perspective and gives the researcher a comparative framework from which to see the results (Denzin, 1989), and according to Fielding and Fielding (1986) it is unlikely to eliminate the problems inherent in each of the methods of data collection. Silverman (2001) illustrated the use of triangulation in multiple ways using a combination of qualitative and quantitative approaches (Table 1.8). Key questions that may assist in decision-making about the appropriateness of a mixed methods design were proposed by Palinkas et al. (2011) and are adapted here:

- What is the rationale for wanting to conduct a mixed methods study?
- How does using a mixed methods approach enhance the quality of the research and the researcher's ability to answer the research question?
- What mixed methods design is appropriate?
- How are the data collection approaches related to each other in time?

The counterfactual to this approach could be, "If I had not used a mixed methods approach, would I have reached the same conclusion?" Mixed methods designs are discussed in more detail in Module 4 of this book.

TABLE 1.7. Mixed Methods Study Designs and Their Characteristics

Study design	Characteristics
Convergent	Collection and analysis of both quantitative and qualitative data at the same time and the comparison for convergence and divergence of results in a single-phase approach to confirm the comparability of findings.
Explanatory sequential	Collection and analysis of quantitative data and thereafter qualitative data, which builds on the results of the former in a two-phase approach to provide depth into the study findings and a deeper explanation and contextual information. A comparison of the findings is not appropriate given the purposive sample for the qualitative study.
Exploratory sequential	Collection of qualitative data initially that informs the development of the survey and data collection instrument followed by administering the survey in a three-phase approach that includes obtaining a deeper explanation of the findings and the contextual information.
Complex	The mixed method involves quantitative, qualitative, or combined data embedded in a larger design, theory, or methodology. If embedded in an experimental design, the qualitative data may be collected independently and used to support or augment the larger quantitative design

TABLE 1.8. Theories at Multiple Levels of Influence of the Socioecological Model

SEM theory level	Examples of theories and models
Individual	Health Belief Model
	Theory of Reasoned Action
	Transtheoretical Model
	Precaution Adoption Process Model
	Information, Motivation Behavioral Skills (IMB) Theory
	Protection Motivation Theory
Interpersonal	Social Cognitive Theory
	Social Support and Social Network
	Stress, Coping and Health Behavior
	Clinician–Patient Communication
Organizational	Stage Theory of Organizational Change
	Community Coalition Action Theory
Community	Social Capital
	Community Organizing and Community Building
	Diffusion of Innovations
Societal	Advocacy Coalition Framework

Incorporating Theory in Applied Research Design

Theories are a generalized way of thinking about the nature of the relationships that exist about a phenomenon. Theories are the product of our thinking. We often call them hunches, and they remain hunches until they are tested using a scientific and systematic approach. As we have more experience with nature and with life around us, some of our predictions are correct; however, that does not make them theories that can be replicated. Theories, however, guide the research enterprise to finding the answers to our questions. Public health has adopted existing theories—most often those from psychology—that help us understand how our populations respond to various stimuli and conditions and how the environment influences behavior and health outcomes. Merriam-Webster defines theory as "a plausible or scientifically acceptable general principle of body of principles offered to explain phenomena." Theoretical and conceptual frameworks are developed as an integral part of the study that shows the relationships among variables as well as being a tool for analysis. The final conceptual framework that is developed following the study contains the variables that are important for defining the outcome.

Public health recognizes the importance of the environment in framing behavior and also the importance of interventions not being limited to the individual predisposing factors. It therefore embraces the Socioecological Model as a framework for situating theories at each level to ensure that in the needs assessment, program planning, and evaluation phases of program planning that theory are incorporated to ensure a holistic environment in which to encourage and achieve behavior change. The constructs from one or more existing theories may be used to support the initial literature review to develop the theoretical framework and then subsequently to create the conceptual framework that guides the needs assessment using qualitative, quantitative, or mixed methods research approaches as described earlier. The variables in the needs assessment become the baseline measures against which changes in the health-related outcome can be assessed. The public health theories from which conceptual frameworks can be drawn are listed as follows. An excellent resource is "Theory at a Glance" (U.S. Department of Health and Human Services, National Cancer Institute, 2005).

Data Collection and Analysis

Creswell and Creswell (2018) propose a philosophical orientation to research as being influenced by the researcher's discipline and influences of their field. Researchers generally embrace four philosophical worldviews, positivism, constructivism, transformative, and pragmatism (Creswell and Creswell, 2018) that then guide the research methodological approach. Quantitative research belongs to the positivism philosophy and qualitative research to constructivism. Transformative research has a political change agenda to confront social oppression and to view transformative research as an act of self-determination and community transformation. It is likely to involve either a quantitative or qualitative approach or both depending on the research question. Indigenous approaches that fall within the transformative paradigm place a high priority on building relationships with commitments to dialogue, self-determination and cultural autonomy and recognize the inherent rights of sovereignty of indigenous persons (Lapan et al., 2012).

Chilisa (2012) provides a focus on "a cultural group's ways of perceiving reality, ways of knowing and the value systems that inform the research process" (p.13) and are more inclined to the constructivist paradigm and qualitative research. Pragmatism embraces all approaches available to understand the research problem and is not committed to any particular philosophy. It emphasizes the importance of continuous learning from mistakes, deliberately seeking new information and possibilities (Broomfield, 2012). It bases its research approach on the practical aspects of research and includes postmodern and theoretical underpinnings as well as reflective social justice lenses (Creswell and Creswell, 2018). The research plan outlines the steps that lead to answering a research question. The approach is always determined by the research question and can involve quantitative or qualitative research methods or a combination of the two in a mixed methods approach (Figure 1.6).

Quantitative data supports an inductive approach to research, whereas qualitative data supports a deductive approach, which is reflected in the philosophical orientation of the researcher. In between these extremes, a quantitative study may have open-ended questions, and a qualitative study may collect data using closed ended questions. A mixed methods research study may be qualitative or quantitative or use an approach that is somewhere in between, but most often studies will have an element of each with a fully quantitative inquiry being at one end of the continuum and a fully qualitative study being at the other end.

A study designated as a mixed methods study is a deliberate combination of the elements of qualitative and quantitative approaches in a systematic way (Figure 1.7). In mixed methods studies, the researcher attempts to offset the limitations of using a fully qualitative method or a fully quantitative method by itself by using them in combination to answer the research question and understand a particular phenomenon. Qualitative and quantitative data also differ in the way they are handled after data collection.

FIGURE 1.6. *From the research question to data collection.*

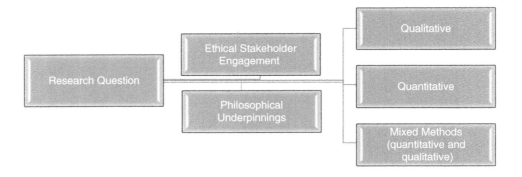

FIGURE 1.7. *Qualitative and quantitative research combined in mixed methods research.*

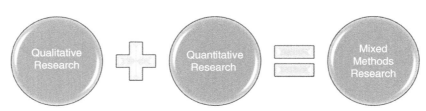

Quantitative data are cleaned, coded, and entered into a quantitative data analysis software such as Excel©, SPSS©, SAS©, STATA©, or R© depending on the preferences of the researcher. Analysis that is conducted is based on the research question and the data that were collected in the survey. Other data (e.g., laboratory, clinical) may be collected and used in the research study. Qualitative data are handled somewhat differently. They are primarily made up of text, unlike quantitative data, which is numerical. Data from interviews, focus groups, and other qualitative research approaches is generally in different forms and the form and format determines how it is handled. For example, data from a focus groups or individual interview may be recorded using an audiorecording device and then transcribed. The transcription is taken through a process of coding and analysis using a range of approaches.

Coding and analysis can be conducted in software such as NVivo©, Dedoose©, and Atlas ti©. The authors have the most experience with NVivo and Dedoose for public health qualitative research, but a number of web-based platforms lend themselves to different levels of functionality. Whether the data are quantitative or qualitative, the software provides the researcher with the opportunity to present the data in diagrammatic formats to allow for easy interpretation of what is often complicated and detailed information. For example, quantitative data are often presented in charts, tables, and graphs, and dashboards, whereas qualitative research is presented in short narratives and quotations. In the latter, researchers also may use heat maps, word clouds, bubble charts, and illustrative diagrams for visualization of their data. Quantitative, qualitative, and mixed methods research designs are covered in more detail in other modules in this book.

Validity and Reliability

The validity of the research study will determine the likelihood that findings can be applied to practice or policy. It is dependent on the soundness of the researcher's plan and the methods that are adopted. The researcher collects accurate, sound, and reliable data to justify the delivery of programs, services, or policy that are considered evidence based.

Quantitative Research

In quantitative research, validity ensures that the research study applies accurate procedures; reliability refers to the quality of the measurement that ensures that the result can be repeated with accuracy. Validity in the results of the research means that instruments used to assess the results must be accurate. The three forms of validity typically expected from instruments are (a) content, (b) predictive or concurrent, and (c) construct. *Content validity* assesses the extent to which the items in the instrument measure what they are supposed to measure. *Predictive* or *concurrent validity* assesses if the instrument can predict a criterion measure (gold standard) or correlate with results from previous studies. *Construct validity* measures the extent to which the instrument is theoretically sound and correlates with the theorized construct. Bias is a deliberate attempt to change the outcome of the study through acts of omission or attempts to highlight something because of a vested interest in the result. On the other hand, reliability in quantitative research refers to the consistency of a measure and is assessed through test–retest reliability, internal consistency across items, and inter-rater reliability across different researchers. These concepts are expanded upon in subsequent modules.

Qualitative Research

In qualitative research, the researcher's experiences and worldviews may influence the questions being explored, so recognizing the influence this has on the data through reflection is a critical part of a qualitative researcher's preparation. The researcher has to keep an open mind and not be influenced, setting aside their own perceptions of the situation or the individual. Validity is replaced with trustworthiness. Consistency (dependability) would be akin to reliability and verifiable through an audit of the raw data and the data reduction process. However, some researchers argue that reliability as a concept is not appropriate in qualitative research.

Suggested approaches for improving the quality of the data include using a constant comparison approach and including deviant cases. Patton (1999) suggests that the credibility of a research study depends on three distinct elements:

- Rigorous data collection methods and techniques and triangulation using a combination of interview, observation and document analysis, multiple observers, theories, methods, and perspectives

- Researcher credibility, training, experience, track record, status, and presentation of self

- A fundamental belief in the qualitative research enterprise that includes naturalistic inquiry, qualitative methods, inductive analysis, purposeful sampling, and holistic thinking

Addressing issues of validity and reliability throughout the research process is critical for ensuring credibility and accurate reporting of findings. Other elements to consider are neutrality of the researcher, transferability, and confirmability (Lincoln and Guba, 1985). Member checking is a feature of qualitative research used to establish credibility and accuracy of the research study findings. A summary of findings or all the findings of the research study are shared with participants of the study. In addition, data are collected until saturation is reached, when among the purposefully selected respondents there is generally a consistency associated with the data (Faulkner and Trotter, 2017).

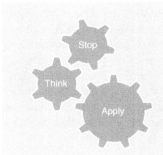

Differentiating Between Validity and Reliability in Research

Describe the characteristics of reliability and validity when applied to quantitative and qualitative research? Devise an acronym or create an image that helps you remember them

Reporting Research Findings

Reporting research data is the last phase of the research cycle and is a responsibility to the funders and to the public's trust. It is a process of presenting findings to the stakeholders as well as to the scientific community at conferences and through research and practice journals and other publication formats. The reader makes the assumption that the research is valid and the report is accurate. Truthfulness in research is the expected standard throughout the process; however, myriad factors result in influencing the integrity and misrepresentation of the research process and finding. These factors are represented in the quality of the research as well as the tacit incentive climate of academia that rewards academics with the longest list of publications.

Tips for Writing up a Research Study

- **Title:**
  - The title should reflect both the spirit and the content of the report.
- **Format:**
  - The document should reflect a clear thread from start to end—from the literature review to the conclusion.
  - Headings in the literature review and the rest of the paper should be consistent with the content discussed within the section.
  - Content should be organized so all parts of the report are properly sequenced to facilitate understanding by the reader.
  - Use the appropriate style for in-text citations and the reference list. List each citation in the reference list.
- **Content:**
  - The thematic approach organizes the themes and subthemes and involves connecting the information into logical, coherent, arguments rather than summarizing each source separately (Box 1.4). In a thematic analysis, each topic or theme is discussed within a section or paragraph. The size of the paragraph or section is determined by the amount of information that is being included.
  - The methodology should describe the study design and the methods clearly and completely so others can conduct the same study independently.

- The analysis must be able to provide the answers to the research questions. If in doubt talk to a biostatistician or statistician.
- The result section summarizes important findings from the study.

BOX 1.4 Thematic Structure of a Section of the Review of the Literature Review Showing Themes and Sub-Themes

Topic: Constructivist Philosophical Underpinnings of Research

Constructivism
- Repertory grid technique
- Analysis of narrative processes of spoken word/text
- Discourse analysis

Social Constructivism
- Discourse analysis
    - Critical ethnography
    - Critical indigenous research
    - Feminist research
- Analysis of rhetoric
- Textual analysis

In this example, each main heading (Constructivism and Social Constructivism) has a subheading (bulleted). In one example, discourse analysis contains addition sub- sub-headings (critical ethnography, critical indigenous research, and feminist research). Each heading or subheading would constitute a paragraph. In the example, if the paragraphs are too short and are more like sentences, they can be rolled up into the next level. So, if there was limited information gathered from a review of the literature for each of the three subheadings under discourse analysis, the sentences could be rolled up into a logical, coherent argument in one paragraph rather than writing about each one separately.

FUNDING RESEARCH

Research is funded using a variety of mechanisms. It may be self-funded by researchers who have an idea about a topic; however, more formal research among a larger group of people, often requires researchers to turn to funding sources. Funding sources are situated within government institutions, universities, for-profit organizations, and their foundations. Access to the funds is directed by the funders and may be restricted to certain categories of research or open to any researcher who is qualified to conduct the research. The institution will generally specify the criteria. The National Institutes of Health (NIH) in the United States, for example, specifies nine different types of funding opportunities that vary from ones representing a new project that has not yet been funded to the resubmission of applications when an unfunded application is modified and resubmitted for review. The agency's website provides the information a researcher needs to know how to apply for a grant. Grant opportunities vary from those directed at new researchers to those for more seasoned researchers. Many of the grants are funded for researchers and allow them to be involved in international research in capacity building and intervention research. Grant information for NIH may be found at their website (U.S. Department of Health and Human Services, National Institutes of Health, n.d.a)

Funders of research are not limited to government. Opportunities for funding large projects may also be provided by private foundations with extensive resources. Information generally available on their websites outlines application expectations, including the criteria for evaluation and the researcher's ability to comply with financial management requirements. For more seasoned researchers, it may include opportunities for additional funds to train and supervise budding researchers.

Funding from private foundations is mission driven and often directed to a specific disease. For example, foundations fund breast cancer, diabetes, and heart disease research, which is often more accessible to those early in their career and who need a relatively small amount of money to undertake a project funders are interested in seeing done. Their funding may also cover the cost of laboratory research to help find a cure for the disease of interest or be broader in its mission, as is the Alzheimer's Foundation of America, which funds dementia-related research. Private foundations may also provide funds to the program that demonstrates creativity and uniqueness to address a need and with potential for replication.

In addition to the larger amounts of funding available for well-established concepts of expensive research ventures, universities and other institutions or organizations may provide seed grants to researchers to explore a new topic that has potential to be funded by one of the larger institutions in the future. This is often an opportunity for a researcher to test a concept or a new idea. Amounts available from these avenues are usually small. Check with research institutions and centers within the university or the research and development arm of an organization or agency for more information. Funding is sometimes restricted to those who have previously submitted a letter of intent.

A letter of intent is a document that specifies what the research is about, and it is the funding entity that requests a full proposal. A call for letters of intent may be sent out from the organization annually to solicit letters that describe intended research. These calls for letters or a full application will appear on their website or other materials or information outlets. The organization will generally provide a list of topic areas it will consider that are in line with the organization's mission. Some organizations and agencies will put out an open call as I have just described, but in other cases the organization will send a call for proposals out directly to the organizations that it is interested in funding. These researchers have often previously been in contact with the funder. This means that a researcher who wants their work to be funded must reach out to the program or research office and develop a relationship with the organization to determine if their interests align and open up opportunities for an invitation to submit a proposal.

BOX 1.5 Components of a Letter of Intent

A summary statement about the intent of the LOI

- The [researcher/research institution] seeks funding to undertake research using an innovative approach to [purpose of the study]. Potential outcomes of this work include: [list potential outcomes]. We are requesting [amount] for a [propose length of study].
- Summarize why the project is needed (one to two paragraphs):
    - What is the issue to be addressed?
    - What makes it an important issue?
    - Who is likely to benefit from the results of the research?
    - Why would the funders care and be interested in funding this study?
- Describe what the research project will entail:
    - Describe the research project in detail and why it is important, different, or expands the base of knowledge in the field/advances the science.
    - Describe the research methodology.
- State the specific outcomes the research project hopes to achieve.
- Describe the credentials of the researchers, the organization, and its partners (one to two paragraphs).
- Provide the budget, including the funding needs for the research and the total amount requested.
- Conclude the proposal:
    - Show interest in discussing the proposal with a staff member.
    - Offer to provide more information.
    - Include appreciation for the opportunity to apply.
    - Provide contact information.
    - Sign appropriately using a organization's signatory—often a research compliance office of the institution.

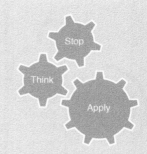

Proposing a Research Study to a Funder

Write a one- to two-page letter of interest to a funder proposing a research study including the following components:

- A summary statement of the project to be conducted including the specific outcomes to be achieved
- A brief description of the approach and methods
- The credentials of the researchers and the organization and its partners
- An estimated budget
- Closing paragraph

SUMMARY

A study is generally based on the review of the literature, the philosophical grounding, and the interest of the researcher and funding considerations. The research plan is the backbone of good research and is dictated by the philosophical underpinnings, the research design, and the specific methods identified by the researcher. The design of the study sets out the specific details of the research study. A faulty design leads to misleading and mislabeled findings. In the absence of a valid study design, results from the study will be dismissed.

Conducting a literature review is a crucial and preliminary step of the research process as it establishes what is known and not known about a given topic. It is used during the entire research process from the topic formulation to the interpretation of the research findings.

A good research question is focused, researchable, relevant, and feasible to answer. The research question may be used to (a) answer a basic scientific question to generate new knowledge; or (b) solve a problem.

Theoretical and conceptual frameworks are developed as an integral part of the study. They show the relationships among variables as well as being a tool for analysis. The results from the study identifies the specific variables that are important for determining the outcome that the study assessed.

Research is funded using a variety of mechanisms. It may be self-funded by researchers who have an idea about a topic; however, more formal research often requires researchers to seek out funders. Funding sources are situated within government institutions; universities; for profit organizations and their foundations.

A letter of intent specifies what the research is about, and the funding entity requests a full proposal should the letter meet its funding priorities. A call for letters of intent may be sent out from the organization annually. The call for letters may also be found on the organization or agency's website.

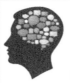

Now that I have reached the end this section, I am able to:

Course Objective	Strongly Agree	Somewhat Agree	Neutral	Somewhat Disagree	Strongly Agree
Outline a research study using the research study design framework					
Discuss validity and reliability					
Describe how research is funded					

SECTION 3: CONDUCTING THE LITERATURE REVIEW

By the end of this section, the learners will be able to:

- Differentiate a traditional (narrative) literature review from other types of reviews
- Describe the literature review process
- Design a traditional (narrative) literature review

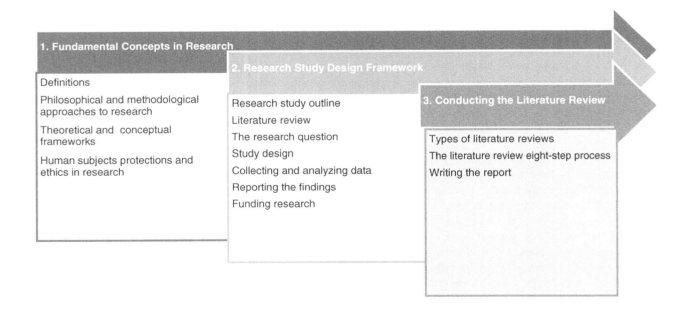

TYPES OF LITERATURE REVIEWS

There are several types of literature reviews, and they vary in purpose, scope, and approach. Table 1.9 summarizes six common types: traditional or narrative, systematic, meta-analysis, meta-synthesis, scoping, and rapid review. Grant and Booth (2009) provide a more comprehensive list of different types of reviews and their respective methodologies.

TABLE 1.9. Types of Literature Reviews

Description	Search and Screening Strategy	Analysis and Synthesis Strategy	Challenges and Limitations
Traditional or Narrative Review			
▪ Identifies, critiques, and synthesizes current literature on a particular topic to establish what is known and not known (knowledge gaps) ▪ Often a chapter in a dissertation or thesis or a section of a journal article to position the study in context	▪ Literature review questions usually not explicitly stated ▪ Does not describe the search, quality assessment, and synthesis strategies ▪ Representative or central: reviews select sources that reflect relevant evidence without being exhaustive ▪ Can be conducted by a single researcher	Narrative or qualitative synthesis using a thematic, content, chronological, or conceptual analysis approach, among others	▪ Potential selection or researcher bias ▪ Cannot be replicated ▪ Not exhaustive or comprehensive
Systematic Review			
▪ A systematic search, appraisal, and synthesis of quality empirical evidence, with an explicitly defined review question, search strategy, data extraction process, and synthesis approach to minimize bias, ensure transparency, and enhance replicability ▪ Often conducted as a stand-alone research project but can also be conducted prior to undertaking further research on a topic.	▪ Answers specific review or research questions ▪ Details a systematic and comprehensive search strategy, specifying databases, search strings, and inclusion and exclusion criteria ▪ Exhaustive: designed to retrieve all relevant literature ▪ Restricted to certain study types that meet the predefined requirements (e.g., experimental studies); requires a quality evaluation of the studies ▪ Requires at least two independent coders	Narrative synthesis with tabular or quantitative summaries	▪ Narrow review questions leave additional questions unanswered ▪ Resource-intensive ▪ Methodological inconsistencies across the studies makes it difficult to draw meaningful conclusions ▪ Potential bias in the screening process related to differences in the interpretation of inclusion and exclusion criteria among researchers involved

(Continued)

TABLE 1.9. (Continued)

Description	Search and Screening Strategy	Analysis and Synthesis Strategy	Challenges and Limitations
Meta-analysis			
▪ A systematic search, appraisal, and synthesis of quantitative studies that includes a complex statistical aggregation/combination of results from the reviewed studies into single quantitative estimates of effect ▪ Can be conducted as part of a systematic review	▪ Starts with a clearly formulated and specific review questions or hypothesis ▪ Details a systematic and comprehensive search strategy, specifying databases, search strings, and inclusion and exclusion criteria ▪ Exhaustive: designed to conduct a search of all relevant literature. ▪ Restricted to certain study types that meet the predefined requirements (e.g., experimental studies); requires a quality evaluation of the studies ▪ Requires at least two independent coders	▪ Explicitly describes methods for analyzing pooled data ▪ Conducts a statistical analysis of the pooled results of estimates of effect to detect patterns or relationships and draw conclusions. ▪ Statistical synthesis in graphical and tabular forms, with narrative summaries	▪ The methodological diversity or heterogeneity of studies challenges statistical integration or aggregation
Meta-synthesis			
▪ A systematic and structured search, critical appraisal, and nonstatistical synthesis of findings from multiple qualitative studies to draw conclusions or formulate novel interpretations or conceptualizations of findings from individual studies **Example:** Wigert et al. (2020)	▪ Starts with a clearly formulated and specific review questions ▪ Details a systematic and comprehensive search strategy, specifying databases, search strings, and inclusion and exclusion criteria ▪ Exhaustive: designed to conduct an exhaustive search of all relevant literature ▪ Requires a quality evaluation of the studies ▪ Requires at least two independent coders	▪ Interpretative analysis techniques (e.g., content analysis, thematic analysis, grounded theory) ▪ Qualitative or narrative synthesis with tabulations and other classification frameworks	▪ The methodological diversity (varied analytic approaches and methodological traditions) of studies challenges their integration and synthesis

TABLE 1.9. (Continued)

Description	Search and Screening Strategy	Analysis and Synthesis Strategy	Challenges and Limitations
Scoping Review			
▪ A preliminary and structured exploration of the nature, volume, and scope of existing literature (including ongoing studies) on a particular topic to identify research gaps and determine the need for a systematic review or primary research ▪ Often used in research proposals (e.g., dissertation/thesis, manuscripts, or journal articles to set the stage for the study) **Example**: Yiu, Rohwer, and Young (2018)	▪ Focused on a broad or general research question ▪ Explicitly describes comprehensive search strategy and study protocol, with changes to inclusion and exclusion criteria as needed ▪ Exhaustive: it includes diverse published or unpublished studies (i.e., gray literature) addressing the central research question, regardless of study designs and methods (e.g., qualitative, quantitative, mixed methods) ▪ Does not require formal quality assessment ▪ Requires at least two independent coders	Does not provide a synthesis of the study findings but uses content or thematic analysis approaches to produce a descriptive account of the size and scope of the existing literature by themes; may include numerical, tabular, or graphical summaries of the size and scope	▪ Time-consuming due to the comprehensive searches and large volumes of results ▪ Potential selection bias since it does not require the appraisal of study quality or risk of bias

(Continued)

TABLE 1.9. (Continued)

Description	Search and Screening Strategy	Analysis and Synthesis Strategy	Challenges and Limitations
Rapid Review			
- A variation of a systematic review that uses a more efficient, accelerated, and streamlined process compared with a traditional systematic review to address urgent information needs for practice or policy - Often conducted as a stand-alone research project **Example:** McLure et al. (2021)	- Answers specific review or research questions - Details a systematic but restricted search strategy, specifying databases, search strings, and inclusion and exclusion criteria - Restricted: Searches are designed to retrieve relevant literature from a few strategically selected databases within a limited timeframe - Restricted to certain study types that meet the predefined requirements (e.g., experimental studies); requires a quality evaluation of the studies - Requires at least one independent coder, with limited involvement of a second coder to check for correctness and completeness	- Narrative synthesis and tabular or quantitative summaries	- Time constraints and restricted searchers limit completeness or comprehensiveness - Methodological inconsistencies across the studies makes it difficult to draw meaningful conclusions - Potential bias in the screening process related to differences in the interpretation of inclusion and exclusion criteria due to the limited involvement of a second coder

THE LITERATURE REVIEW PROCESS

The literature review is an ongoing and iterative process that begins during the conceptualization of the research study and is refined as the study progresses or as new themes emerge (Easterby-Smith et al., 2008; Steeves et al., n.d.). While we describe several types of literature reviews, our focus is on conducting a traditional (narrative) literature review as part of a thesis, dissertation, and other research studies. We propose an eight-step road map for conducting a traditional literature review, categorized into the following three stages (Figure 1.8): (a) planning the review; (b) reviewing the literature; and (c) writing the review report. Our traditional or narrative review process incorporates some elements of a systematic review to improve the quality, breadth, and strength of the review (Mallett et al., 2012). This review process is discussed and illustrated using type 2 diabetes mellitus as an example. For participatory or collaborative research projects, the key stakeholders should be actively engaged throughout the literature review process, most importantly in the planning and writing stages.

FIGURE 1.8. *The three-stage literature review process.*

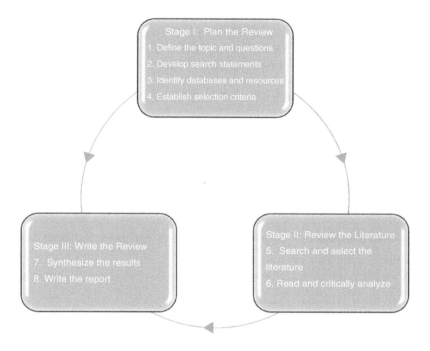

Stage I: Planning the Literature Review

The *planning stage* is the initial stage of the literature review process, where the review's focus and search strategy are established. This stage comprises four major tasks:

- Define the literature review topic and questions.
- Develop search statements.
- Identify databases and resources.
- Establish selection criteria.

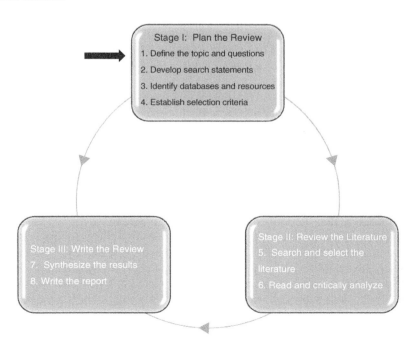

1. Define the literature review topic and questions.

    A literature review should begin with a clear formulation of a review topic and questions. Randolph (2008) makes a distinction between *literature review questions* (i.e., questions to be addressed by a review of existing literature) and *research questions* (i.e., questions to be addressed by an empirical research study). Note that for a stand-alone literature review, the review questions are the research questions. Literature review topics and questions are often inspired by numerous factors including exploratory searches and preliminary readings of relevant literature, brainstorming, or concept mapping with colleagues or advisors, scientific presentations by experts, or professional and personal experience. While many start with a broad topic or question, these preliminary exploratory readings often reveal relevant subtopics and research gaps that gradually lead to more refined and focused review questions (Efron and Ravid, 2019). Review questions that are too broad may produce an overwhelming number of results from the search of the literature that is not easily manageable, whereas very narrow questions may exclude potentially useful sources (Cronin et al., 2008). The questions in Box 1.6 are general questions that can be used as a starting point for formulating more specific literature review questions on a topic.

BOX 1.6 Guiding Questions for Formulating a Topic for the Literature Review

1. What are the origins and definitions of the topic?
2. What are the key concepts, variables, and themes about this topic, including relationships among these concepts?
3. What are the main questions that have been addressed on this topic?
4. What are the theories or models that have been applied to this topic in practice or in research?
5. What methodological approaches have been used to study this topic, including the strengths and limitations? Are there alternative approaches that have not been used?
6. What are the major issues, debates, and inconsistencies about the topic?
7. What are the gaps in knowledge, theory, and methods on the topic?

Adapted from Hart (1998, 2018)

---

2. Develop the search statement.

    Having defined the review questions, the next step is to develop the search statements that will be used to retrieve relevant literature from search engines or databases. The researcher begins by identifying and listing the main concepts of the topic including the synonyms and related words. Preliminary or exploratory readings of relevant literature (e.g., systematic reviews) often reveal key concepts related to the topic. In addition, some databases have searchable thesauri with controlled vocabulary or subject terms that help in identifying additional relevant terms for the search.

    To build precise search statements, the search terms or key words can be connected using *Boolean operators*. These operators are simple words that combine search terms to expand or narrow the search. The three most commonly used Boolean operators are AND, OR, and NOT. The operator AND narrows the search by identifying sources containing all the specified words or phrases. This is the default setting in many databases when search terms are entered without specifying an operator. In contrast, using OR expands the search by retrieving articles containing at least one of the specified words or phrases. Finally, the Boolean operator NOT narrows the search by excluding a specified word or phrase. The search terms and Boolean operators can be enclosed within parentheses to ensure that they are combined and interpreted effectively, in which case the database processes the information starting from the innermost (within parentheses) to the outermost statement (outside of parentheses).

    In addition to Boolean operators, various symbols can be used to produce focused or comprehensive search results. *Truncations* (also known as stemming) and *wild cards* expand the search by capturing variations of a word. While truncation and wild card symbols vary by database, the most frequently used symbols are *, ?, $. When entered next to a root word, the truncation symbol instructs the database to identify articles with variable endings of the root word. On the other hand, wild cards substitute one letter of a word with a symbol to capture alternative spellings of the word. Some databases (e.g., PubMed) do not support the wild card function but automatically produce variable spellings of a word in the search. Using quotation marks around a phrase such as "type 2 diabetes" identifies sources containing the exact phrase. The researcher should always check each database's search tips or tutorials, library guidebooks, or consult the librarian to ensure the appropriate use of search terms, Boolean operators, and symbols in different databases. Table 1.10 presents examples of searches using each Boolean operator, quotation marks, and parentheses to demonstrate their effects on the search.

TABLE 1.10. Symbols and Operators Used in Building Search Statements for a Literature Review

Operator/ symbol	Description	Examples	
		Search term	PubMed results
AND	Finds sources with all the specified words or phrases	type 2 diabetes AND socioeconomic	311 articles with both *type 2 diabetes* and *socioeconomic*
OR	Finds articles with at least one of the specified words or phrases	type 2 diabetes OR socioeconomic	144, 117 articles with either *type 2 diabetes* alone, *socioeconomic* alone, or both *type 2 diabetes* and *socio-economic*
		(type 2 diabetes OR non–insulin-dependent diabetes OR diabetes mellitus) AND socioeconomic	969 articles
		compared with:	
		type 2 diabetes AND socioeconomic	311 articles
NOT	Excludes the specified word or phrase	diabetes NOT type 1 diabetes	639,104 articles, excluding any article with the phrase *type 1 diabetes*
		compared with:	
		diabetes	676,411 articles
Parentheses: ( )	Ensures an effective interpretation of the search statement by instructing the database to process the information from the innermost (within parentheses) to the outermost terms (outside parentheses)	(type 2 diabetes OR non–insulin-dependent diabetes OR diabetes mellitus) AND (socioeconomic or social compared with: type 2 diabetes OR non–insulin-dependent diabetes OR diabetes mellitus) AND socioeconomic or social	13,271 articles that contain any of words in the first statement (i.e., *type 2 diabetes, non–insulin-dependent diabetes,* or *diabetes mellitus*) together with any of the words in the second statement (i.e., *socioeconomic* or *social*) 850, 552 articles

(Continued)

TABLE 1.10. (Continued)

Operator/ symbol	Description	Examples	
		Search term	PubMed results
Quotations: " "	Finds sources containing the exact phrase	"type 2 diabetes" Compared with: type 2 diabetes	115,736 articles with the exact phrase *type 2 diabetes* 167,881 articles containing *type* and *2* and *diabetes* (similar to using the operator AND)
Truncation: *,?, $	Finds documents with variable endings of the specified root word	diabet*	715, 524 articles with any of the following: diabetes, diabetic, diabetogenic, diabetologist...etc.
Wild card: *,?, $	Finds documents with alternative spellings of the same word	organi?ation	Not supported by PubMed but yields results containing the spellings *organization* and *organisation* in other databases

Developing search statements is an iterative process of pilot testing and revising the search terms until satisfactory results are produced. During this step, it is important to document the initial and final search statements, including their respective results to avoid repeating unproductive searches, to justify and describe the development of the search statements, and to ensure that the search can be reproduced in the future.

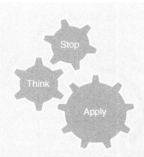

Formulate Search Terms for a Literature Review

Your professor has asked you to conduct a literature review on a topic you are interested in. Identify this topic and provide the following information:

1. Write one question that you would like your literature review to answer (i.e., the literature review question).
2. Based on the literature review question you have formulated, develop two search statements that you can use in retrieving the literature on your topic.

Discuss your responses with a classmate or instructor.

3. Identify the databases and other resources for the search.

Another important aspect of the planning stage is to identify the databases and additional resources from which the literature can be retrieved. Grewal et al. (2016) outline three main methods for identifying the literature to be reviewed:

- Electronic or hand searching of relevant databases or journals
- Snowballing or checking the reference lists of useful articles
- Drawing from existing theories and scholars and experts on the topic

Technological advances have facilitated access to online search engines, websites, and databases containing a wealth of literature including journal articles, books, government reports, organizational reports, conference papers, and theses and dissertations on a variety of topics. Selecting appropriate databases depends on several factors including the research/review topic, the database's coverage or subject area, and its accessibility. Some databases are multidisciplinary and cover a variety of subject areas, whereas others are subject or discipline specific. Ideally, the search should cover multiple databases—both multidisciplinary and subject-specific—to gain a deeper understanding of the topic. Librarians and library websites often compile comprehensive lists of databases arranged in alphabetical order or by subject area. The researcher should read the descriptions of each database to assess its relevance to the topic. Some databases and resources are free to individual users while commercially licensed databases are only accessible to those associated with institutions that have purchased the membership or subscription (Creswell and Creswell, 2018; Efron and Ravid, 2019). While the accessibility of the database itself should be taken into consideration, the search should not be limited to databases with full-text articles only since full text articles can be alternatively accessed through the interlibrary loan or in print in the library. Johns Hopkins University's Welch Medical Library (n.d.) website presents a comprehensive list of health and public health-oriented databases, some of which are described in Table 1.11.

TABLE 1.11. Common Databases for Public Health Research

Database	Description	Discipline	Link
PubMed	Contains biomedical and life sciences literature	Biomedicine and health fields, and related life sciences (behavioral sciences, chemical sciences, and bioengineering)	https://pubmed.ncbi.nlm.nih.gov
CINAHL (Cumulative Index of Nursing and Allied Health Literature)	Contains literature for nursing and other health professions such as biomedicine, alternative medicine, nutrition and dietetics, physical therapy, and occupational therapy	Nursing and allied health professions	https://www.ebscohost.com/nursing/products/cinahl-databases
Cochrane library	A collection of databases of systematic reviews and meta-analyses on effective health care interventions	Medicine, nursing, allied health professions	https://www.cochranelibrary.com
Embase	A database of biomedical and pharmacological literature, with s focus on drug research, pharmacology, toxicology; also covers alternative therapies, occupational therapy, and physical therapy	Biomedical and pharmacological sciences	https://www.embase.com

(Continued)

TABLE 1.11. (Continued)

Database	Description	Discipline	Link
Global health	Contains international medical and public health research	Public health, tropical medicine, and other biomedical and life sciences	https://www.cabdirect.org/globalhealth
ERIC (Education Resources Information Center)	A database of education literature and resources	Education	https://eric.ed.gov
Scopus	A major multidisciplinary database for the social sciences, life sciences, health sciences, physical sciences, and arts and humanities	Multidisciplinary	https://www.elsevier.com/solutions/scopus
PyscINFO	Major database for behavioral and social science literature	Psychology, psychiatry, medicine, education, behavioral, and social sciences	https://www.apa.org/pubs/databases/psycinfo
Web of science	Indexes literature in the sciences, social sciences, arts, and humanities	Multidisciplinary	https://login.webofknowledge.com

Not all sources are indexed in databases, thus nonindexed or nondatabase sources should be identified to ensure a more comprehensive literature review. The *gray literature* refers to the literature produced in commercial publishing channels, such as reports from government agencies and professional organizations, conference papers and proceedings, dissertations and theses, technical reports, bulletins and fact sheets, and policy documents outside of peer reviewed academic journals. The gray literature can be identified through searches on common search engines (e.g., Google) and specific government (ending in .gov) and organizational websites (ending in .org or .edu), gray literature databases, or in the library (i.e., print versions). The gray literature is a valuable source of information, particularly when there is a dearth of peer-reviewed resources on the topic. However, literature that has not undergone a formal peer-review process should be used in light of this limitation or critically evaluated and validated against other sources. Additional sources can be identified through snowballing, which consists of scanning the bibliographies or reference lists of relevant articles (e.g., systematic reviews) to identify additional sources for the literature review.

4. Establish selection criteria: inclusion and exclusion criteria (filters)

Establishing the selection (inclusion and exclusion) criteria for the literature search helps optimize the search and selection process to capture high-quality and useful sources. These criteria should be selected based on the review purpose and questions (Stage I), the overall research objectives, as well as the specific guidelines outlined by a research grant, discipline, or institution. Systematic reviews require the explicit articulation of the selection criteria for transparency, consistency, and replicability purposes. While this is not required for traditional or narrative reviews, we recommend defining and documenting the selection criteria for the same reasons.

Some inclusion and exclusion criteria can be applied as filters during the database searches to produce more focused results, while others can be evaluated by the researcher during the screening and selection process (Stage II-step 5). The databases described in the previous section offer several filters that can be applied to refine searches. Box 1.7 provides examples of selection criteria for a literature review.

> **BOX 1.7** Examples of Selection Criteria for a Literature Review
>
> - Publication date:
>   - Usually, no older than 5–10 years except for seminal, foundational, or historical literature
> - Types of publication:
>   - Primary: original research/work (usually included in dissertation literature reviews)
>   - Secondary: evaluation or synthesis of original research (e.g., systematic review)
>   - Tertiary: synthesis of secondary sources (e.g., textbooks)
>   - Peer-reviewed (usually preferred in dissertation and thesis literature reviews) or non–peer-reviewed sources
> - Publication language
> - Participants' sociodemographic characteristics
> - Research design
> - Setting or geographic location
> - Exposure or outcome of interest

Phase II: Conducting your Literature Review

Once the literature review topic, questions, search terms, databases, and selection criteria are established, the next phase of the literature review process involves the search, selection, critical reading, and analysis of the retrieved sources.

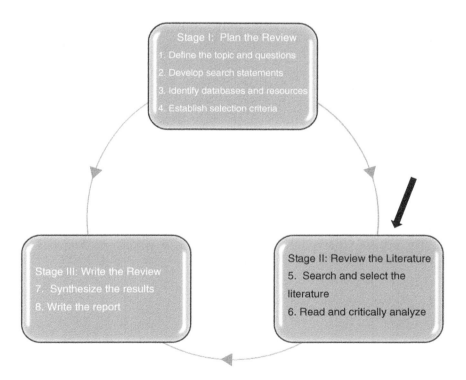

5. Search, screen, and select the literature.

The literature search is an iterative process that is ongoing until information saturation is reached, where subsequent searches no longer produce new sources or new information and the review questions have been answered (Efron and Ravid, 2019; Rennison and Hart, 2019). Applying the pre-defined search statements (Stage I-step 2) to the selected databases (Stage I-step 3) will produce search results that are then screened by the researcher in two main rounds. First, the researcher begins with a preliminary screening of the titles, abstracts, or sections of the initial search results to assess their relevance to the review questions (Stage I-step 1) as well as their eligibility based on the pre-defined selection criteria (Stage I-step 4). This initial title-and-abstract screening process enables the researcher to narrow the list of articles for consideration by removing irrelevant and ineligible sources. The second screening, which can also be conducted in conjunction with the next step (Stage II-step 6), involves scanning sections or full texts of the remaining sources before engaging in critical and analytical reading. The lack of full-text articles should not deter their consideration for inclusion into the review since they are often accessible upon request from a librarian or through an institution's interlibrary loan. Researchers should contact the librarian to inquire about accessing such articles.

While the volume of the search results can render this process overwhelming and time-consuming, there are several tools to optimize and organize the search and selection process. One such tool is the PRISMA Diagram (Figure 1.8). This diagram is used to ensure transparency and replicability in systematic reviews and can also help in maintaining a structured record of the search and selection process in traditional literature reviews.

FIGURE 1.9. *Preferred Reporting Items for Systematic Reviews and Meta-Analyses (PRISMA) Flow Diagram.*

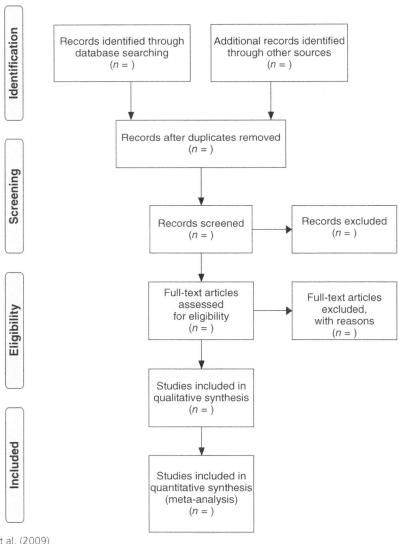

Reprinted from Moher et al. (2009)

Another useful tool is reference management software, which can be used to store and organize the sources into folders, as well as to generate automatic citations in different citation styles when writing. There is a wide variety of reference management tools, some of which require individual or institutional subscriptions for members of academic or research institutions. Some common reference management software include Zotero (www.zotero.org; free), Mendeley (www.mendeley.com; free), Papers (www.papersapp.com; subscription), EndNote (https://endnote.com; subscription), and RefWorks (www.refworks.com; subscription). The majority of electronic databases discussed in Stage I-step 3 provide options to save, email, or export retrieved sources to a reference management software, among other locations (Efron and Ravid, 2019).

6. Read and critically analyze the literature.

Once all the sources are identified and stored in the reference management tool, the researcher evaluates each source using a critical and analytical lens. Critical and analytical reading is *not* summarizing nor merely accepting the literature. It involves higher-order cognitive skills such as appraising, comparing, contrasting, questioning, critiquing, and organizing. The critical reader performs the following tasks: (a) examines the literature to gain a deeper understanding of the major concepts and their relationships; (b) critiques, compares, and contrasts findings across sources (i.e., consistencies, conflicts/contradictions); (c) critiques methodological approaches and theoretical applications; and (d) identifies gaps in the findings, methods, and theories. During this process of reading and rereading, the researcher critically evaluates each source's research questions, assumptions, methods, central findings and conclusions, strengths and limitations, and recommendations for future research. Reading should be intentional, strategic, and purposeful in that it seeks to answer the review questions defined in Stage I-step 2. Screening continues in the reading phase, where nonuseful sources can be excluded from the review, and the PRISMA flowchart (Figure 1.9) can be revised accordingly. Box 1.8 outlines guide questions for the critical reading of the literature.

BOX 1.8 Critical Reading Questions for a Literature Review

The following are examples of questions to ask when reading each literature review source (Efron and Ravid, 2019; Rennison and Hart, 2019):

- What research problem or gap, questions, or hypotheses does this study address?
- What are the key assumptions, and how can they affect the study?
- In what context was this study conducted? How does the context compare with other sources?
- What are the methods and theories used? Why? Strengths and limitations?
- What are the central arguments, findings, and conclusions of the study?
- What is the evidence to support these findings and conclusions? Are there alternative explanations for the findings? Are the conclusions strongly supported by the results?
- How does this study compare (agreements, disagreements) with other literature on the topic?
- Overall, what are the stated and unstated strengths and limitations of the study?
- What are the study's recommendations for future research?
- What is my interpretation of this study? How does it advance my understanding of the topic? How does it relate to my study?

In practice, reading, note-taking, and organizing take place concurrently. As the researcher critically reads each individual source, they take notes of pertinent findings, arguments, or conclusions including their critical evaluations and comments. These notes can be organized under categories and themes and subcategories and subthemes and cited using the reference management tools discussed in the previous section. These themes can be predetermined or emerging from the literature in the form of recurrent ideas, patterns, and trends. The following are common note-taking methods for a literature review (California Polytechnic State University n.d.; Murdoch University n.d.):

- *The outline method*: Note-taking using bullet points organized under main themes (headings) and subthemes (subheadings) emerging from the literature (see Resource A)

- *The Cornell method*: Note-taking in a two-column table, with the key concepts and themes in the left column, the main findings in the right column, and the researcher's reflections in the bottom row (Pauk, 2001) (see Resource B)

- *The chart method:* Note-taking in a multicolumn table with some of the following common column headings: source (author, year), study purpose and research questions, study setting and context, participants, methods, main findings, limitations, contribution to the review, and comments and reflections
- *The mapping method:* Graphical or visual representation of key concepts from the literature and their connections or relationships
- *The sentence method:* Writing each main idea or argument from the literature as a separate line or sentence, and numbering or grouping lines or sentences under appropriate headings or subheadings

Regardless of the note-taking method, the researcher should differentiate between the information extracted from the literature and their critical interpretations of each source to ensure transparency and avoid plagiarism later in the writing stage. One simple technique to prevent plagiarism is to keep salient excerpts from the literature in direct quotations with appropriate citations when reading and note-taking and paraphrasing them later in the writing stage (Napitupulu et al., 2019).

After reading and taking detailed notes from the literature, the next step is to organize the notes in preparation for the writing stage. This process involves cleaning up and rearranging the notes from the previous step by strategically grouping (copy and paste) related arguments or concepts into appropriate thematic and sub thematic areas to depict their connections and relationships. This saves time and enables the researcher to flow smoothly when writing their synthesis of the literature. In addition, concurrent reading, note-taking, and organizing enables the researcher to assess whether information saturation has been reached and to fill gaps in the thematic areas through additional refined searches as needed.

Phase III: Write the Literature Review

Once the literature has been critically appraised and organized around key themes and subthemes, the researcher can begin writing the literature review report. An embedded literature review report generally contains an introduction, body, conclusion, and a reference or bibliography section. A stand-alone review may include an abstract and a methods section in addition to the aforementioned sections. When writing the literature review report, we recommend starting with the body or synthesis of the literature (step 7) before completing the remaining sections of the report (step 8).

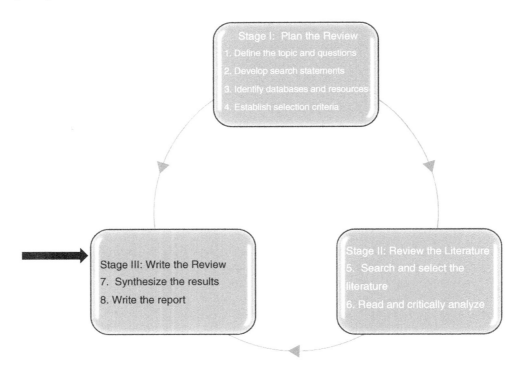

7. Synthesize the review findings.

The synthesis of the literature forms the body of the literature review report (see full report in step 8). The synthesis is an integrative, comparative, and evaluative discussion of the reviewed literature (University of West Indies, 2019). It involves connecting the information from the reviewed literature into logical, coherent, and original arguments or conclusions rather than summarizing each source separately. Overall, this synthesis presents a scholarly conversation between authors, one that captures their agreements and disagreements (Oregon State University, 2020). The researcher's unique interpretation of the literature positions the researcher within this scholarly dialogue on the topic while building a solid argument for their own study (Efron and Ravid, 2019). The synthesis should answer the literature review questions formulated in Stage I.

Before writing the synthesis, the researcher outlines its structure. The following are common structures for the synthesis (body) of the literature (Carnwell and Daly, 2001), from which the researcher can select one or a combination depending on the review purpose or questions, field or discipline, and institutional requirements:

- *Thematic:* Organizes the review or synthesis into themes and subthemes that reflect recurrent patterns in the literature—described in the previous sections since it is the most common format in public health literature reviews

- *Chronological or historical:* Organizes the synthesis by time periods, with a critical discussion of the development or evolution of the concept or phenomenon over time—pointing to future research directions, drawing from the historical progression of the topic

- *Methodological:* Organizes the review around various methodological approaches used in the reviewed studies, with critical comparisons of their findings, overall strengths, and limitations—facilitates the identification of alternative methodologies

- *Theoretical:* Organizes the review around key theories and models used in investigating the topic, including their strengths and limitations—usually informing the development of a theoretical framework for the study

Regardless of the structure of the synthesis, it should be organized into sections (themes) and subsections (subthemes), with each paragraph focusing on a single main idea. Inspired by the MEAL (main idea, evidence, analysis, and linkage) approach adapted by Rennison and Hart (2019) and the 5 C approach (cite, compare, contrast, critique, connect) for writing a literature review (Edith Cowan University, 2008), we propose that the synthesis include the following elements for each theme and subtheme:

- Introduce the main idea or thesis or topic statement.

- Discuss, compare, contrast, and cite the evidence: similarities or agreements, contradictions or inconsistencies, debates, and controversies.

- Present your critique or analysis of the evidence: strengths, limitations, and possible or alternative explanations for inconsistencies.

- Link or connect the evidence to the review questions, to your research, and to the next section or subsection (use transitions).

The narrative or synthesis should gradually and logically build toward the research agenda (topic or questions) of the thesis or dissertation.

8. Write the full literature review report.

Once the researcher has all the necessary elements, they engage in several rounds of outlining, drafting, proofreading, and editing to produce the full and polished literature review report. This section outlines a full literature review report, summarizing the key contents of each section: introduction, body, conclusion, and references or bibliography (Box 1.9).

> **BOX 1.9** Sections of a Literature Review Report
>
> I. *Introduction*: Provides an overview of the topic and establishes the purpose and methods of the literature review
>   - Define the main topic or problem and its significance.
>   - Describe the overall state of evidence on the topic, highlighting major research gaps and areas of conflict and debate.
>   - State the rationale, purpose, and objectives of the literature review, the review questions, and its potential contribution to the current evidence on the topic.
>   - Describe the review methods, including the search statements, databases, selection criteria, and synthesis and analysis process.
>   - Describe the organization of the literature review section and report.
>
> II. *Body*: Synthesizes the reviewed literature and is organized into headings and subheadings with variations by structure (i.e., thematic, chronological, methodological, theoretical)
>   *Heading/Theme 1*
>   - Introduce the main point (i.e., thesis or topic statement).
>   - Discuss, compare, contrast, and cite the evidence: similarities and agreements, contradictions and inconsistencies, debates, and controversies.
>   - Present your critique or analysis of the evidence: strengths, limitations, and possible or alternative explanations for inconsistencies.
>   - Link or connect the evidence to the review questions, to your proposed research, and to the next section or subsection (use transitions).
>
>   *Subheading*
>   - Introduce the main argument related to the subtheme (i.e., thesis or topic statement).
>   - Discuss, compare, contrast, and cite the evidence: similarities and agreements, contradictions and inconsistencies, debates, and controversies.
>   - Present your critique or analysis of the evidence: strengths, limitations, and possible or alternative explanations for inconsistencies.
>   - Link or connect the evidence to the review questions, to your research, and to the next section or subsection (use transitions).
>
> III. *Heading/Theme 2* (repeat previous structure as needed for all the themes and subthemes)
>   *Conclusions*: Summarizes key findings (agreements, disagreements), gaps, and new research directions
>   - Summarize the main conclusions in response to the review questions.
>   - Summarize the strength or quality of current evidence on the topic.
>   - Reiterate key limitations or gaps in the current evidence (i.e., limited, inconclusive, contradictory findings, theories, or methods).
>   - Provide recommendations for future research based on the limitations and gaps.
>   - Discussion of the position, significance, or potential contribution of your research to the current evidence base.
>
> IV. *References*: All sources are cited using the appropriate citation style (see Module 5).

Length of the Report

One common question when undertaking a literature review is, "What is the expected length of the report?" There is no single answer to this question since the length of the literature review depends on several factors including the nature of the topic, type of project or paper, level of study (e.g., undergraduate, masters, doctorate), scope of the available literature, or the institution or advisor's requirements. The literature review report is often a full chapter of a traditional thesis or dissertation report or a short section of a journal article (i.e., background or introduction section). It is important to consult the advisor or institution's guidelines/handbook to determine the expected or required length of a literature review.

> **BOX 1.10 Tips for Writing an Effective Literature Review**
>
> - *Be critical and analytical*: Do not merely summarize or synthesize other authors' arguments and conclusions but instead present your critical and informed analysis and interpretation.
> - *Write concisely*: Express yourself in the fewest words necessary to convey your critical synthesis; use short sentences and paragraphs.
> - *Avoid overciting*: Be focused and selective. Include only sources that are most relevant and useful in answering your review questions and informing your proposed research.
> - *Limit direct quotations*: Paraphrase, integrate, and synthesize the sources. Direct quotations should be reserved for emphasizing information that is pertinent, memorable, or hold special significance.
> - *Be objective and unbiased*: Do not only include supportive sources but also discuss competing or opposing views or arguments rather than being one-sided.
> - *Avoid plagiarism*: Ensure that all ideas acquired from other sources are accurately cited and referenced.

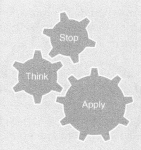

Critique of a Literature Review Report

In pairs, identify a published or unpublished literature review on your topic of choice (preferably a thesis or dissertation report). Read the literature review section and independently respond to the following questions, after which you will discuss and compare your responses in your pairs.

Introduction
1. What is the topic of the review?
2. What is the purpose or objective of the review?
3. What questions does the review address, if any?
4. What were the methods for selecting the sources?
    - What were the search terms/statements?
    - Which databases were searched? Was it a comprehensive search?
    - What were the inclusion and exclusion criteria?

Body
5. Is the review organized in a logical manner?
6. What is the structure of the synthesis (i.e., thematic, chronological, methodological, theoretical)?
7. What is your overall assessment of the synthesis of the literature (i.e., strengths and weaknesses)?
    - Does the review provide a critical and analytical synthesis of the literature?
    - Is the synthesis unbiased or objective (i.e., does it include diverse or conflicting viewpoints)?
    - Does the review include a critique of the study designs and methodologies?
8. Were the review questions answered or was its purpose fulfilled?
9. List the gaps, limitations, or unresolved issues that are highlighted in the report.

Conclusion
10. Does the conclusion clearly reiterate or emphasize the main gaps or unresolved conflicts?
11. What are the author's recommendations for future research?
12. Does the author make a connection between the review and their proposed research?
13. Does the review provide a strong justification or rationale for the proposed study?

SUMMARY

The literature review is an ongoing and iterative process that begins during the conceptualization of the research study and is refined as the study progresses or as new themes emerges. While we describe several types of literature reviews, our focus is on conducting a traditional (narrative) literature review as part of a thesis, dissertation, and other research studies. The eight-step roadmap for conducting a traditional literature review is categorized into the following three phases: (a) planning the review, (b) reviewing the literature, and (c) writing the review report.

Developing search statements is an iterative process of pilot testing and revising the search terms until satisfactory results are produced. During this step, it is important to document the initial and final search statements, including their respective results to avoid repeating unproductive searches, to justify and describe the development of the search statements, and to ensure that the search can be reproduced in the future.

Critical and analytical reading is *not* summarizing nor merely accepting the literature. It involves the higher-order cognitive skills of *analysis*, *evaluation* and *creating* categories.

Note-taking can be done using the outline method (notetaking using bullet points), the Cornell method (notetaking in a two-column table), the chart method (notetaking in a multicolumn table), the mapping method (visual representation of key concepts), or the sentence method (writing each main idea or argument as a separate line or sentence).

There are several methods for reporting the literature review findings. The thematic method organizes the review or synthesis into themes and subthemes that reflect recurrent patterns in the literature. The chronological or historical method organizes the synthesis by time periods, with a critical discussion of the development or evolution of the concept or phenomenon over time. The methodological strategy organizes the review around various methodological approaches. The theoretical method organizes the review around key theories and models used in investigating the topic.

Once the researcher has all of the necessary elements, they engage in several rounds of outlining, drafting, proofreading, and editing to produce the full and polished literature review report.

Now I have reached the end this section I am able to:

Course Objective	Strongly Agree	Somewhat Agree	Neutral	Somewhat Disagree	Strongly Agree
Differentiate a traditional (narrative) literature review from other types of reviews					
Describe the literature review process					
Design a traditional (narrative) literature review					

REFERENCES

Aarons, D. (2018). Research in epidemic and emergency situations: A model for collaboration and expediting ethics review in two Caribbean countries. *Developing World Bioethics*, *18*, 375–384.

Bartlett, L., & Vavrus, F. (2017). *Rethinking Case Study Research*. New York: Routledge.

Boaz, A., Hanney, S., Borst, R., O'Shea, A., & Kok, M. (2018). How to engage stakeholders in research: design principles to support improvement. *Health Research Policy Systems, 16*(60), 2–9. http://doi.org/10.1186/s12961-018-0337-6

Brookfield, S. D. (2012). *Teaching for critical thinking. Tools and techniques to help students question their assumptions*, San Francisco, CA: Jossey-Bass.

Calba, C., Goutard, F. L., Hoinville, L., Hendrikx, P., Lindberg, A., Saegerman, C., & Peyre, M. (2015). Surveillance systems evaluation: a systematic review of the existing approaches. *BMC Public Health, 15*, 448. https://doi.org/10.1186/s12889-015-1791-5

California Polytechnic State University. (n.d.). Note taking systems. https://content-calpoly-edu.s3.amazonaws.com/asc/1/documents/StudySkills/NoteTakingSystems.pdf

Carlson, R. V., Boyd, K. M., & Webb, D. J. (2004). The revision of the declaration of Helsinki: Past, present and future. *British Journal of Clinical Pharmacology, 57*(6), 695–713. https://doi.org/10.1111/j.1365-2125.2004.02103.x

Carnwell, R., & Daly, W. (2001). Strategies for the construction of a critical review of the literature. *Nurse Education in Practice, 1*(2), 57–63. http://doi.org/10.1054/nepr.2001.0008

Casado, B. L., Negi, N. J., & Hong, M. (2012). Culturally competent social work research: Methodological considerations for research with language minorities. *Social Work, 57*(1), 1–10.

Center for Social Justice and Community Action. (2012). Community-based participatory research. A guide to ethical principles and practice. UK: Durham University. http://www.dur.ac.uk/resources/beacon/CBPREthicsGuidewebNovember20121.pdf

Charmaz, K. (2014). *Constructing grounded theory* (2nd ed.). Sage.

Chilisa, B. (2012). *Indigenous research methodologies*. Sage.

Christopher, S., Watts, V., McCormick, A. G., & Young, S. (2008). Building and maintaining trust in a community-based participatory research partnership. *American Journal of Public Health, 98*, 1398–1406.

CITI. (n.d.). Research Ethics and Compliance Training. https://about.citiprogram.org/en/homepage

Coughlin, S. S. (2009). *Case studies in public health ethics*. American Public Health Association Press.

Council for International Organizations of Medical Sciences (2002). International Ethical Guidelines for biomedical research involving human subjects. CIOMS: Geneva.

Creswell, J. W., & Creswell, J. D. (2018). *Research design qualitative, quantitative, and mixed methods approaches*. Sage.

Cronin, P., Ryan, F., & Coughlan, M. (2008). Undertaking a literature review: A step-by-step approach. *British Journal of Nursing, 17*(1), 38–43. http://doi.org/10.12968/bjon.2008.17.1.28059

Denzin, N. H. (1989). *Interpretive biography*. NewburyPark. https://doi.org/10.4135/9781412984584

Easterby-Smith, M., Thorpe, R., & Jackson, P. (2008). Doing a literature review. In *Management research* (3rd ed., pp. 29–53). Sage.

Edith Cowan University. (2008). Literature review: Academic tip sheet. https://intranet.ecu.edu.au/__data/assets/pdf_file/0011/20621/literature_review.pdf

Efron, S. E., & Ravid, R. (2019). *Writing the literature review: A practical guide*. Guilford Press.

Ember, C., & Ember, M. (2009). *Cross-cultural research methods*. AltaMira Press.

Faulkner, S.L. and Trotter, S. (2017). The International Encyclopedia of communication Research Methods. https://doi.org/10.1002/9781118901731.iecrm0060

Fink, A. (2019). *Conducting research literature reviews: from the Internet to paper* (5th ed.). SAGE.

Frier, P. (2018). *Pedagogy of the oppressed*. Bloomsbury Academic.

Glanz, K., Rimer, B. K., & Viswanath, K. (2015). Theory, research and practice in health behavior. In K. Glanz, B. K. Rimer, & K. Viswanath (Eds.), *Health behavior and health education theory, research and practice*. Jossey-Bass.

Graham, R.W. (2005). Illustrating triangulation in mixed methods nursing research. Nurse Researcher, 12 (4), 7-18 DOI. 10.7748/2005.04

Goodman, M. S., & Thompson, V. L. S. (2017). The science of stakeholder engagement in research: Classification, implementation, and evaluation. *TBM, 7*, 486–491.

Grant, M. J., & Booth, A. (2009). A typology of reviews: An analysis of 14 review types and associated methodologies. *Health Information and Libraries Journal, 26*(2), 91–108. http://doi.org/10.1111/j.1471-1842.2009.00848.x

Grewal, A., Kataria, H., & Dhawan, I. (2016). Literature search for research planning and identification of research problem. *Indian Journal of Anaesthesia, 60*(9), 635–639. http://doi.org/10.4103/0019-5049.190618

Harris, M. J. (2017). *Evaluating public and community health programs*. John Wiley and Sons, Inc.

Hart, C. (1998). *Doing a literature review: releasing the social science research imagination*. Sage Publications.

Hart, C. (2018). *Doing a literature review: Releasing the research imagination* (2nd ed.). SAGE Publications.

Hlongwa, P. (2016). Current ethical issues in HIV/AIDS research and HIV/AIDS care. *Oral Diseases, 22*(s1). http://doi.org/10.1111/odi.12391

Huang, G. D., Bull, J., Mckee, K. J., Mahon, E., Harper, B., & Roberts, J. N. and CTTI Recruitment Project Team (2018). Clinical trials recruitment planning: a proposed framework from clinical trials transformation initiative. *Contemporary Clinical Trials, 66*, 74–79. https://doi.org/10.1016/j.cct.2018.01.003

Johns Hopkins University. (n.d., May 19, 2020). Public Health Resources. https://browse.welch.jhmi.edu/public_health/public_health_literature_sources

Jones, J. H. (1993). *Bad blood: The Tuskegee Syphilis experiment*. Free Press.

Kumar, R. (2014). *Research methodology, a step-by-step guide for beginners*. Sage.

Lahman, M. K. E. (2018). *Ethics in social science research. Becoming culturally responsive*. Sage.

Lincoln, Y. S., & Guba, E. G. (1985). *Naturalistic inquiry*. Sage.

Lapan, S. D., Quartaroli, M. T., & Riemer, F. J. (Eds.). (2012). *Qualitative research: An introduction to methods and designs*. Jossey-Bass/Wiley.

Love, P., Laws, R., Hesketh, K. D., Campbell, K., & J. (2019). Lessons on early childhood obesity prevention interventions form the Victorian infant program. *Public Health Research & Practice, 29*(1), 3–6.

Mallett, R., Hagen-Zanker, J., Slater, R., & Duvendack, M. (2012). The benefits and challenges of using systematic reviews in international development research. *Journal of Development Effectiveness, 4*(3), 445–455. http://doi.org/10.1080/19439342.2012.711342

McLure, M., Eastwood, K., Parr, M., & Bray, J. (2021). A rapid review of advanced life support guidelines for cardiac arrest associated with anaphylaxis. *Resuscitation, 159*, 137–149. https://doi.org/10.1016/HYPERLINK

Merriam, S. B. (2009). *Qualitative research: A guide to design and implementation*. Jossey-Bass.
Mertens, D. M., & Wilson, A. T. (2019). *Program evaluation theory and practice. A comprehensive guide* (2nd ed.). Guilford Press.
Miles, M. B., & Huberman, A. M. (1994). *Qualitative data analysis: An expanded sourcebook* (2nd ed.). Sage Publication.
Mir, R., & Watson, A. (2000). Strategic management and philosophy of science: The case for a constructivist methodology. *Strategic Management Journal*, *21*(9), 941–953.
Moher, S., Liberati, A., Tetzlaff, J., & Altman, D. G. (2009). Preferred Reporting Items for Systematic reviews and meta-analyses: The PRISMA statement. *PLoS Medicine*, *6*(7), e1000097. http://doi.org/10.1371/journal
Murdoch University. (n.d.). Literature Reviews - Research Guide. https://libguides.murdoch.edu.au/LitReview
Napitupulu, S., Napitupulu, F. D., & Kisno (2019). *Research methodology in Linguistics and Education*. Deepublish Publisher.
Ndebele, P. (2019). *African Governments need to fund research ethics training*. University World News.
Oparah, J. C., Salahuddin, F., Cato, R., Jones, L., Oseguera, T., & Mathews, S. (2015). By us, not for us: Black women researching pregnancy and childbirth. In A. J. Jolivette (Ed.), *Research justice methodologies for social change*. Policy Press, The University of Chicago Press.
Oregon State University. (2020). Researching the literature review. https://guides.library.oregonstate.edu/literaturereview
Palinkas, L. A., Horwitz, S. M., Charmerlain, P., Hurlburt, M. S., & Landsverk, J. (2011). Mixed methods design in mental health services research: A review. *Psychiatric Services*, *62*, 255–263.
Patton, M. Q. (1999). Enhancing the quality and credibility of qualitative analysis. *Health Services Research*, *34*(5), 1189–1208.
Pauk, W. (2001). *How to study in college* (7th ed.). Houghton Mifflin Co.
Perez, M. A., & Luquis, R. R. (2008). *Cultural competence in health education and health promotion*. Jossey-Bass.
Pratt, B. (2019). Constructing citizen engagement in health research priority setting to attend to dynamic of power and difference. *Developing World Bioethics*, *19*(1), 45–60.
Randolph, J.J. (2008). *Multidisciplinary methods in educational technology research and development*. Available at: https://scholarworks.umass.edu/pare/vol14/iss1/13
Reichel, M., & Ramey, M. A. (1987). *Conceptual frameworks for bibliographic education: Theory into practice*. Libraries Unlimited.
Rennison, C. M., & Hart, T. C. (2019). Conducting a literature review. In *Research methods in criminal justice and criminology* (pp. 62–97). SAGE.
Resnik, D. B. (2015). What is Ethics in Research & Why is it Important? National Institute of Environmental Health Sciences. Retrieved 9/25/2022. https://www.niehs.nih.gov/research/resources/bioethics/whatis/index.cfm
Saxe, J.G. (1873). The Blind Man and the Elephant. Common Lit CCBY-NC-4.0 license li https://www.commonlit.org/en/texts/the-blind-men-and-the-elephant
Sbaraini, A., Carter, S. M., Evans, R. W., & Blinkhorn, A. (2011). How to do a grounded theory study: A worked example of a study of dental practices. *BMC Medical Research Methodology*, *11*(1), 128. http://doi.org/10.1186/1471-2288-11-128
Shah, S. R., Ahmed, F., & Khan, R. (2018). Writing a critical review of literature: A practical guide for English graduate students. *Global Language Review*, *3*(I), 136–153. http://doi.org/10.31703/glr.2018(III-I).09
Silaigwana, B., & Wassenaar, D. (2019). Research ethics Committees' oversight of biomedical research in South Africa: A thematic analysis of ethical issues raised during ethics review of non-expedited protocols. *Journal of Empirical Research on Human Research Ethics*, *14*(2), 107–116. http://doi.org/10.1177/1556264618824921 . Epub 2019 Jan 24
Silverman, D. (2001). *Interpreting qualitative data*. Sage.
Steeves, K., Williams, J., and Clarke, S. (n.d.). Writing a literature review: introduction. In McMaster University's Graduate Thesis Toolkit, McMaster University.
Strekalova, Y. A. (2018). Defining research: The effect of linguistic choices on the intentions to participate in clinical research. *Clinical Nursing Research*, *27*(7), 790–799.
U.S. DEPARTMENT OF HEALTH AND HUMAN SERVICES National Institutes of Health (2005). Theory at a Glance. A guide for Health Promotion Practice. Retrieved 9.25.2022. https://cancercontrol.cancer.gov/sites/default/files/2020-06/theory.pdf
U.S. Department of Health and Human Services. (n.d.b). The Belmont Report, Ethical Principles and Guidelines for the Protection of Human Subjects of Research. https://www.hhs.gov/ohrp/regulations-and-policy/belmont-report/index.html
University of West Indies. (2019). The literature review. https://libguides.uwi.edu/c.php?g=11323&p=59138
Wigert, H., Nilsson, C., Dencker, A., Begley, C., Jangsten, E., Sparud-Lundin, C., Mollberg, M., & Patel, H. (2020). Women's experiences of fear of childbirth: A metasynthesis of qualitative studies. *International Journal of Qualitative Studies on Health and Well-Being*, *15*(1), 1704484. https://doi.org/10.1080/17482631.2019.1704484, https://scholarworks.umass.edu/pare/vol14/iss1/13
Woolf, S. H. (2008). The meaning of translational research and why it matters. *JAMA*, *299*(2). 211–213. http://doi.org/10.1001/jama.2007.26
Yiu, K. C., Rohwer, A., & Young, T. (2018). Integration of care for hypertension and diabetes: A scoping review assessing the evidence from systematic reviews and evaluating reporting. *BMC Health Services Research*, *18*, 481. https://doi.org/10.1186/s12913-018-3290-8

CHAPTER

MODULE 2: QUANTITATIVE RESEARCH

This module provides the learner with a more detailed coverage of the research process from the perspective of quantitative research. Qualitative research is covered in Module 3 of this textbook. This module, with its focus on quantitative approaches, builds on the foundation provided in Module 1 and expands the learner's understanding of research concepts. It covers the design of the research study, the development of a survey instrument, and the collection of data. It provides an overview of data analysis and includes the fundamental concepts of conducting a literature review along with ethical and cultural considerations, and it gives the learner an opportunity to apply research concepts to a strategy for developing a research grant from a call for proposals. The module is divided into three sections: (1) Basic Principles of Quantitative Research; (2) Designing and Implementing the Research Study; and (3) Pulling It All Together, an overview of grant writing. Section 2 is further divided into four sections (A–D).

By the end of the module, learners will be able to:

- Discuss philosophical, ethical, and cultural underpinnings of research
- Design a survey research study
- Construct a data collection instrument and collect the data
- Describe the informed consent process and design an ethically responsible research study
- Discuss data analysis and reporting of survey research
- Write a successful grant proposal

Integrated Research Methods In Public Health, First Edition. Muriel Jean Harris and Baraka Muvuka.
© 2023 John Wiley & Sons, Inc. Published 2023 by John Wiley & Sons, Inc.
Companion website: www.wiley.com/go/harris/integratedresearchmethods

Module 2: Quantitative Research

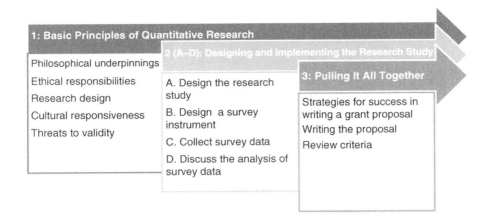

SECTION 1: BASIC PRINCIPLES OF QUANTITATIVE RESEARCH

By the end of the section, learners will be able to:

- Describe three to four approaches for conducting a research study
- Discuss ethical and cultural factors influencing research
- Discuss threats to internal and external validity in the context of quantitative research

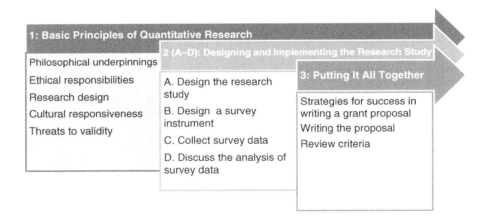

INTRODUCTION

This section provides basic principles fundamental to the quantitative research enterprise. It provides the learner with an understanding of the philosophical principles associated with quantitative research and discusses ethical and cultural principles that undergird valid public health research. It gives an overview of the different research methods and threats to validity in research.

PHILOSOPHICAL UNDERPINNING

The postpositivist view is that scientific reasoning is essentially the same process as commonsense reasoning, except that with the former scientists follow specific procedures very closely. This approach studies a reality while recognizing the possibility of errors in measurement and leveraging multiple observations (known as triangulation) to keep them to a minimum. It also recognizes the importance of peer review and critique and the evaluation of knowledge. In the postpositivist deductive approach, the research methodology is described as being controlled, rigorous, systematic, verifiable, and empirical and has the ability to withstand critical scrutiny (Kumar, 2014). Over the course of scientific inquiry, views have changed, and papers have been corrected and retracted as studies have been found not to meet the highest scientific standards or have not used the most appropriate scientific methods. Scientific findings are subject to peer review and scrutiny, and science gets corrected. The fact that science changes as new information comes to light means that scientists learn and adjust all the time.

The postpositivist research approach requires a well-thought-out, structured, and prescheduled set of procedures with an emphasis on the measurement of variables. Variables are identified during the literature review, based on the researcher's experience or in consultation with experts in the subject area. This view relies on the substantiation of the outcomes from the use of large sample sizes and determining generalizability. The expectation is that the results of a large heterogeneous study population in postpositivist research will apply to other populations and places, a term known as *generalizability*. Large studies are usually expensive to conduct, so it is helpful to engage larger institutions, which maintain the infrastructure to receive large grants. All research, however, must be conducted based on a set of procedures that guide scientific research and form the basis for the research plan.

ETHICAL RESPONSIBILITIES

A study may be considered unethical if it is scientifically unsound, breaches an individual or a community's confidentiality, or wastes resources. Ethical issues in the *creative relationship framework* in culturally responsive indigenous research require the researcher to continually reflect on their demographic profile and how it might limit understanding of the issues in the study. In addition, it recognizes the importance of commitment to co-participants, ongoing consenting of the participants, and mutual respect and reciprocity (Chilisa, 2012).

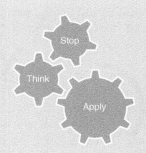

Understanding the Impact of Cultural Differences on Research

The Creative Relationship Framework requires the researcher to continually reflect on their demographic and cultural characteristics. Discuss how these characteristics could affect the research process and the issues associated with engagement. How can the principles of co-participants and ongoing consent from members of the community inform the research methodology?

While ethical review is required for all research studies and ethics or institutional boards have a mandate to review and approve applications, the researcher has the ultimate responsibility to determine that the study is ethical and meets required standards to protect human subjects. Research ethics have their foundation in four fundamental principles (Childress and Beauchamp, 2001): (1) respect for persons, (2) beneficence, (3) maleficence, and (4) justice.

Respect for persons requires that people are treated as autonomous and capable of making their own decisions. It also requires that persons who are emotionally disabled, young children, prisoners and others who have diminished capacity to make decisions are to be protected by society. In addition, they should be included in research studies only under specific circumstances since they are unable to give true informed consent. The United Nations Convention on the Rights of Persons with Disabilities (CRPD) has elevated research on disabilities as an ethical and human rights issue and a priority for global research. Guidance for ethical disability health research provides recommendations for their protection (Durhan et al., 2014). This ethical principle is informed by an *ubuntu* worldview that promotes compassion, care, togetherness, empathy, and respect that allows for mutuality between participants and a tolerance for each other's language and opinions (Mkabela, 2005). Ubuntu is a term of the Bantu people that means "I am because we are." It speaks of our humanity toward others.

Beneficence is based on the principle that requires researchers to do no harm. In that vein, researchers must ensure that research procedures and interventions must not place individuals at physical or psychological harm through mistreatment. Researchers must minimize risk and maximize the benefits. *Maleficence* is essentially the opposite of beneficence and is less often seen in the literature. Merriam-Webster defines it as "the act of committing evil."

Justice addresses issues of fairness. Researchers must consider the fairness of the request for marginalized and vulnerable populations to participate in research and yet not benefit from the products of the research. Individuals who are marginalized and belong to vulnerable populations may not be in a position to give true informed consent and are also less likely to opt out of a study. They often do not fully understand what it means to participate voluntarily.

In the course of obtaining ethics clearance to conduct a research study involving human subjects the Board must be assured that the participant has the opportunity to give informed consent. The research is categorized based on assumed risk and for the purposes of review may be approved as exempt, expedited, or full review. When there is even minimal risk, the individual who participates in the research must have the benefit of knowing their level of risk through an *informed consent process* that must follow ethics and institutional board review guidelines.

Research with Persons with Disability

Research involving persons with disability requires researchers to understand the cross-cultural context and engage early with disability organizations and local researchers to understand the Convention of the Rights of Persons with Disabilities (CRPD) requirements to ensure that disability inclusive rights–based language is used. This includes assessing competence for individuals to give initial informed consent but with subsequent agreement as the research proceeds, using the principle of justice to protect from disproportionate research burden, avoiding stigmatization, engaging in critical reflection, not projecting values into the process, and making all research decisions transparently (Durhan et al., 2014). The CRPD aims to promote and protect those with long-term physical, mental, intellectual, and sensory disabilities and ensure they have full protections, equal human rights, and individual freedoms. (United Nations, 2006).

CULTURAL RESPONSIVENESS

Valid research requires the researcher to be authentic and to possess cultural skills, the ability to work effectively, and develop meaningful relationships with people of various cultural backgrounds. It is evident that the person who initiates the research, is the principal investigator (PI), or the lead researcher on the team, must be true to their own personality, spirit, or character. *Culture* includes the customs, social interactions, and institutions of a people or other social group. Thus, in conducting research, we step into another culture. Appreciating and embracing cultures different from our own facilitate an environment in which trust can be built.

Power and privilege play important roles in the validity of the research because these dynamics affect both sides of the continuum and the ability for each party to be authentic. They exist across multiple domains irrespective of the country in which the research is being conducted and occur across race, gender, age, sexual orientation, and class. However, in his book *Privilege, Power, and Difference*, Johnson (2001) describes privilege as more about social categories and as primarily focused on the people we identify as reference groups in quantitative, postpositivist research that we use to ascribe values of good or bad, high or low. As a result, to improve the authenticity and validity of the research, researchers must strive to identify and incorporate stakeholders who can work effectively and provide a cultural bridge to the work.

Drawing on the principles of community-based participatory research, engaging the community to be part of the study throughout is a critical part of a culturally responsive research methodology. It differs from traditional postpositivist methodologies by intentionally incorporating cultural values and recognizing their impact on study participation, retention, and trust in the process (Chilisa, 2012). However, their underlying practice of engagement is one that could be incorporated in all research to increase the validity of the research irrespective of the study design.

RESEARCH DESIGNS

Public health research takes advantage of a variety of research designs and approaches that are described next. Description and analytical studies are the two primary approaches to conducting epidemiological studies.

Descriptive Studies

A descriptive study describes the prevalence of a situation, problem, or phenomenon systematically providing information to the researcher related to questions that ask *what, where, when,* and *how much of* the situation, problem, or phenomenon is found or takes place within the population and the population sample. Descriptive studies generally include surveys that provide information about the distribution of particular characteristics of interest to the researcher. These studies may be done at the population level or through the use of samples that can be extrapolated to the population. They may include population estimates of disease, disability, or demographics or may assess access to and utilization of services. They are incorporated in a wide range of research approaches and are used to describe the demographics or other characteristics of the study population in a research study. Results from a descriptive analysis are reported as frequencies and categories. These study approaches are described individually; however, note that they can be combined in any given study. For example, a cross-sectional study may be exploratory using either primary or secondary data.

The Cross-Sectional Study A cross-sectional study is an observational study that provides data on a sample or population without manipulating the environment (as in an experimental study). It allows the researcher to compare different populations and their characteristics at a point often referred to as a snapshot. This type of study primarily assesses who does and does not have the disease or the problem. While it cannot provide information regarding the cause and effect of disease or public health outcome, it can, over an extended period, provide information that allows the researcher to identify risk factors for the disease leading to more conclusive research methodologies. Cross-sectional studies use surveys either alone or in conjunction with other tests to assess prevalence of the exposure to the disease or of the disease itself and are useful for planning and monitoring public health programs and health service delivery.

Similarly, cohort studies that are also cross-sectional studies identify individuals with the exposure or risk factors associated with the disease or health outcome. Unlike cross-sectional studies, in a cohort study, individuals are followed over time. Cohort studies can be combined with other studies such as an experimental design.

The Longitudinal Study A longitudinal study, like a cross-sectional study, is an observational study, with the difference being that the longitudinal study gives the researcher the opportunity to collect cross-sectional collect data using several observation points over time. In this design, the researcher may see changes in the population either in the risk factor associated in the disease or in the health outcome.

The Retrospective Study A retrospective study compares two groups of people, identifying cases (those with the disease), and controls (those without the disease). The study involves using medical histories or a survey since it looks backward in time to assess factors that influenced the health condition that has already occurred at the time of the study. A retrospective cohort study looks at associations between the health condition and the exposure and explores possible relationships, but it does not allow the researcher to specify a causal relationship between the risk factors and the health condition.

A case control study is a retrospective observational study, designed to help determine if an exposure to a particular substance/element is associated with a specified outcome of interest. In this study, the cases are identified first, and then a set of controls that are free of th e outcome are identified based on predefined characteristics. The purpose of the study is to look back in time, determine which of the subjects in the study were exposed, and then compare the frequency of the exposure in each group—the cases and the controls. In a case control study, it may be difficult to pinpoint past exposures and the time sequence between the exposure to the risk factors and the outcome.

The Exploratory Study An exploratory study, which is often described as a pilot study, is undertaken in quantitative research when little is known about the subject. It can help in determining the research design, sampling, or data collection method for a more conclusive and larger study. Their value can be limited for decision-making when small sample sizes are used that do not adequately represent the larger population and are not generalizable. However, exploratory studies save time and resources if used to determine the types of research worth pursuing and how to use limited resources in population level studies. Exploratory studies are an intentional design in mixed methods research when they often feature as qualitative research. They are discussed in a later module.

The Correlational Study The correlational study attempts to discover the existence of a relationship or association between two sets of variables, independent and dependent variables. The study may occur within other study designs such as in a cohort study. Correlation studies determine if an increase or decrease in one variable (independent variable) results in the increase or decrease in another variable (dependent variable). In a correlation study, the relationship between two variables does not infer a cause and effect. Predictions may be made in the form of hypotheses that are derived from theories that predict or explain the relationship between interrelated sets of concepts. Correlation exists when measures vary together, and it is possible to predict the value of one variable by knowing the values of another. A positive correlation exists between two variables when an increase in one variable leads to an increase in the other variable or a decrease in one variable leads to a decrease in another. A negative correlation exists when an increase in one variable leads to a decrease in the other. The correlation coefficient determines how well the measures covary and is a measure of the strength of the correlation and ranges from −1 to +1 with zero being in the middle. When there is a strong positive correlation the correlation coefficient is +1; when there is a strong negative correlation the value of the coefficient is close to −1. A value of zero means that the variables are not correlated.

Survey Research

Survey research is one of the groups of descriptive research designs that uses questionnaires and interviews to collect data from participants. While surveys often stand alone as the research method, they also form a part of any of the research designs. Surveys are often the first response when researchers think about answering the research question on the observations, attitudes, feelings, experiences, behavior, and opinions about a population of interest (Hox and Boeije, 2005). Survey research is found across a range of research designs in descriptive and analytic studies research and is by far the most often used approach for collecting data. Surveys can range from being a short series of questions to obtain individuals' preferences, to a longer and detailed survey using a rigorously designed study instrument in a variety of forms and formats. They are incorporated in studies from the simplest and most modest cross-sectional studies to the most sophisticated and complex experimental and quasi-experimental studies as well as in clinical trials. They have historically been used to collect data in large population-based studies and are the basis of census data as well as large health databases. They are administered in a variety of ways taking advantage of every avenue possible to reach individuals, whether face-to-face or electronically. Like other research, if not conducted with utmost care, the data can be misleading and unreliable.

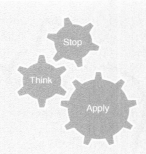

Selecting a Research Approach to Assess Prevalence of Disease

Researchers are studying the prevalence of diabetes. Which research approach would be most appropriate for this study? What factors will affect the measurement of the existence of the disease among the population over time. Explain your reasoning.

Analytical Studies

Analytical studies focus on assessing the cause of a particular outcome. They try to clarify the *why* and *how* the variables exist in a relationship within an experiment. Causes related to disease outcomes may include genetic predisposing factors, infectious agents, and physiological or physical risk factors in places where we live, work, and play. The risk factors can occur at multiple levels—individual or environmental (interpersonal, community, organizational, and policy). Alternative explanations for the outcomes we observe may result from events that occur by chance, bias, or the presence of a confounding variable. Prior to an analytical study, the researcher develops a hypothesis describing the assumed relationship between the independent and the dependent variables that can then be tested within the study to determine if there is sufficient evidence to support the hypothesis. An intervention study is effectively an experiment that can be designed to assess the effect of an intervention. Experimental designs employ a random assignment of the study subjects to the intervention or control group, while a quasi-experimental design takes on a variety of arrangements to minimize the treats to validity.

Experimental designs have randomly assigned intervention, and control groups and quasi-experimental designs do not.

Experimental Research Designs The use of experimental design studies is often indicated following observational studies. However, they are rarely conducted in public health, and when they are they are related to randomly selected entities, such as for example schools or communities, if they meet the required criteria. The use of experimental research designs is covered in other texts.

Quasi-experimental Research Design Quasi-experimental designs the more often used designs in public health to demonstrate relationships. They are referred to as nonequivalent group designs and were introduced to address the concern that experimental designs are often not appropriate in a public health arena. They can use data that has been collected retrospectively as well as prospectively and can be used to assess the impact of program or policy interventions (Schweizer et al., 2016). Like experimental studies, quasi-experimental designs include control groups that assist in accounting for some of the biases; unlike experimental designs, the control groups are not randomly assigned. Two or more groups constitute the control groups, but they do not receive the intervention/treatment and include pre-/post-intervention measurements. The fact that the groups in the quasi-experimental designs are not randomly assigned, results in the difference between the two research designs. There are a number of approaches defined as quasi-experimental designs, including pre-experimental designs such as a single sample postintervention only and single-group pre-/post-intervention designs. Like often described in clinical trials, blinding can occur in quasi-experimental designs to reduce the risk of either the researchers or the participants from knowing what the intervention is and therefore contaminate the study (Shadish et al., 2002). Designs that are more usually identified as quasi-experimental designs include the nonequivalent control group design, single group interrupted time series, and a control group interrupted time series design (Schweizer et al., 2016). The interrupted time series design, which incorporates a control group and follows the study subjects over an extended period taking multiple observations, addresses many of the threats to validity that plague human subjects' research (Table 2.1).

TABLE 2.1. Quasi-Experimental Designs

Name of design	Definition of design	Notations for design x = intervention O = observation/measure	
Single sample post only	Measures occur only after the intervention	Sample A	x O
Single or group sample pre/post	Measures occur before and after the intervention	Sample A	O x O
Nonequivalent control group	Nonrandomized intervention and control groups with pre- and postintervention measures	Sample A Sample B	O x O O O
Single group interrupted time series	Multiple pre- and postintervention measures	Sample A	OOO x OOO
Control group interrupted time series	Multiple pre- and postintervention measures of both the nonrandomized intervention and the control groups	Sample A Sample B	OOO x OOO OOO OOO

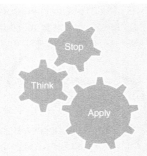

Describe an Experimental or Quasi-Experimental Designed Study

Take a few minutes to consider the following exercise and make a few notes. Conduct a literature review to identify an intervention that incorporated an experimental or quasi-experimental design. Write a one-page summary of the intervention and the research design that was used to assess the intervention. Make sure to cite the reference.

Secondary Data

One of the options open to researchers in quantitative research is the use of existing data. Existing data can be incorporated into any study design as a means of analyzing data to answer a research question. Existing data may be found at the offices of other researchers. For example, health data can usually be obtained from health departments and agencies and hospitals, and economic data may also be found at ministries of finance, labor, housing, economic affairs. International organizations and nonprofit research centers are another source of data that is available for use. Forms of secondary data include official statistics, census data, administrative and medical records, and public health data produced in large population-based surveys. Data repositories like the Inter-University Consortium for Political and Social Science Research (ICPSR) stores, curates, and provides access to scientific data that accessed through its website.

In selecting an existing instrument to answer questions, the researcher recognizes that the instrument was collected for a purpose that might be different from their research. Likewise, if the researcher selects an existing database built from a previous study or data collected without a specific research question in mind, the data in the database may not have all the desired variables and conceptualization for the current research study. It may also be the case that the data were constructed using a limited demographic sample, again not appropriate for the current study. Therefore, in both cases there may be limitations in answering the research questions. If secondary data are to be useful, they must have information regarding why, how, when, and where they were collected and who was included in the data set. In addition, any biases should also be noted. Unlike primary data, which is collected by the researcher, the context in which the data were collected is usually not as well-known, and drawing valid conclusions may prove difficult.

An existing database may have been collected for local, regional, or national use previously and involve either very small data sets and samples or very large sample sizes. In either case, this must be considered when designing the research study since the size of the data set and the representation of the population may have consequences with regards to both internal and external validity. In using secondary data, the researcher may be working backward from the database to craft an appropriate research question. While this is feasible, it takes a certain level of skill to ensure the same level of rigor in the process to reach valid conclusions. Of course, as pointed out, the limitations from the instrumentation and data collection are inherent in the study. Using secondary data may save time and effort compared to collecting primary data, but it may also be more difficult to use by the beginning researcher without the necessary data analysis skills if it is a large population-based data set. In clinical settings, patient records or an existing database may constitute secondary data and form the basis of a clinically based study that requires the use of patient- and hospital-related data to answer the research question. Developing surveys for the purpose of collecting primary data that is specific for the research study and using secondary data both have their own challenges that must be considered in the context of the research question that is being answered (Table 2.2).

The data analysis procedure is summarized as follows, but the reader is referred to other texts that describe the analysis of quantitative data in more detail:

TABLE 2.2. A Comparison of Primary and Secondary Survey Data

Primary data	Secondary data
Data collected primarily to answer the research question	Data collected for another purpose and not primarily for answering the research question
The researcher has access to the descriptions of the methodology, sampling design, and weights	Can be difficult to locate relevant and adequate descriptions of the methodology used for its collection such as sampling design, and weights.
The researcher has the opportunity to collect data that is free of systematic bias	The data may not be of the required quality for the research study free from systematic bias
All changes made between the data collection and the data entry should be well documented and records maintained	It may be difficult to get information about the data set and any changes to the survey data during the data entry and process for data analysis
Validation of survey tool is required	Validation of survey tool may not be known and is required

Adapted from Hox and Boeije (2005).

- Assign a number to the value for entry into the database (e.g., Excel©, SPSS©, R©, SAS©, STATA©, Qualtrics©).
- Check the data for missing variables and wrongly entered dates.
- Recode data as required.
- Establish a code book to provide a definition for each variable.
- Explore the data using data visualization such as descriptive analysis (mean, modes, medians, range, variance, quartiles and standard deviation, skewness, and kurtosis as appropriate for the type of data).
- Run appropriate inferential statistics.
- Make sure the correct statistical test is selected based on the type of variables, the scale of measurement, the distribution of the data, and the types of questions.
- Assess the results against the established alpha value (*p*-value) that assess the probability that the findings of the test did not occur by chance. The lower the value the more likely the researchers are that the findings of the research are genuine.

THREATS TO VALIDITY

In the absence of a control group, researchers are generally concerned about potential bias in drawing conclusions about the relationship between the independent variables and the dependent variable. These biases are described as threats to validity, either internally or externally. A research study with internal validity accurately measures what it intends to measure. The threats to validity challenge a researcher's ability to conclude that the independent variables did cause the outcome of interest. It is important that during the design phase of the study the researcher identifies potential biases/threats to validity and takes precautions aimed at minimizing the threats whether the threats are at the sampling, data collection, or analysis phases of the study (Table 2.3). The research design most likely to minimize the threats to internal validity is the experimental design with its randomly assigned control and intervention groups

The other threat to validity in research is the threat to external validity. This threat is related to the ability of the researchers to generalize their results to the larger population. A study has to first have internal validity for it to have external validity, and if the sample is not sufficiently heterogeneous it will affect it generalizability. Generalizability is

TABLE 2.3. Threats to Internal Validity

Threat to validity	Description
Attrition	A disproportional loss of participants in the intervention or control group resulting in a different profile of the participants in the postintervention measures compared to the preintervention measures. Often those who drop out have different in characteristics and the results of the study may have been different if they had stayed in the program.
Hawthorne Effect	When individuals know they are being studied they change their behavior and adopt atypical behaviors causing a bias in the measurement.
History	Events take place outside the intervention that could affect change the relationship between the variables making it difficult to conclude that the intervention caused the outcome of interest. Such events could cause inflation in postintervention results.
Instrumentation	Changes occur to the instrument that affect the measurements related to the research due to the instability of the measure.
Maturation	Changes in the participants due to natural or physiological changes that occur over time. These changes may be biological, emotional, or intellectual, which may be misinterpreted as changes due to the intervention.
Selection	Individuals drop out of an intervention that was previously equivalent; individuals are not randomly selected, or individuals self-select, and the sample is not representative of the population.
Statistical Regression to the Mean	This threat is related to individuals having extreme high or low scores in the pretest measures that migrate closer to the mean in the posttest measurement. This artifact in the measurement mimics a real change in the scores.
Type 1 errors	In setting the alpha level of significance for a study at $p \leq 0.05$, the researcher may find significant differences occurring just by chance that are not due to the intervention and reject a hypothesis when it should not have been rejected.
Type 11 errors	To avoid Type 1 errors the researcher may set the alpha at $p \leq 0.01$. In this case, they do not reject the hypothesis when they should have rejected it (and accept the alternative hypothesis).

affected by the bias in selecting the sample and the size of the sample. Conclusions drawn on research conducted using small or nonrandomly selected samples lack external validity. Similar to selection bias, sampling bias results in samples of individuals that are different in important and measurable ways from those who do not participate and do not represent the population from which the sample was drawn. Research conducted online may be at greater risk of not being able to have a random sample and must rely on purposive or convenience samples. Internal and external threats to validity must be kept in mind as the research study is being designed since it is in the design of the study that threats to validity are minimized.

SUMMARY

The postpositivist view believes that scientific reasoning is essentially the same process as common-sense reasoning, with the difference being primarily in scientists following specific procedures very closely. It believes that there is a reality that can be studied; however, there is also the recognition that there could be errors in measurement, and multiple observations are required. It considers the need for multiple methods to try to minimize the error. This process is known as *triangulation*. It also recognizes the importance of peer review and critique and the evaluation of knowledge. In the postpositivist deductive approach, the research methodology is described as being controlled, rigorous, systematic, verifiable, and empirical and has the ability to withstand critical scrutiny

A study may be considered unethical if it is scientifically unsound, breaches an individual or a community's confidentiality or wastes resources. Ethical issues in the *creative relationship framework* in culturally responsive indigenous research, requires the researcher to continually reflect on their demographic profile and how it might limit understanding of the issues in the study. In addition, it recognizes the importance of commitment to co-participants, ongoing consenting of the participants and mutual respect and reciprocity (Chilisa, 2012).

Everybody identifies with one or more cultures, since culture is defined as being the customs, social interactions, and institutions of a people or other social group. The culture of others could be that of themselves, their family, or their community making it important to always consider cultural aspects of the work. Appreciating and embracing cultures facilitates an environment in which trust is built and is conducive to a person's growth and development.

Description and Analytical studies are the two primary approaches to conducing epidemiological studies that include a range of approaches in public health that include observational and experimental design studies.

In the absence of a control group, researchers are concerned about potential bias in drawing conclusions about the relationship between the independent variables and the dependent variable. These biases are described threats to internal or external validity. A research study that has internal validity, is one in which the study accurately measures what it intends to measure. The threats to validity challenge a researcher's ability to conclude that the independent variables did in fact cause the outcome of interest.

Now that I have reached the end this section, I am able to:

Course objective	Strongly agree	Somewhat agree	Neutral	Somewhat disagree	Strongly agree
Describe three to four approaches for conducting a research study					
Discuss ethical and cultural factors influencing research					
Discuss threats to internal and external validity in the context of quantitative research					

STEP 2A: DESIGNING AND IMPLEMENTING THE RESEARCH STUDY

By the end of this step, learners will be able to:

- Describe the process for conducting a research study
- Develop a problem statement and research question
- Discuss sampling in research

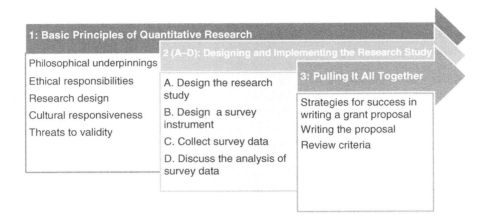

INTRODUCTION

The postpositivist research approach follows a well-thought-out, structured, and prescheduled set of procedures with an emphasis on the measurement of variables. Variables are identified during the literature review and are based on the researcher's experience or in consultation with experts in the subject area. It relies on the substantiation of the outcomes from the use of large sample sizes and determining generalizability. Many of the research studies conducted in public health are smaller and may or may not be generalizable, yet the goal of the researcher is to develop measurement instruments that meet the criteria for valid and reliable research. This is particularly true of evaluation research (Harris, 2010). Irrespective of the size of the sample, the researcher ensures that the best approach is used for sampling.

PLANNING FOR RESEARCH

The best research is a planned systematic approach to answering the research question. Key considerations in planning research studies include asking and answering the following questions:

- Who will be engaged in the research study?
- Why is this study important to me, to the field of public health, and for whose benefit?
- What philosophical, ethical, and cultural underpinnings, and what research design will be most appropriate for answering the research question?
- What methodological approach is most suitable?
- What will it take to collect, analyze, and report on valid and reliable data?

The planning process unfolds with identifying the answer to the first question, who will be engaged in the research study? A researcher or a team of researchers generally initiates the process of identifying the need for the research, conceptualizing the study and determining the research question; they collect, analyze and interpret the results and report them to the larger population. The roles of the researchers are determined by the research team; however, their skill sets likely determine their activities within the team.

Culturally and ethically responsive research includes those who belong to the specific population on whom the research study will focus. The research team may include residents of the community included in the research, colleagues across multiple professional areas, and staff of organizations, universities, and agencies. Ideally, stakeholders are involved in public health research throughout the process and have critical roles and responsibilities including giving voice to the study population. If the study is about homeless individuals, there should be representatives of the homeless population engaged in the planning and other aspects of the study. Similarly, if the study is about racial minority or other disadvantaged groups, they should be invited to participate in the research study from the beginning to ensure that the study is culturally responsive and incorporating cultural values, recognizing its impact on study participation, retention, and trust in the process (Chilisa, 2012). In the Designing a Public Health Research Study, the first step in the research planning process is assembling the research team, which is then followed by the steps that facilitate a systematic response from researchers. The subsequent steps are described in this section (Figure 2.1).

FIGURE 2.1. *Overview for designing a public health research study.*

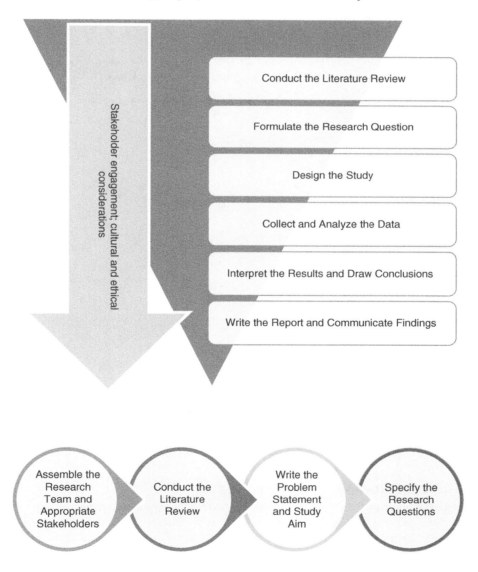

Assemble the Research Team

The research team is made up of a group of skilled researchers with a range of experience. Generally, the PI is responsible to the funder for the implementation of the study and the team brings a range of skills that support the achievement of the research goals. In addition, other stakeholders may be invited to be a part of a team that initiates or implements the research in a variety of roles such as conceptualizing the study and determining the research question, collecting the data, serving as participants in the study, and being be instrumental in the data analysis and interpretation of the results. Roles are determined by the research team. Stakeholders in public health research could include but not the limited to residents of the community that is included in the research, colleagues across multiple professional areas, staff of organizations, universities, and agencies. Among residents of the community, a culturally responsive research study should also identify those belonging to the specific population about who the research study will be focused. For example, if the study is about homeless individuals, there should be representatives of the homeless population engaged in the planning and other aspects of the study. Ideally, stakeholders are involved in public health research throughout the process and have critical roles and responsibilities.

The terms of reference (ToR) for a research study is an explicit statement of personnel and resources for the project that includes roles, responsibilities, and the processes that the research team establishes at the outset. It lays out the formal expectation of the project. Researchers recognize however, that a ToR serves as a contract or may be perceived as such with positions on the team being often organized in a hierarchical structure. Truly collaborative research teams would design the ToR together clearly outlining:

- The purpose and goals of the research team
- The processes for conducting the research and accomplishing the research task
- Communication among and between the team and outside individuals and agencies
- Roles and responsibilities
- Confidentiality statements
- Milestones
- Publication agreements and authorship

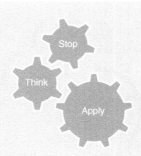

Writing a Terms of Reference

As a researcher interested in conducting a study related to refugee health, who would you identify as stakeholders to include on the research team? Write a TOR for one member of the research team. Carefully describe the role they will play in the study.

Conduct the Literature Review

Determining the topic or question for the research requires completing a literature review with its steps for planning, conducting, and writing the review (Figure 2.2). See Module 1 for a more detailed discussion of how to conduct a literature review. The literature review in public health and for journal publications is best written as an integrative literature review. The integrative literature review provides a critical analysis of the literature that tells a story about the phenomenon, with the goal of carefully identifying the components of the problem being researched by synthesizing the literature across multiple authors. A synthesis of the literature helps the researcher identify patterns that reflect new perspectives and a conceptual framework for the study and the research agenda (Torraco, 2005). It allows the

FIGURE 2.2. *Overview of the steps for conducting a review of the literature.*

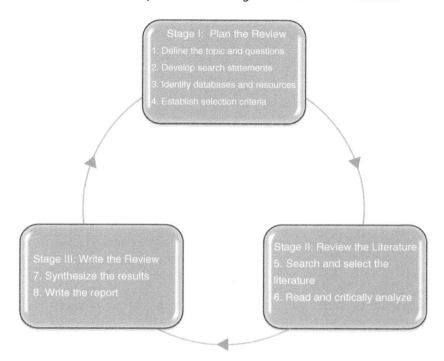

researcher to identify gaps in the literature more readily, as well as key contributions, strengths, weaknesses, and deficiencies (Torraco, 2005). The thematically organized review has headings and subheadings that describe the independent variables in relationship to the dependent variable in the study with each combination of variables (independent and dependent) being compared across the literature. An important benefit of a thematic organization of the literature is that it reduces the risk of plagiarism.

Literature relevant to the research topic may cover two types of information: (1) very general about the topic; and (2) more specific to the research question. The literature review begins with the general information and narrows down to the more specific information. It allows the researcher to review existing literature to understand what previous researchers have found and know about the topic of interest. By this step of the research process, the researchers have defined a broad topic area to focus the literature review (e.g., women's health during pregnancy, quality of life of individuals with disability, refugee mental health).

Check List
- Organize information.
- Be succinct.
- Ensure references are complete.
- Capture only research findings.
- Examine each reference critically.
- Write the review.

Reviewing the Literature

- Provides an understanding of the theoretical frameworks across multiple disciplines that have guided the research of previous studies
- Clarifies ideas and establishes the basis for the research
- Helps to identify gaps in existing research and to conceptualize their research problem clearly
- Provides information about new research ideas and directions and references to new ideas and unanswered questions
- Provides insights into approaches and methodologies that have been used to answer similar research questions

The literature review provides the researcher with a clear justification for the study and situates it within the field as relevant and important and provides a firm foundation for posing the researcher's study question. When the study is based on previous research and built from identified gaps in the literature, it is of greater value to the field. It is tempting to step right into research without taking the time to conduct a literature review. The problem with not conducting a literature review is that understanding can be limited or lacking and critical issues can be overlooked. Near the end of a published article or in the abstract, the researchers will often point out areas of study that their research did not cover or questions that their study was unable to answer suggesting areas for further research, leading to:

- New and unexplored areas of the topic
- Expanded population studies
- Alternative research designs and methodologies
- Expansion of an existing study from what is currently known

Writing an Integrative Literature Review

While there are many approaches for writing a literature review, the literature in public health and for journal publication are best written as integrative literature reviews. The integrative literature review provides a critical analysis of the literature that tells a story about the phenomenon with the goal of carefully identifying the components of the problem that is being researched. A synthesis of the literature in an integrative approach helps the researcher identify patterns that help identify new perspectives and a conceptual framework for the study and the research agenda (Torraco, 2005). In a thematic review, the researcher organizes and discusses the literature from the search based on themes or theoretical concepts. The concepts are generally related to the overall theme or subject area of the research study. It starts with a question, and the question guides the literature search. The themes are the constructs for the study, so they are organized in paragraphs and the different references are discussed. For example, a researcher writing about prenatal care among displaced women may discuss the literature in the context of the social determinants of health; the individual paragraphs will discuss the differences and similarities in the findings from the literature in separate paragraphs that cover factors at the individual, interpersonal, community, organizational, and policy levels. It allows the researcher to identify gaps in the literature more readily as the problem is being investigated. It also lets the researcher identify key contributions, strengths, weaknesses, and deficiencies that allow the researcher to specify a research topic that will more likely expand the field of study (Torraco, 2005).

Theoretical Frameworks in Research

The initial research of the literature allows the researcher to construct the theoretical framework that provides a stronger foundation for the research. When considering the individual and the individual's behavior in a postpositivist research study, the factors that operate to achieve the various outcomes that are measured, do so at multiple levels. The socioecological systems perspective considers elements at the individual and environmental levels and integrates theories and models (Figure 2.3). It dictates that it is not sufficient to assess outcomes at the individual level but also must consider the organizations, community access, societal norms, and laws and regulations that operate at local, national, and international levels. Determinants at these levels influence physical, emotional, and mental health outcomes. The World Health Organization (WHO) defines health as a state of complete physical, mental, and social well-being and not merely the absence of disease or infirmity, a definition that was adopted in 1948. However, in postpositivist research in public health, there is an increasing focus on the measurement of the aspects of well-being influenced by socioenvironmental factors. Structural and systemic racism and social exclusion weigh heavily on Black, Brown, and other racially, sexually, educationally, and economically excluded individuals and result in many of the poor health outcomes and the enormous disparities that we measure today.

The Centers for Disease Control and Prevention (CDC) and the WHO have both endorsed the need to include the social determinants of health as drivers of health status and in 2019 called them out explicitly in many of the sustainable development goals (SDG). The SDGs provide myriad opportunities for public health research to adopt an integrated approach to addressing the social policies and conditions that influence where we live, work, play, and age (CSDH, 2008). In intervention- or outcome-related research, a range of theories drives the assumptions associated with the behavioral outcomes with precursors to the behavior operating within multiple spheres and represented by the social-ecological model (Figure 2.4).

Conceptualizing the framework of the research within the socioecological model allows the researcher to identify a more complete set of variables in the conceptual map as the basis for the study. Incorporating established and published theories within its multiple levels increases the likelihood that concepts and constructs known to influence the behavior and drive the health and well-being outcomes included in the research study. For example, individual-level theories such as the theory of planned behavior (Fishbain and Ajzen, 1975) or the health belief model (Hochbaum, 1958)

FIGURE 2.3. *Socioecological perspective model reflecting the dynamic relationship between the individual and the factors that influence health outcomes.*

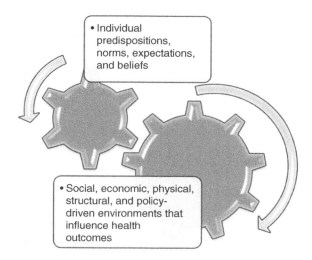

FIGURE 2.4. *Socioecological model.*

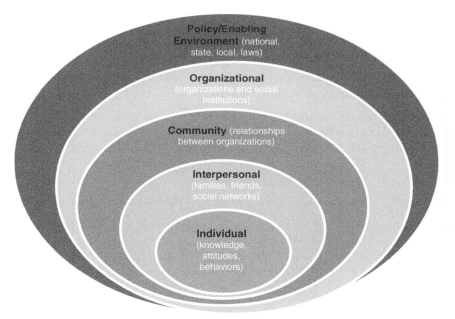

Adapted from Brenfenbrenner (1977)

operate in the smallest sphere influencing behavioral and health outcomes of individuals, based on their knowledge, attitudes, and skills or what the social cognitive theorist Bandura (1986) refers to as predisposing factors. Otherwise, we miss critical components for understanding the factors associated with disease mechanisms or health-seeking and health-related outcomes. Improving mortality and morbidity related to heart disease is unlikely to be influenced by medical interventions alone but instead to rely on individuals living in socially, economically, and politically supportive environments that decrease the risk of sustained levels of stress.

A 1997 study of the global burden of disease predicted the increase in mortality and disability would be determined by factors such as socioeconomic development, education, technological developments, and exposure to environmental hazards (Murray and Lopez, 1997). Almost 15 years later, a review of social and economic policies found physical and mental health or health care effects of social and economic policies for 72% of low-income populations in four domains: (1) housing and neighborhood; (2) employment; (3) family strengthening and marriage; and (4) income (Osypuk et al., 2015). In their model of development to assess socioeconomic disparities, Galama and Kippersluis (2018) found that individuals with higher socioeconomic status (SES) also have better health and lived longer, primarily due to their greater access to wealth, earnings, and education that ensured less physically and psychologically demanding working conditions. These findings reinforce the importance of considering the effect of multiple variables on health outcomes and the use of theoretical and conceptual models in the assessment of health outcomes and the design of public health research. Drawing on the work of Black feminist researcher Crenshaw (1989), Krieger (2012) reminds us that our research must integrate the intersecting factors in the same way they interact to produce health and the social conditions in which individuals live, work, and play, and they cannot be stratified into individual parts, which needs to be respected and reflected in our research.

The Problem Statement

While the literature review provides the evidence, the problem statement provides a brief overview of the major issues associated with the research area as identified by the literature. The major issue addressed in the problem statement is the question that the research will answer. It includes gaps in the literature and provides the justification for the study. It is completely objective and focuses only on the facts without including any subjective comments or commentary. It provides a clear indication of the significance of the problem, who it impacts, what the impacts are, and opportunities to address it. The components of the problem statement are conceptualized in a summary statement that includes:

- What is already known about the specific problem
  - What the problem is and why it matters
  - The risk factors associated with the problem at multiple levels of the socioecological model
- The major gaps in knowledge in the literature
- The proposed study and its relevance in addressing the gap
- The benefits to understanding or resolving the problem that should be significant enough to contribute to the existing body of research and lead to further research

The problem statement does not include any reference to the research question. It provides the justification for the study from the perspective of the literature. Once the problem is clearly stated, the researcher writes a statement that gives the reader an insight into how the problem that has been articulated through the literature review, is leading to the research study.

The aim provides this insight. The aim is written such as:

The aim or purpose of this study is to determine/explore/understand/investigate/examine. . .

Example: The aim of the study is to examine the factors associated with disaster preparedness among older adults who reside in an assisted living facility.

The next step is to develop the research questions.

Writing Problem Statements and Specifying the Study Aim

1. Write down a research question or public health issue that will guide the literature review
2. Draw a table with four columns labeled Construct, Theory, Reference, and Notes to summarize the literature and keep track of the readings (see example following).

3. Conduct a literature review based on the public health issue in step 1, and fill in the columns to provide a summary of the literature and record the references concurrently. The literature review may turn up constructs that are not specifically aligned with a theory. That is okay. List the construct, the reference, and the notes that show how the construct is relevant to the study's independent and dependent variables. The theory column helps to keep track of how the construct was used and strengthens the evidence base for including it.
4. Once the literature review is complete, the table contains a list of the concepts that other researchers have identified as relevant for the research topic.
5. Using the table as a guide, write a thematically organized literature review highlighting the similarities and differences in the various studies. Include citations and a reference list.
6. Write a problem statement and specify the aim of the study.

Construct	Theory	Reference	Notes—study results
Intention	Theory of reasoned action	Fawzy and Salam (2015)	Intention (independent variable) had a positive effect on consumer's adoption of mobile technology (dependent variable)
Intention		Pepper et al. (2019)	Neither the exposure to the factual message nor a message that added uncertainty to the factual message (independent variable) impacted intention to try vaping soon or to stop vaping in the next six months (dependent variable)

The Research Question The question that gets answered is about the relationship between various factors and the public health problem being investigated. The relationships between the risk or protective factors are based on a researcher's theory that may have their foundations in public health–related fields as well as business, psychology, sociology, or biology. The theoretical framework outlines the theories that have been suggested that provide an understanding of the topic from multiple perspectives and helps guide the researcher to the research question. Once the research question is decided on, the researcher has the additional task of developing a conceptual framework. The literature review discussed earlier provides the information the researcher needs with respect to the variables to be measured, but there may still be a need to return to the literature periodically during the entire research process to identify new research findings and to further explore the issue. This may be especially true, if the review of the literature was not exhaustive or had been conducted a while ago since research is a dynamic area with new research being published frequently. Other important aspects of the research question are related to the marketability of the research idea for being competitive in a grant review.

The research question guides the study design and the methodology, so make sure it is comprehensive yet specific enough to give the researcher a road map for the study. If the aim of the study requires multiple questions, then each question must meet the same criteria. The research proposal in a grant application will be more likely to be reviewed favorably if the research question suggests an overall impact of the study findings, the public health significance, and an innovative idea. An example of a research questions is, "When Ebola enters a home, a family, and community: A qualitative study of population perspectives on Ebola control measures in rural and urban areas of Sierra Leone." A carefully crafted question may suggest the study design and the likely data management and analysis strategy. A good research question has many qualities that make it satisfying to study, contributes to advancing knowledge in the field, and is essential to guide the research. Research questions must be:

- Clear, concise, and specific
- Focused on the public health problem
- Feasible to answer given the time frame, financial resources, and access to the study population or data required to answer it
- Complex enough so that it requires thought and analysis

- Able to reflect the purpose of the study
- Relevant to the field of study and contributes to the development of research or practice

Careful and thoughtful planning, which can take three to six months for a thesis of dissertation, ensures that the results are a direct product of the research study and consistent themes can be traced from the literature review through to the discussion at the end of the report or manuscript. For research findings to be fully embraced by the field, the research has to be of a standard that is replicable. Having a well-thought-out study plan provides the blueprint that may result in a much greater likelihood of the study being replicated and the results of the study being recognized as valid. A well-conceptualized project starts with a research question, which provides the impetus for the research design.

DESIGNING THE STUDY

The design of the research study starts with the literature review and is followed by the research question, which then helps the research identify the specific approach to the research. Building the conceptual framework is the next step in the process.

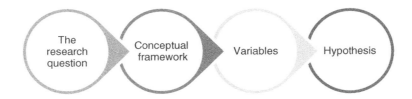

The Conceptual Framework

The conceptual framework provides the boundaries for the study in that it defines the focus of the research. Kumar (2014, p. 77) describes a conceptual framework as a "framework of reminders" since it represents the relationships of the variables to each other and reminds the researchers of important components to be covered.

> The conceptual framework builds from the gap in the literature that the research will address

Suppose for argument's sake that the research study is being conducted by physicians. They may elect to focus on the *causes of mortality from the CODID-19 pandemic*. A public health researcher on the other hand, may be more interested in *prevention strategies that may apply to future epidemics*. The literature review conducted by the public health framing of the topic, explores the risk and protective elements associated with COVID-19 Infection and strategies that have been used to reduce risk factors. In researching the literature, the researcher identifies specific areas that are under researched. In addition to exploring the research literature for purposes of getting to the research question, the researchers may engage cultural ambassadors to discuss local and cultural factors that influence the infection and prevention measures that were promoted and adopted. Engaging stakeholders during this process helps provide a cultural lens in developing the conceptual map that ensures that all possible elements are considered and helps to ensure a fuller exploration of the literature. In engaging cultural ambassadors during the 2014–2015 Ebola epidemic in Sierra Leone, anthropologists and public health found that rural residents associated Ebola with witchcraft and the individual's death with the use of chlorine to sanitize the ambulances (Kinsman et al., 2017). Indigenous or local research is often labelled as false or of less value and not recognizing the focus of western knowledge as defining global research agendas without engaging with the local community. Chilisa (2012, p. 78) provides an example of this:

> *The meanings given to HIV/AIDS differed given the context of the illness. If it was the middle aged and elderly who were sick, HIV/AIDS was called Boswagadi. In Tswana culture, anyone who sleeps with a widow or widower is afflicted by a diseased called Boswagadi. For the majority of the young, AIDS is Molelo wa Badimo (fire caused by the ancestral spirits) and for others, AIDS is Boloi (witchcraft).*

Social justice-based research examines the relationships and intersections between what people know and what is represented in the literature. It seeks to transform structural inequities and strive for critical engagement with communities, especially those of color and marginalized peoples. Social justice-based research allows researchers to develop a conceptual map of the relationship among *experiential, mainstream,* and *cultural* and *spiritual knowledge* (Jolivette, 2015) (Figure 2.5).

FIGURE 2.5. *Conceptual map of elements of the research.*

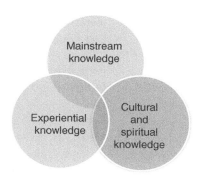

A conceptual map represents the framework for the proposed study, and it illustrates the relationships between the variables. It is a useful tool in the early stages of conceptualization of the research study. Concept maps may be developed simply with a paper and pencil on a sheet of paper (Figure 2.6) or using computer software such as CMap, Buzan's iMindMap, or Microsoft Visio. Microsoft Visio software can be downloaded from the internet. Shapes may be used to distinguish independent concepts.

The literature review that was conducted earlier in the process was based on the initial research question; however, once the literature review was complete and the gaps identified, the study that emerged is likely different from the original study that was envisaged. It is time to specify the literature that supports the newly assumed relationships that have emerged from the problem statement and the research question to ensure that the study is fully conceptualized and to determine how the research study and specifically the conceptual framework is supported by the literature. The variables that are included in this map may also be variables that are conceptualized as important for this study, but not having previously been tested as part of a public health–related study. However, these variables may exist in other fields of study and have been included in research studies in different ways than is intended for this study. The inclusion of researchers from other disciplines and community members increases the likelihood of expanding the public health lens to new and exciting horizons. For example, trust may not have been previously included in studies related to work in program and policy development in public health, but it was proven to be an important variable in the business literature and may be introduced by a new opportunity to conceptualize the variables that could potentially contribute to achieving the outcome. This hypothesized relationship could lead to trust being included in the study as an independent or dependent variable.

A table that summarizes all the relevant literature necessary to build the framework from the literature review is a helpful approach to putting together the major components of the literature and keeping track of the references and the relationships between the variable. An example is provided in Table 2.4, where column 1 lists the construct, column 2, the theory associated with the construct (if known), column 3, the reference to the peer reviewed article, and column 4 provides relevant information for the study. This approach has three advantages for the researcher: It (1) provides a

FIGURE 2.6. *Capturing the elements in a conceptual framework.*

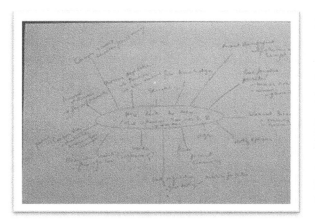
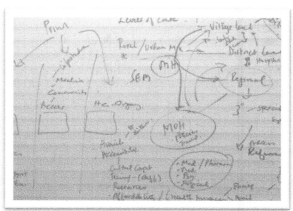

TABLE 2.4. Summarizing Findings from the Literature Review

Construct	Theory	Reference	Notes (participants, study design, measures, and findings)
Causal Attribution	Attribution	Rose, M.K., Costabile, K.A, Boland, S.E, et al. (2019). Diabetes causal attributions among affected and unaffected individuals. BMJ Open Diab Res Care, 7:e000708	**Participants:** 692 adults **Study Design:** Random Assignment of participants into 3 groups (Type 1, Type 2 diabetes, a control group) via web-based tools. **Measures:** open-ended questions assessed diabetes knowledge and 8-Likert Scale items that measured causal attributions. **Findings:** Individuals attributed both Type 1 and Type 11 diabetes to genetics. Individuals with Type 1 diabetes were more likely to attribute a germ or virus as a cause for Type 1 diabetes compared to individuals with Type 11 diabetes.

clear understanding of the underlying theoretical framework; (2) provides a quick reference to the relationship between the variables; and (3) reduces the risk of plagiarism. Once this process is complete, an updated concept map may be needed to guide the development of the next stages in the process.

The Methodology

The next step in the process is *formulating the methodology plan*. The methodology draws on all the components of the research study that have already been considered so far to determine how the research question will be answered.

- The literature review
- Ethical and cultural considerations
- The philosophical underpinnings
- The research designs
- The theoretical and conceptual frameworks
- The variables that have been identified

The previously formulated or revised research question must be clear, succinct, and address a gap in the literature, for which the justification has already been provided in the assessment of the gaps in the literature and the problem statement. In quantitative research the question that is framed may suggest a descriptive/observational or analytical study. A descriptive/observational study will lead the researcher to ask what approach will be most appropriate, a cross-sectional, retrospective, or prospective study or possibly a question, what risk factors influence a disease or health outcome? If, however, it is to assess an outcome of an intervention and therefore an analytical study, the question that might be asked is, whether an experimental design or a quasi-experimental design is more appropriate. Studies may focus on people, problems, or a variety of phenomena. In public health where people and problems are often associated with programs, programs may also be the focus of the research. The research question determines the relationship of the research question to the research design and suggests what variables are most relevant to measure, the data collection strategy, the sample size and strategy for sampling the study population. The clearer the research question, the easier are the next steps. Additional considerations for the research study to progress may include the researcher's expertise, the magnitude of the task, availability of data and resources, access to the study population, and the relevance of the topic for the purposes of advancing the academic discipline and our understanding of the world.

The methods section of the research study is probably the most important aspect of the research as it defines exactly how the research question is going to be answered and the expectation of the reader is that the study can be reproduced with the assumption that the same or a similar answer will be obtained if the same conditions are followed. At the end of the study, the researcher must be able to clearly describe the following components (Kliewer, 2005) so it is important to ensure that good notes are maintained throughout the research study:

- Research questions and hypotheses
- The study population and its demographics
  - Sample size and its calculation
  - Inclusion and exclusion criteria
  - How the sample was selected for the study including methods of recruitment
- Procedures that were undertaken for the study
  - Data collection methods
- Measures and definitions that were used
- The validation procedures for the instruments used in the study to assure data quality
- The statistical tests that were undertaken. Studies will usually include a descriptive analysis of the study sample, specific tests that show the association between the independent and dependent variables, global and specific tests that compare the population samples, and any specialized tests required for answering the research question. The *p*-value that was used for testing significance must also be specified.

The importance of the research question for ensuring an appropriate study cannot be overemphasized. Table 2.5 shows examples of the relationship between the research question and the research study design.

TABLE 2.5. Relationship of the research design to the research question

Research design	Examples of research questions	
Correlational	What is the relationship between two variables?	What is the relationship between wealth and health?
Descriptive	What are the characteristics of a public health issue?	<ul><li>What are the features of a community that has recently experienced the effects of climate change?</li><li>What are the socio-demographic differences between individuals who tested positive for COVID-19 and those who did not?</li><li>What is the risk of Human Immunodeficiency Virus Disease (HIV) following exposure through a needlestick injury?</li><li>What are the risk factors for urinary tract infection during pregnancy?</li></ul>
Evaluation	How effective is the intervention?	To what extent was the intervention provided to individuals with disability effective in increasing their access to services?
Explanatory	Does one variable have an effect on another?	What impact does race have on the health of individuals?
Exploratory	What are the factors that influence the public health outcome?	How does exercise influence sleep patterns in women during pregnancy?
Intervention	How can the outcome be achieved?	What strategies are most effective for increasing health seeking behaviors to reduce the risk of heart disease?

The rest of this chapter will focus on the use of survey research to answer a research question and will not delve into the different designs specifically.

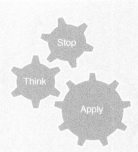

Formulating Research Questions and Hypotheses

1. What public health/health topic is of primary interest to you?
   - Why do you choose this topic area for your study? How do you justify selecting it? What provides the basis for you to explore this topic?
   - What does your research topic/question contribute to the field of health/public health?

2. List the variables that may need to be defined in your literature review? Draw a conceptual model that reflects your current thinking.
   - What theory or model might help you ensure a complete set of variables for this study?
   Refine your conceptual model once you complete your literature review.

3. Formulate your research questions.
   Formulate the H_o and H_A hypotheses for this study.

SURVEY RESEARCH DESIGN

The survey research design uses questionnaires and interviews to collect data from participants. Though surveys often stand alone as an approach to answer a research question, they may form some part of other research designs. Therefore, the rest of this module will be devoted to surveys as a methodology and a data collection tool. Surveys for data collection are either previously developed but adopted for use in a current study or are specifically developed for a research project. Using a previously validated instrument is often preferable over developing a new instrument by saving valuable time and resources. However, in adopting the approach to use an existing instrument, the literature review will help the researcher identify instruments that have been previously validated, but in wanting to use the instrument with a different population, the researcher may need to first ensure it is valid and reliable for their population. Assessing an existing survey tool means determining its purpose, audience, context and measurement qualities. The COSMIN (COnsensus-based standards for the selection of health Status Measurement INstruments) database contains over 300 systematic reviews of measurement properties of various instruments measuring health outcomes. Instruments that have been used in research projects and published are either available free or for a charge. This will usually be stated. Researchers should be contacted to provide information about the tool if it is not documented. A review of the psychometric properties of the instrument and the population to which they apply will provide the researcher with the information necessary to decide which instrument works best for their research. Existing surveys may not be valid and reliable in cross-cultural research since they may not be culturally and linguistically appropriate.

Surveys are made up of only closed-ended questions or a combination of closed and open-ended questions. Closed-ended questions allow the researcher to ask a variety of questions although styles of questions limit the responses that the respondents can give by selecting only answer from a predetermined set of responses. Possible responses could be yes–no, a Likert-type scale, or a range of options from which respondents choose the answer that they believe is correct. Examples of closed-ended question are:

- Do you enjoy doing research?
- What method did you use the last time you collected data?

Open-ended questions allow the researcher to ask questions that require more than one word or short phase answers and can be in sentences or longer. For example, asking the respondent to explain their previous response elicits details and greater depth to the answer. So going back to the previous example, asking the question, "Do you enjoy doing research?" may result in the answer yes or no. A follow-up open-ended question that asks for an explanation gives the respondent an opportunity to explain why they enjoy doing research. Surveys have a number of advantages and disadvantages that include the amount of data that can be collected, the time and effort associated with developing them, their suitability, and how much data can be collected (Table 2.6).

Survey research is subject to a few of the threats to validity described earlier, although most of them are in the context of intervention research. However, in collecting data for survey research, the validity of the research is assessed based on the data collected, with the potential for errors accruing from survey development through data analysis. The potential bias in survey research results from the measurement errors that are associated with the validity and reliability coupled with the data collection and the extent to which the sampling approach has resulted in a biased sample. The loss of participants in a pre-/post-sample results in conclusions based on a biased sample as does a sample from a flawed sampling approach. Also, the Hawthorne effect is limited to individuals that are being observed and the survey data may not reflect the extent to which the responses were influenced by this phenomenon, a factor that may also result in measurement error. Therefore, to consider concurrently the design of the study and the implementation of survey research strategy in reducing threats to internal validity is critical to drawing valid conclusions (Table 2.7).

External validity is the extent to which the researcher is able to generalize the findings of the research beyond the sample that was studied to others (people, settings, situations) and a broader context. There is always a trade-off between internal validity and external validity. Internal validity is the extent to which the researcher is confident that the relationship that is being measured is real and cannot be explained by other factors. Yet to achieve the external validity means having a broader population representation in the sample making it more difficult to control for factors that are not directly related to the study. Some of the threats to external validity are similar to the threats to internal validity (selection bias, history, instrumentation, Hawthorne effect), but external validity includes characteristics of the respondents and the time, place, setting, and conditions of the study. One aspect of being able to claim generalizability is in replication of the study across multiple populations and settings with the same results (Morton and Williams, 2008).

TABLE 2.6. Advantages and Disadvantages of Survey Research

Advantages of survey research	Disadvantages of survey research
Researchers can collect large amount of data in a relatively short time	The results can be affected by an unrepresentative sample if a careful sampling strategy is not utilized
While valid surveys necessitate a lot of work to develop, they are fairly quick to analyze	Poor survey development process could result in poor survey questions and invalid results
Compared to other data collection methods, it is fairly easy to train data collectors	Inappropriate and adequate training for data collection results in poor quality data
It is less expensive than other data collection methods	A very large sample size could incur significant financial cost
Survey instruments may be already available that have been tested and validated in previous studies	Previously developed instruments may not be appropriate for the study

TABLE 2.7. **Minimizing Threats Internal Validity in Survey Research**

Threat to internal validity	Description	Important to address in survey research yes/no
Attrition	A disproportional loss of participants in the intervention or control groups resulting in a different profile of the participants in the postintervention measures compared to the preintervention measures.	Yes. Optimize relevance and value; provide reminders and incentives; frequent contacts; incentives
Hawthorne Effect	When individuals know they are being studied they may change their behavior and adopt atypical behaviors causing a bias in the measurement.	Yes. Reduce the pressure and individuals feel less likely to act unnaturally.
History	Events take place outside the intervention that could affect (contaminate) the relationship between the variables making it difficult to conclude that such events did not cause inflation in the survey results.	Yes. Keep good records of events that may influence the results of the study.
Instrumentation	Changes occur to the instrument that affect the measurements related to the research due to the instability of the measure (interviewer, survey characteristics).	Yes. Instruments not valid and reliable and are administered differently across the study sample
Maturation	Changes in the participants due to natural or physiological changes that occur over time. These changes may be biological, emotional, or intellectual, which may be misinterpreted as changes due to the intervention.	Yes. Important in comparing different age groups, races, cultures, and different times
Selection	Individuals drop out of an intervention that was previously equivalent; Individuals are not randomly assigned, or individuals self-select; the sample is not representative of the general population and favors a particular segment of the population.	Yes. Results in sampling error. Adjust for loss in sampling; clearly defined study population; randomization; incentives/prizes; well-designed questionnaires; sampling approach
Statistical Regression to the Mean	This threat is related to individuals having extreme high or low scores in the pretest measures that migrate closer to the mean in the posttest measurement. This artifact in the measurement mimics a real change in the scores, although it is an artifact.	Yes. May also affect single measures when they may be identified as outliers but subsequent samples from the population may be closer to the mean. Use good study design and appropriate statistical methods not selecting the most extreme cases.

TABLE 2.7. (Continued)

Threat to internal validity	Description	Important to address in survey research yes/no
Type 1 errors	In hypothesis testing, if the analysis of the data in the sample shows a difference from the hypothesis, we reject the hypothesis. The null hypothesis (H_0) states that there is *no statistical difference in the means between the two variables*. A type 1 error is the probability (likelihood) of rejecting a null hypothesis (H_0) when it is true. This is denoted by α (the significance level- p-value). In public health research this is usually set at 0.05 (5%).	Yes. A small or skewed sample may result in inaccurate conclusions based on the sample observations of the data. Pick a smaller α (0.01)
Type 11 errors	A type 11 error is the probability of not rejecting (failing to reject) the null hypothesis (H_0) when it is false and there is in fact a difference in the means. This is denoted by β. Increasing the power of the test reduces this error. In a hypothesis, it is stated as H_A	Yes. A small (underpowered) or skewed sample may result in inaccurate conclusions about the research findings. Use a larger sample size.

Variables

An earlier reference to the research question suggested its importance in guiding the research and being clear concise and specific as well as being feasible yet complex enough to provide direction for the study. The clarity in the research question also provided direction for the variables that would be included in the study. For example, the question, "What is the level of disaster preparedness among older adults?" The dependent variable was conceptualized as two questions related to preparedness measured on a four-point Likert scale. The independent variables were social support, community participation, community trust, and demographic characteristics. Each one constituted a variable that was measured. For example, social support was found in the literature to be associated with emergency preparedness and was assessed through a single item: "During a crisis, I receive adequate help and support from family, friends, or neighbors" (Kim and Zakour, 2017).

The elements that are identified in the literature as describing an individual, a situation, or a phenomenon and can be measured using one of several scientific approaches, are generally referred to as variables. A diabetes study could assess knowledge, causal attributions of diabetes such as diet, physical activity, environment, and aspects of prevention. In addition to being measured, variables can be manipulated or changed over the course of intervention. There are two main types: independent and dependent variables. Additionally, two variables—extraneous and intervening—interfere with the research study in ways that are not always known. In a descriptive study, the focus is on the factors associated with the condition of interest. For a cause-and-effect study, such as an experimental or quasi-experimental designed research study, however, the researcher would also be interested in the relationship between the independent and outcome-dependent variables and how the extraneous and intervening variables influence and the case of the extraneous or confounding variable may distort the relationships. Age is often cited as confounding variable since at an older age individuals will exhibit different behaviors than younger individuals. For example, if age is not taken into consideration in looking at health-related outcomes that are influenced by the level of physical activity, then the true relationship between physical activity and heart disease may be missed (Figures 2.7 and 2.8).

FIGURE 2.7. *Types of variables and their influence on the research.*

Independent	Dependent	Extraneous	Intervening
• Factors that bring about change on each other and on the dependent variable	• The result of the interactions of the independent variables	• Factors that increase or decrease the effect of the independent variable (s) on the dependent variable; also known as confounding variables	• Factors required for the independent variable to have an effect on the dependent variable but cannot be directly measured; also known as mediating variables

FIGURE 2.8. *A conceptual map showing the hypothesized relationships among variables.*

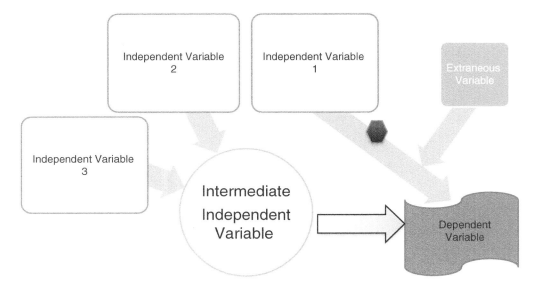

The Hypothesis

The research question specifies what is to be researched and suggests what methods are most relevant, the variables to measure, and the relationship between the variables. The researcher may have sufficient evidence from the literature to be somewhat confident in a relationship between the variables and be prepared to develop hypotheses. A hypothesis is simple, specific, clear, and measurable and should test only one relationship at a time. There are two types of hypotheses: the null hypothesis and the alternative hypothesis. The null hypothesis is stated as there being no difference between the two groups and no association in correlation tests and is depicted as H_0 while the alternative hypothesis is depicted as H_A or H_1 and specifies that there is a difference between the groups or outcomes (Kumar, 2014). The null hypothesis formally describes the behavior of the data treated as valid unless the actual behavior of the data as determined by the test contradicts the assumption. The alternative (H_A) is never proven; the researcher either rejects or accepts the null (H_0) hypothesis. The main purpose of this test is to determine if an observed difference between the means is statistically significant and a measurable probability that the sample statistics are good estimates of the population parameters (Marusteril and Bacarea, 2010). The significance level is defined as the probability of making a decision to reject the null hypothesis when it is in fact true (type 1 error). It is generally set at alpha (α) of 5%, 1%, and 0.1%, corresponding to a confidence interval of 95%, 99%, and 99.9%, but most often it is set at 5% ($p \leq 0.05$) (Marusteril and Bacarea, 2009) (Table 2.8).

The level of statistical significance is expressed as the *p*-value. If the difference between the mean score is significant and did not occur by chance, the strength of the difference is represented by the *p*-value. A *p*-value of 0.03 means that there was 3% chance of finding a difference as large as the one in the study given that the null hypothesis is true

TABLE 2.8. Comparing The Null Hypothesis with The Alternative Hypothesis

Null hypothesis (H_0)	Alternative hypothesis (H_A/H_1)
There is no difference between group A and B - Consuming fruits and vegetables have no effect on obesity levels - Social support had no effect on preparedness	There is a significant difference between group A and B - Consuming fruits and vegetables have a positive effect on obesity levels - Social support has a positive effect on preparedness

and there is no difference in the means. Testing is designed to assess the plausibility that the sample difference reflects a true population difference or is due to sampling fluctuation. The alpha level (α) is established before the tests are run representing the cutoff between the high and low probabilities, and the findings from the test statistic are compared with it. When α is set at 0.05 (5% chance) given the previous example ($p = 0.03$; 3% chance), the null hypothesis would be rejected, and the alternative hypothesis would be accepted. While α is often set at 0.05, it could also be set at 0.01 reflecting a 1% or less chance of rejecting the null depending on the study and the researcher's confidence in the results. The error of rejecting the null hypothesis when it is in fact true is a type 1 error, and the error of accepting the null hypothesis when there is in fact a true difference exists in the population is a type 2 error (Suen and Ary, 1989).

SAMPLING

The sampling strategy is developed during the planning process and the design of the research study. The sampling strategy is determined by the research question and the research design. In survey research, probability sampling, where each person in the population has an equal chance to be selected to participate in the study, is preferred to ensure that the results from the study are generalizable to the larger population. Obtaining a random sample of individuals or units can be achieved using a range of approaches including random, stratified, and systematic sampling. The sample design has implications for cost associated with collecting the data for the study and the researcher's ability to draw valid conclusions. Probability sampling provides the researcher with confidence in knowing that the conclusions that are drawn about the study population are credible and reproducible and limits the errors associated with measurement. However, if individuals drop out of the study or do not respond to the survey, the loss of these individuals results in a smaller sample size increasing the sampling bias due to attrition and nonparticipation. This is particularly problematic in studies with control groups, where there could be a disproportionate loss of participants either from the intervention or treatment group or the control group from attrition resulting in a selection bias and threat to validity.

Random Sampling Design

Simple random sampling is the mechanism by which researchers attempt to achieve a probability sample. It is assumed to be unbiased and is the most rigorous of all the probability sampling methods. Each individual has an equal chance of being selected. It requires a priori determination of a careful selection process for including individuals within the sample. Small sample sizes have a larger sampling error than larger samples, whereas a sample size of over 400 has negligible error. The first step in probability sampling is identifying the sampling frame, or the population from which the survey sample is drawn. The population sampling frame is drawn from a list that includes all the individuals or units in the population. The most common approach is using a random number table or a computer random number generator or a fishbowl technique to draw the appropriate and predetermined sample size (Kumar, 2014). National and local census or population level data can be used to identify segments in the population that can be used to design the sampling frame.

Stratified Sampling

An alternative approach to achieving a heterogeneous sample based on the principle of being able to achieve greater accuracy of the estimate is by using a stratified sample (Kumar, 2014). In this approach, the population is divided into subgroups called strata and individual or units are randomly selected from each stratum. Strata can be created by using demographic profiles of the individuals, race, gender, communities, or any other characteristic important to the research. For example, if strata were the design of choice for a study that involved all adults, one might decide on the strata a priori and randomly select individuals from the designated stratum to ensure representation of each age group. The next consideration is the size of the groups. In proportionate stratification, the size of the sample is determined by the proportion of the characteristic in the population from which the sample is drawn, while in disproportionate sampling there is no such consideration, and the sample size may be the same from each group (Figure 2.9).

Cluster Sampling

In a larger population stratified random sampling is more difficult, so an alternative sampling approach is to divide the populations into clusters that are made up of designated units based on identifiable characteristics called clusters (Kumar, 2014). A school district for instance could form one of many school districts in the town, so rather than conduct the study in all school districts; the strategy would randomly select say 50% of the school districts for the study, potentially reducing the number of schools in the sample by half. This process could continue through different stages by considering the needs of the study, the total sample size required and the number of resources available. If the study originally focused on high schools, for example, then clusters would be limited to high schools through the process. The final sample could be selected using the stratified random sampling technique (Figure 2.10).

Systematic Sampling

Systematic sampling involves selecting a random starting point from a numbered list and using a fixed interval to select successive individuals or units in the list. Although the starting point is selected randomly, the subsequent individuals are not. If, however, a different element is selected within each interval, then it is possible to have a resultant random probability sample (Kumar, 2014). A list of athletes in each school may be the population of interest,

FIGURE 2.9. *Diagrammatic representation of stratified sampling.*

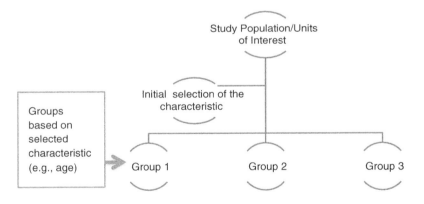

FIGURE 2.10. *Randomly selected clusters (1 and 4) were used for the final sample.*

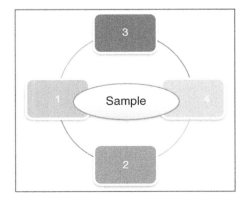

> **BOX 2.1** **Multi-stage Cluster Sampling**
>
> Using a combination of approaches the population for a health equity–based nutrition study of food outlets, the district was first divided into three zones A, B, and C. Within the three demarcated zones there were 211 food outlets: 61 in zone A; 83 in zone B; and 67 in zone C. Using a sample size calculation, the total number of food outlets required to be sampled for the study was determined to be 40. However, since the goal was to achieve a sample that would be suitable for drawing population-level inferences, proportional sampling was used to calculate the final sample size from each zone using
>
> $$n_h = \frac{N_h}{N} \times n$$
>
> where
>
> n_h = sample size of stratum h (that is the sample size for each zone)
> N = Total size of population
> n = Total sample size
> N_h = Population size of stratum h (population size of each zone)
>
> The sample taken from each zone was then calculated as
>
> $$\text{Zone A} = \frac{61}{211} \times 40 = 11$$
>
> $$\text{Zone B} = \frac{83}{211} \times 40 = 16$$
>
> $$\text{Zone C} = \frac{67}{211} \times 40 = 13$$
>
> Given the number of units required from each zone, a simple random sample using the fish bowl draw identified 40 ($n = 40$) food outlets that participated in the study.

but to reduce cost and keep a somewhat unbiased sample, every fifth individual maybe selected. So instead of having a sample of 1,000, the final sample size is much smaller but could be smaller still if within each interval, every person who is second is then selected.

Step 1: Prepare a list of all the elements in the study population

Step 2: Decide on the sample size

Step 3: Determine the size of the interval (total population/sample size)

Step 4: Select one position within the interval

Step 5: Select the same position for each subsequent interval

Convenience Sampling

Often the researcher identifies a sample for the study based on nonprobability sampling, and the results generally cannot be applied to the general population. The problem with convenience samples is that the respondents are not randomly selected and the final sample for analysis may be biased in ways that are not understood and violate the assumptions of many of the statistical tests. It is the least expensive way of arriving at a study sample, but it does not result in a sample that can be generalized to the general population. A study sample is defined as a convenience sample when the individuals selected for the study volunteer and are easy to reach but there is not specific rationale for including them in the study besides the fact that they were easily available. In addition, the population characteristics could be unique to that location.

In purposive sampling the researcher takes advantage of this ease of meeting people but selects specific individuals who may be appropriate for their study purpose and who are easily identified based on predefined characteristics. It can also be used in assessing specific criteria phenomena. A purposive sampling approach may be used to select respondents from a refugee population who had previously resided in a particular country or region since the group may be small or large but fairly spread out. Other terms include quota sampling when the researcher also chooses the study sample based on predefined criteria.

Snowball sampling is a method of data collection that has individuals who have already participated in the study to identify others like them. It relies on networks to identify study participants until the required sample size is reached. It is generally adopted as a sampling approach when the research involves difficult-to-reach, marginalized, or stigmatized populations and similar to purposive sampling produces a specialized sample. Individuals with a rare disease, disability, or other outcome may have to be identified this way. The sampling approach produces limitations for generalizability to the larger population. Snowball sampling falls into the category of nonrandom sampling but specifically may also be referred to as purposive sampling, which aims to get into the research study a particular sample. In a research study conducted among low-income families in attempting to understand challenges related to access to healthy foods and safe places for physical activity, while families were not explicitly recruited using this technique many were referred by their family and friends to participate in the study. It became very difficult to say no (Table 2.9).

TABLE 2.9. A Summary of Sampling Approaches and Descriptions

Sampling approach	Description of approach	Advantages/disadvantages
Cluster sampling	In-tact groups are selected for the sample, and individuals within the sample and entered into the study	More time and cost-efficient than probability sampling, but clusters may not represent the population as a whole.
Convenience sampling	Choosing groups, individuals or settings with no clearly defined strategy and the researcher relies on individual's willingness to participate	Convenient, but nonprobability sampling and may give biased results that cannot be applied to the entire population so unable to generalize the results.
Purposive sampling	Selecting individuals to participate based on specific characteristics. Includes homogenous, deviant, and case sampling.	Prone to researcher bias but can be useful depending on the purpose of the study and based on clear criteria for selection of study participants. Often used in qualitative research.
Simple random sampling	Every member of the population has an equal chance of being selected and included in the final sample for the study. Each person is selected independently.	Since every member of the population has an equal chance of participating, it is reasonable to generalize the results. Difficult to get a complete list of members to ensure and representativeness and not generally it is not available for a large population.
Snowball sampling	Individuals are recruited into a study based on recommendations from others	It is impossible to generalize the results since the sample has not been based on a random selection but is representative of the population being studies. Particularly useful with hard-to-reach populations.
Stratified sampling	Homogenous groups based on one or more criteria are set up and a random sample is selected from each stratum in a number proportional to the size of the group when compared to the population.	Provides a sample that is representative of the population and allows for generalizations. The entire population must be divided into the homogenous groups.

TABLE 2.9. (Continued)

Sampling approach	Description of approach	Advantages/disadvantages
Systematic sampling	Individuals are selected from a list or drawn in a systematic predetermined manner. The selection of the first sample determines the subsequent drawing.	The sample may be compromised if the samples drawn based on this approach also result in a trait that introduces a bias that affects the representativeness of the sample. Ensures a more even spread of the sampling across the population.

SAMPLE SIZE CALCULATIONS

When planning a research study, the researcher must consider the number of individuals required for the sample, however, the sample size calculation may be different depending on the type of study (Charan and Biswas, 2013). Calculating the sample size allows the researcher to obtain a smaller segment of the population for testing that is representative of the population, although the sample that is drawn only provides an estimate and predicts the population parameters. The larger the sample, the closer the results are likely to be in predicting the population parameters, represented by a tight the confidence interval (Jacobson, 2012). The most appropriate sample is a random sample, although there is still an error associated with the estimate for which the formula provides a correction. A random sample requires that each person in the population has an equal and independent chance of being selected. The size of the sample and the extent to which the sample differs from the normal distribution of the characteristics of the population affect the inferences that can be made from the sample to the population (Kumar, 2014). A small sample does not have sufficient statistical power to answer the research question. A random sample can be obtained by a variety of methods including using a table of generated numbers, computer program, and a fishbowl approach were each person/item within the population of interest is numbered and put into a bowl or some other approach that achieves the same purpose. Each number that enters the sample is randomly drawn from the bowl/basket/box until the calculated sample size is reached.

To be able to accurately determine the sample size the researcher must specify the level of confidence, the degree of accuracy and the estimated standard deviation. The larger the sample, the more accurate is the estimate of the population. The sample size for a cross-sectional study that estimates the prevalence of a characteristic within the population would use the following formula (Charan and Biswas, 2013).

$$\text{Sample size} = \frac{Z_{1-\alpha/2}^2 \, p(1-p)}{d^2}$$

where $Z_{1-\alpha/2}$ = Error rate set at ($p < 0.05$) and 1.96
P = expected proportion of the trait in the population based on previous studies or pilot studies
d = absolute error or precision—decided by the researcher.

The sample size depends on:

- The acceptable level of significance ($p \leq 0.05$)
- Power of the study
- The expected size of the difference (the effect size)
- Underlying rate of the factor/event in the population
- Standard deviation in the population

Free software and calculators for sample size calculations are available online for calculating sample size and power. For example: Qualtrics ^{XM} can be used to calculate sample sizes when using stratified random sampling.

Using Existing Instruments in Survey Research

Developing an instrument takes time and a fair amount of effort and resources especially with regards to ensuring the items are designed to answer the research questions and the instrument is both reliable and valid for the population being studied. Using an existing instrument often seems attractive until the researcher finds that the survey does not contain all the questions required for a particular study or that it was validated for a different population. However, there is some value in first trying to identify an appropriate instrument or questions that can be used in designing a new questionnaire. It is worth noting that the researcher may have to pay for the use of an existing survey instrument. There are publicly available surveys such as those developed using federal grants, which are free. A list of sources that include the National Survey on Drug Use and Health and the General Social Survey can be found on the American Psychological Association Website.

There are three steps in determining if an existing instrument is appropriate:

1. Specify the purpose and the needs of the study.

2. Explore existing measurement instruments that are appropriate for the study purpose.

3. Review the instrument and determine its suitability based on its psychometric properties; the comparability of the study population in characteristics such as gender, race/ethnicity, and education level; and previous use (through a literature review).

Instruments are generally concerned with measuring knowledge, attitude, ability, personality, and behavior. A helpful tool for assessing the methodological quality of the measurement properties of a health status instrument that reports patient outcomes is the Consensus-based Standard for the selection of health Measurement Instruments (COSMIN) checklist (Mokkink, Terwee, Patrick, Alonso, Stratford, Knol, Bouter, and deVet, 2020).

Once the instrument is determined to be suitable for the existing study, the next steps are to pilot test it with the intended population. If it is suitable after these steps are completed satisfactorily, the instrument may be adopted. If it is not suitable after pilot testing, careful notes need to be taken to help build a new instrument or identify an alternative previously developed instrument.

Given that there are number of different options for the delivery of surveys whether they were based on existing surveys or are developed specifically for the present study, careful consideration needs to be given to a variety of factors that are likely to influence how the researcher gathers survey data. These factors include the survey development and processing and survey distribution features. Historically, reminder postcards have been used for mail surveys and in a study where a mailed postcard was compared with sending a second questionnaire package found that the second package yielded a higher response rate (Becker et al., 2000). In the present internet era, prenotification by mail postcards or text messages influenced the recognition of the sender when web-based surveys were sent out, increasing survey completion (Keusch, 2015).

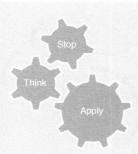

Reviewing Existing Surveys

Search for and locate an existing survey in the public health field. Write a one-page summary describing the survey and provide information about its characteristics, the study population, and its psychometric properties. Read through the survey and discuss what you liked and disliked about the format and style of presentation.

STEP 2B: DESIGNING AND IMPLEMENTING THE RESEARCH STUDY

By the end of this step, learners will be able to:

- Outline the process for survey development

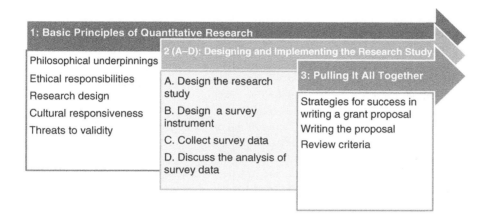

DESIGNING A SURVEY INSTRUMENT

Developing surveys, using clear guidelines will increase the likelihood of individuals completing it accurately and of the researcher conducting valid survey-based research. Since poor processes used in developing instruments will result in a lack of rigor that leads to poor quality data and misleading conclusions (Boyton and Greenhalgh, 2004), start by having a rationale for using a survey; develop the survey based on a well-conducted literature review; pretest and pilot test the instrument prior to full implementation in an effort to reduce measurement error. In collecting primary data using a survey, the researcher is able to explicitly solicit information to answer the research question. The research design that incorporates a survey may have its particular needs for information. For example, a survey that compares those individuals who have the disease with those who don't and needs to track risk factors would need to ensure that the data that is required to distinguish particular groups or categories are included in addition to demographic questions that form the basis for any survey.

Collecting primary data requires careful consideration of the survey methodology, including the development or adaptation and proper validation of the data collection tool. Pretesting and pilot testing the tool is critical to ensure the survey is appropriate for the study population both culturally and linguistically. Once the data are collected and archived it becomes secondary data for use by other researchers. As pointed out earlier, it is important that careful notes are taken and saved about the content and psychometric qualities so that anybody wanting to use it in the future would have access to that information (Figure 2.11).

FIGURE 2.11. *The nine-step survey development process.*

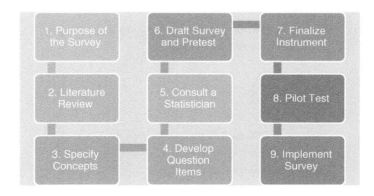

Step 1: Clarify the purpose of the instrument

The purpose of the survey is based on the research question and the survey's appropriateness for answering the question. It includes the need to understand perspectives from a population and any of its sub-groups. The purpose may also be to provide basic demographic information and patient profiles in the case of clinical research studies. A survey can be used to test a theory, or to develop or evaluate a program or policy. However, not all questions can be answered by a survey. For example, the question, "How do women who seek care and communicate their concerns with their health care provider in my city?" may be more appropriate for a qualitative research study. If, however, the question reframed as, "Do health disparities in access to health care exist for immigrant women in my city?" is more likely to lend itself to a quantitative study using a survey to collect the data. An alternative question that could lend itself to a survey with psychometric properties and built on a series of scales could be, "What attitudes of immigrant women influence access to health care?" In general survey research can be used to measure the diversity, extent and intensity of the phenomena with larger sample sizes than qualitative research will allow.

Taking cultural aspects of the respondents into consideration during this stage of the research is critical in identifying important concepts that might apply to the study. In the previous example, immigrant women may think about access to health care in very different ways that may be influenced by their past experiences. A recent study of immigrant and refugee women found that they were influenced by their cultural background, socioeconomic factors, and social stigma when making decisions about health care practices (O'Mahony et al., 2013). In a culturally responsive research study, it is important to think about context from the very beginning recognizing the importance of engaging marginalized groups from the beginning in order to facilitate genuine and lasting change and embrace research participants as members of the research family and not just as study participants (Jolivetté, 2015). So, what do we gain from including immigrants or indeed other marginalized populations in our study? We gain the advantage of not allowing our biases to influence the research and ensure closer attention to the voices of the participants (Freeman, 2015). Culturally sensitive researchers ensure that their research is designed to be independent of their personal views but reflect closely the voices of the participants. They understand their own cultural beliefs and values and strive to understand the preferences, assumptions, and stereotypes that could influence their work.

The philosophy of inclusion must be reflected throughout the research study

Step 2: Define the research question and the objectives of the study.

Define the research question that supports the survey development and define the objectives of the study, the availability of resources and access to the survey population.

Only if the objectives can be met, is a survey a good use of time and finances. Conduct a literature review to identify the concepts and constructs related to the research question. We return to our plan for conducting a literature review. The literature review consists of a set of articles that support the concept (topic or question) being assessed. More detailed coverage of conducing a literature review is provided in Module 1. An overview of the planning and conducting the literature review is provided in Figure 2.12.

  Literature review process Phase I and 11.

Phase I. Plan the review
1. Define the topic or question
2. Develop the search terms
3. Identify databases and other resources for the search
4. Establish the screening criteria

Phase II. Conduct the review
5. Search and select the literature
6. Read and analyze the literature
7. Identify the constructs and concepts to measure

In public health research, and especially in behavioral research, incorporating a theory is critical for future program planning and development. Incorporating a theoretical framework provides a basis for understanding the factors that influence the behavior and how specifically to intervene. It helps to identify targets to set for the intervention and the theory-based survey can be used to develop baseline data from which to measure changes that occur as result of the intervention when the evaluation is conducted. The literature is an important source of the information to provide a framework for the survey.

Constructs and concepts from the selected theory as well as concepts thought to be important for study but not contained within any recognized theories are important to consider. Many of these concepts may come from other work that might have been done such as qualitative research as a precursor to developing the survey as in sequential mixed methods studies. The additional concepts may come from working with the extended family of stakeholders that represent the community from which the study data will be drawn. These are all important for ensuring a well-developed and well-rounded research study. It also reduces the likelihood that there are gaps in the conceptualization of the survey instrument. So conduct the literature search, read and analyze the literature, and synthesize the literature identifying the important concepts for your study. Rather than writing a full report of the literature, instead list the concepts that are important to include in answering the research question. Drawing a concept may provide a reminder of which constructs need to be included. A list or a concept map organized in themes will help to clarify this task also. A study of teamwork in health care identified 39 surveys that measured teamwork of which 10 met the criteria for having psychometric properties (Valentine et al., 2015).

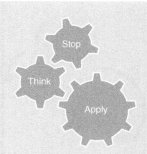

Designing a Survey Instrument—Step 1

Write down the purpose of the survey. Select a research topic and conduct a literature review. Make a list of all the constructs and concepts that relate to your topic from 7 to 10 carefully selected articles, so you have sufficient information to work with. Draw a concept map or make a list of all the concepts you identify and note anything about them that would be important for you to keep track of. Write a short reflection on the activity.

Step 3: Specify the concepts that are important to include for answering the research question.

Define each concept and subconcept that will be measured making sure each is distinctly different. A core concept of the transtheoretical model (Prochaska, 1984) is *environmental reevaluation*, defined as realizing the impact of the unhealthy behavior or the positive impact of the healthy behavior on one's social and physical environment. This was followed by defining the concept and then the survey question. In the 2012 study, one item used in the survey by Blaney et al. (2012) was, "I think that regular exercise plays a role in reducing health care costs" (Figure 2.13). Survey design requires that consideration is given to each type of error that is likely to occur and minimize the errors. One such error is not appropriately defining the concepts and the measures for the study.

Step 4: Write appropriate questions/items needed to measure the concept accurately.

Each item contains only one concept (core or sub-core). Consider cultural and linguistic factors that may influence the question and the response categories.

In the 1930s Likert created a new approach for measuring people's attitudes. In his approach to survey development, the participant's attitude is measured on a five-point agreement scale from strongly disagree to strongly agree with neither agree nor disagree (neutral) at the mid-point. This approach of combining items to measure specific concepts is now used across multiple studies although the scales that are used are inappropriately referred to as Likert

FIGURE 2.13. *Going from the concept to the survey item.*

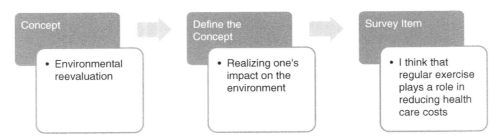

scales. There are three types of scales to measure attitude—the Likert scale, the Thurstone scale, and the Guttman scale. All of these are used to measure attitudes, although the most widely used and easiest to build and analyze is the Likert scale. Each item is developed as either an open-ended or a closed-ended question. It is also important to recognize the measurement levels associated with each scale. The Likert scale requires *ordinal data*, the Thurstone requires *interval data* and the Guttman scale depends on *ratio data*. Other resources such as DeVellis and Thorpe (2021) and Boateng, Neilands, Frongillo, Melgar-Quinonez, and Young, S. (2018) provide more detailed accounts of scale development.

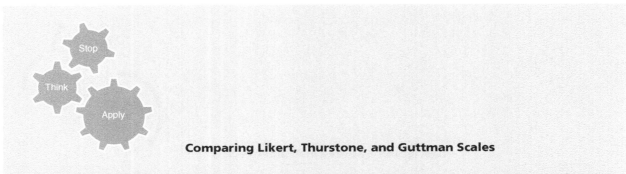

Comparing Likert, Thurstone, and Guttman Scales

Write a short paragraph describing each of the following scales Likert, Thurstone, and Guttman scales. Give one to two examples of questions that would be appropriate for each of scale.

In writing the items for the survey the wording for each question must be:

- Clear and unambiguous
- Recognize that most survey questions rely on individual's memory so time frames must be reasonable or tied to a specific memorable event
- Use short and simple phrases and active voice
- Avoid using metaphors and colloquialisms that may be unfamiliar to the respondents

Tips for creating a valid survey instrument are provided in Table 2.10.

Step 5: Organize the questions into an instrument that flows smoothly and does not irritate the respondent and create unintended bias.

Sudman et al. (1996) proposed a cognitive model for survey development and its associated cognitive process. The process of survey item development recognizes that individuals go through a process of question interpretation, information retrieval, forming a judgment about the question, forming the response, and finally answering the question (Figure 2.14). The brief, relevant, unambiguous, specific and objective model (BRUSO) (Peterson, 2000) suggests that surveys should be brief, relevant, specific, and objective, and items in the survey should be easy to interpret. In addition, questions must not include the word NOT, and answer categories must provide variability. For example, vary the responses to questions across the survey to include true–false, yes–no, categorical, or numerical scales, and measurement levels of the data are ordinal, interval, and ratio.

TABLE 2.10. Tips for Creating A Valid Survey Instrument

Survey instrument design tips Each question is:	Practice in survey design	
	Good	Poor
Brief and contains only one concept or idea	x	
Clearly defined and precise so the respondent knows exactly what the question is asking	x	
Consistent with a time frame that respondents can remember	x	
Culturally and linguistically appropriate	x	
Is in the first (birth) language of the respondent	x	
Loaded, emotional, evocative, or threatening		x
Not reflective of how the respondents think and talk		x
Organized in a logical sequence	x	
Relevant to answering the research question	x	
Worded to avoid unintended bias in the response	x	
Written so it leads the respondent to their best answer to the question	x	

FIGURE 2.14. *Cognitive processing for answering a question.*

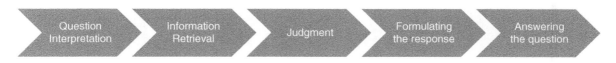

Question Interpretation → Information Retrieval → Judgment → Formulating the response → Answering the question

Step 6: Consult with a statistician to ensure that the response categories are appropriate for the proposed data analysis to answer the research question.

Step 7: Develop the first draft of the survey instrument, reading through each question carefully and checking that it meets the criteria of a good survey outlined in Step 4.

Over half of the studies that used scales to detect, minimize, and correct for socially desirable responses were influenced by social desirability (van de Mortel, 2008). Therefore, Latkin, Edwards et al. (2017) suggest addressing the motivations for socially desirable responses in data collection by first asking questions related to aspirational or perceived normative levels of behavior before asking about actual behavior potentially producing a more accurate estimate of behavior.

The survey design can be structured or semi-structured, with semi-structured surveys containing opportunities for the respondent to explain their responses to open-ended questions. As mentioned previously, the most appropriate method to use for the study is the one that is best for answering the research question. The methods reviewed in this section are appropriate for collecting survey data that asks questions primarily about getting facts. Most surveys are developed as structured instruments. They allow little flexibility and focus on *who, what,* and *how,* rarely asking *why* only when an additional question is asked to get an explanation. The development of semi-structured surveys with the inclusion of open-ended questions has become more commonplace. They provide the researcher opportunities to get a deeper understanding of the respondent's perspective in open-ended questions. The types of questions (closed-ended) allow only a certain type of response, and the response category must be closely matched both the type of question but also the type of analysis that is required to answer the research question (Table 2.11).

In addition, the survey format should be appropriate for the mode of data collection, whether it is deployed through in-person or telephone interviews or self-completed in a printed or online version. Online options may include email, web, or social media. Research suggests that low response rates are often due to participants being unable to read or follow the survey. Questions should be short enough for the respondent to understand the question, but not so short that it is perceived as abrupt (Boyton and Greenhalgh, 2004). In designing the survey, an important consideration is the appearance and layout of the instrument.

The instrument's psychometric properties of an instrument are an important element in ensuring that the survey instrument measures what it says it is measuring (validity) and is stable (reliability) when it is administered. At a minimum, a good survey performs well when it has the following traits: internal consistency, interrater reliability, and structural and content validity (Valentine et al., 2015). If an instrument that sets out to measure the level of physical activity measures the type but not the amount, then the assessment of the instrument is not it is not valid.

TABLE 2.11. Examples of Question Types and Response Categories for Surveys

Question type	Question	Possible response category
Numeric	What is your weight	_____ lb. or kgs
Yes/No	In the last week, have you consumed more than 2 glasses of beer?	☐ Yes ☐ No
Categorical	What is the highest level of education you have obtained	☐ less than high school ☐ high school ☐ some college ☐ college degree ☐ postgraduate
Likert scale	On a scale from 1 to 5, with 1 being strongly disagree and 5 being strongly agree, how would you rate your level of agreement with the statement. "Climate change is an important issue to focus on"	☐ Strongly agree ☐ Disagree ☐ Neutral ☐ Agree ☐ Strongly agree
Rank order	How would you rank the following in order of importance to you?	number 1 = most important number 4 = least important _____ vacation _____ climate change _____ family _____ personal security

BOX 2.2 Recommendations for the Format of a Survey Instrument

- Questions must be typed.
- Instructions should be clear.
- Questions should be spaced so that there is sufficient white space to make it pleasing to the eye.
- For uniformity keep response categories to the right of the page with the questions on the left and numbered sequentially.
- Leave more sensitive questions and questions that require more consideration to later in the questionnaire. Start with easy and more straightforward questions.
- Consider how the survey will be used: guided and completed by the interviewer or filled out by the study participant.

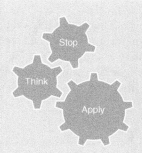

Designing a Survey Instrument—Step 2

Using the concepts you included in the concept map, develop a set of questions with their response categories that together will help you answer your research question. Make sure that each question is related to the overall research question or the aim of the study.

Survey Instrument Validity

The broad definition of *validity* as it applies to measurement is the instrument's ability to measure empirically what it is designed to measure and adequately reflects the real meaning of the concept under consideration. Structural validity refers to the instrument's items in a scale having a high covariance and reflects the construct they are measuring and assesses the number of dimensions of the concept are being measured (Babbie, 1989; Valentine et al., 2015). To assess the number of dimensions in the scale the instrument is subjected to factor analysis that provides an assessment of the number of distinct factors and the values of the factor loadings, eigenvalues, and goodness-of-fit statistics (Valentine et al., 2015).

There are three main types of validity: content (face), construct, and criterion validity. Content and face validity are the easiest to assess, although the assessment may be based on individual's interpretation of logic of the relationship between the item and the research question or study objective. Construct validity is a measure of the quality of the survey instrument and is based on statistical procedures that assess the contribution of each item to overall construct being measured. It is the degree to which a group of items in a survey represent the construct that is being measured. The more abstract the concept, the more difficult it to determine its construct validity. Criterion validity is measured against an observable criterion or gold standard to determine how well it compares. Predictive validity is the degree to which the instrument can predict the outcome being measured when compared with the gold standard. Concurrent validity is the degree to which the newly developed instrument compared to the existing instrument against which it is measured (Table 2.12).

There may be multiple scales within a survey, although it is important to remember to minimize fatigue for the respondent. Very long surveys increase fatigue and result in measurement errors that could affect the reliability of the data. Another factor that could alter the final results of the research study is related to changing the order of the questions. Egleston et al. (2011) suggest that the effect of changing the order of questions is related to the goals of the study. For example, survey fatigue could affect data in longitudinal studies if the order of questions is changed. However,

TABLE 2.12. Standards of Validity in Instrument Design

Standard	Definition
Content validity	The extent to which the items are representative of the research question and the objectives of the study
Construct validity	The extent to which the items measure what the researcher intends to measure
Criterion validity	The extent to which the items can be compared favorably with a known standard

given the difficulty in separating content from length, Rolstad et al. (2011), in their meta-analysis of 20 papers, suggested focusing on the content of the survey to ensure content validity rather than the length.

Once a tool has met the criteria for reliability and validity for one population, it does not mean that it is valid and reliable for another population. Therefore, it is important to confirm the study population for the initial psychometric testing. In the use of previously developed instruments, confirming cross-cultural validity is critical. Cross-cultural validity is critical and refers to the extent to which the original measure and the adapted measure are equivalent following their adoption for a new culture or their translation into a different language (Polit, 2015).

Survey Instrument Reliability

Reliability refers to the accuracy, stability, and predictability of the survey instrument. Reliability is assessed as the degree of consistency between administrations of the survey instrument when it is administered repeatedly under the same or similar conditions. Multiple factors affect the measurement of reliability of a survey instrument. These factors result in errors, including:

- Ambiguity of the wording
- Changes in the setting
- Changes in the respondent or the interviewer
- Regression toward the mean of the respondents in the study if the means started out by being very high or very low

Test–retest reliability is a measure of the stability of the instrument. Other means of assessing reliability of an instrument is using parallel forms of the same test procedure and split-half technique, where half of the instrument is designed to correlate with the other half of the instrument. When surveys in the social sciences are developed using multiple questions in Likert scales, a measure that indicates internal consistency of the items as they relate to an overarching latent concept is Cronbach's alpha (α). A sample size of 50 is considered adequate for assessing reliability (Terwee et al., 2007). It is a coefficient of reliability and reflects the consistency of the scale. Increasing the number of items in the scale increases α, yet a high alpha can also indicate redundancy in the items. It is important that each scale measures only one latent variable. The number of latent variables can be assessed separately by conducting a factor analysis (Price, 2016, and Brown, 2015) The acceptable range for Cronbach's alpha (α) is 0.6–1.0. An alternative test for assessing reliability with dichotomous or binary variables is the Kuder-Richardson-20 test. It should be used only if there is a correct answer for each question; therefore, it is not suitable for Likert scales. The scores for KR-20 range from 0 to 1, where 0 means no reliability and 1 means perfect reliability. Refer to a statistical manual for more details about all the tests mentioned in this section. As noted already, once a tool has met the criteria for reliability and validity for one population it does not mean that it is valid and reliable for another population, so it is important to confirm the study population for the initial psychometric testing and if necessary, repeat it.

Use a previously validated survey when available and feasible

Step 8: Finalize and pretest the instrument.

The pretest can be completed with colleagues and peers. They check for appropriateness of the questions and the instrument for measuring the expected outcomes of the study, redundancy in the questions, and flow of the items. A well-designed survey generally has:

- An introduction providing the purpose of the survey
- Instructions at the beginning and throughout as appropriate so the respondent understands how the questions are to be answered (e.g., "Circle all that apply")
- Questions organized in a logical order with the least important questions at the end
- Mutually exclusive response options for answering each question to minimize confusion

To limit bias in responses to a scale-type instrument, keep the response options going in the same direction, from negative to positive. Changes in direction increases measurement error as respondents may not notice the change. For example, consider a Likert scale where the first five questions have responses that are 1 = strongly disagree and 5 = strongly agree and then questions 6–8 have 1 = strongly agree and 5 = strongly disagree. It is quite likely the respondent will not notice the switch resulting in questions 6–8 possibly being responded to differently from the true intention of the respondent.

Once all the items are written, confirm the readability of the survey instrument. This can be done easily in Microsoft Word© with the Flesch-Kincaid Grade Level Test. Here are instructions for how to conduct a readability score:

- Go to File at the far left of the ribbon at the top of the screen
- Go to Options
- Select Proofing
- Check "check grammar with spelling"
- Check "show readability statistics"
- Press OK at the bottom right corner of the screen to enable the feature
- Go back to the document
- Highlight the section of the document that is to be reviewed
- Click Review on the ribbon at the top of the page
- Click the ABC Spelling & Grammar button on the far left of the ribbon. Review the guidance and make changes as necessary
- The reading level is displayed after the spelling and grammar function is complete
- Save any changes to the document

Readability is based on the average number of syllables per word and the number of words per sentence. The more syllables there are and the longer the sentence, the higher the equivalent grade level. Surveys for the general public should be at the same reading level as newspapers, so a score of 6 means that a sixth grader (middle school/junior high) can understand the survey. If the readability score is high, considering rewording the items to achieve a lower reading level.

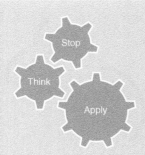

Designing a Survey Instrument—Step 3

Organize the questions from the earlier assignment into a survey instrument so they flow and form a progressive sequence. Add a set of demographic questions so you are able to describe your respondents. Number the questions and provide a title and instructions for how individuals should answer the questions. Consider the guidance that is provided in this section.

Step 9: Pilot test the instrument with a sample of the intended respondents or similar, but not the sample that will ultimately be drawn for the research. The primary reason for selecting a different group of individuals for the initial pilot testing of the survey is repeating the survey could result in an error in the measurement if the respondent remembers the questions or any feedback from discussing it and changes their answer. This is considered a threat to internal validity. In conducting the pilot test, each person who participates should be debriefed to ensure they understand the purpose of the exercise. The researcher asks participants to respond to questions about each question and the survey as a whole and compares their responses with their original survey response. Questions for the pilot test may include their response to the length of the survey, the instructions, the clarity of the questions, and their understanding of the questions. They are also asked to suggest any gaps in the topics they may have noticed and how well the layout of the questions helped them complete the survey (Box 2.3).

BOX 2.3 Pilot Test Questions

- How long did it take you to complete the survey?
- Were the instructions for completing each question clear? If not, how could the instructions have been clearer?
- Were any of the questions unclear or ambiguous? If yes, can you explain why?
- What do you believe the question was asking about?
- What came to mind as you read/heard the question?
  - If different from the original intent of the question, consider revising the question after further probing and understanding underlying concerns
- How did the question make you feel?
  - Allows the researcher to gauge the respondent's response to sensitive questions
- What made you select the answer to any particular question?
- Were any important topics left out in trying to achieve the purpose of this study?
- Did the layout help make the process easier or difficult to answer the questions?
  - If it made the process difficult, what suggestions do you have for improving the layout?

If the answers are not consistent, the research must clarify their understanding of the question and make changes to any words that might have been misinterpreted or not understood. Once the pilot testing process is over and all the formatting is complete, the finalized version of the survey is now ready for use, retaining all versions of the survey for future reference.

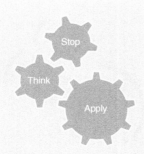

Designing a Survey Instrument—Step 4

Pilot-test the instrument you have developed and using their feedback revise your survey. Check over the survey. Conduct at least one psychometric check on the survey. Make sure it is complete, and have two to four people you know complete it and give you feedback using questions for conducting a pilot test in Step 9.

TRANSLATING SURVEY INSTRUMENTS

In cross-cultural research, using instruments that have been translated into the local language and taking into consideration the culture of the respondents is critically important. Accurate translation is required in the measurement of the concepts of the study with scales and constructs created in one language not always being able to describe the experience of individuals in another culture. Translation is a deliberate and iterative process that involves individuals who speak the language of the instrument and the language to which the translation is required. Google translate or other machine-based translation is not considered to be appropriate for survey translation given their inability to appropriately translate language accurately or reliably. In many languages there may not be a literal translation of a word or phrase, and often actions are expressed in more nuanced terms than is used in the English language. Common issues with translation have been identified as demanding a deep understanding of both the grammar and the culture associated with the study. There are challenges during the translation that include the differences in:

Surveys must be appropriate for the intended population

- idioms and expressions,
- inclusion of compound words, and
- words that may be more appropriately stated as phrases in the target language

One procedure that can be used to translate an instrument taking into consideration the needs to ensure that there is appropriate translation of the survey instrument is known as back-translation, where there are two individuals who are both familiar with both the language and the culture (Marin and Marin, 1991). The survey is translated into the target language, then is independently translated back to the language of the original survey, and the two versions are compared for inconsistencies in language and meaning that reflects cultural gaps. This may lead to revision of the translated version.

In McGorry (2000), she recommended the following guidelines for accurate cultural and linguistic revision of a survey:

- Use short and simple phrases and active rather than passive voice.
- Use at least two independent translators.
- Have a translator present during data collection.
- Obtain verbal feedback on any problems associated with completing the survey.
- Run preliminary statistics to investigate the characteristics of the data. (Figure 2.15)

FIGURE 2.15. *Summary of the process for translating and adopting an instrument.*

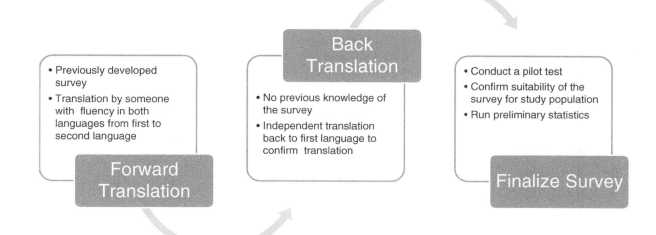

In order to reduce the error associated with poorly translated instruments, translations should be:

- Conceptually equivalent in words and phrases
- Simple, clear, and concise
- Easily understood by survey respondents
- Devoid of jargon, technical terms and vernacular that is specific to only one group
- Devoid of derogatory and racially or culturally discriminatory terms

Reference: Survey Center (2016)

The Informed Consent Form and Process

Before survey data are collected from individuals participating in research, informed consent to participate must be obtained either written or verbally, although a signed consent form is required in any invasive research or research that is classified having more than minimum risk to the respondent. The foundation of the Informed Consent is the ethical principle of *Respect for Persons*. It acknowledges the values of autonomy and agency of the individual. Informed consent is given by individuals to participate in a research study and follows guidelines provided in *IRB Regulation for the Review of Research to protect the rights and welfare of study subjects* The informed consent process communicates information about the proposed research project to the prospective study participant that outlines the project description, the study sample size, the risks and benefits associated with the study and contact information for the researchers and others who can be contacted to discuss concerns about the research study.

The research process requires the prospective participant to understand the informed consent document, trust the process and not anticipate any harm from participating. However, it often provides the information in terms that are complex, technical and specialized (Kadan, 2017) even though the goal is to ensure that the information is provided at the reading level of the study participant. The consent form is generally in the form of written consent, but when this is not possible as in telephone surveys or if the individuals are unable to sign their names, then appropriate methods are used to ensure documentation of the process. Specific and unfamiliar language and terms may be confusing to individuals and communities that have low reading and comprehension levels and experiences. Challenges to satisfactory implementation of the informed consent process include the complexity of the information, poor readability, and comprehension that is influenced by demographics, intellectual ability, and anxiety (Kadan, 2017).

Fundamentally, the informed consent process is a communication process between the researcher and the prospective participant in the study. However, Chilisa (2012) argues that the individualistic approach that primarily reflects Western values and emphasizes a one-on-one contract between the researcher and the participant also requires the individual to represent the entire community without the community having input into the process. In her model, the community would provide responses based on a discussion of the research and where membership of the circle is "informed by an intricate web of connections" (p. 195).

Working with indigenous communities poses challenges for getting informed consent. In the author's experience, working in Sierra Leone and in Ghana, the chief of the village is first consulted who calls the elders of the village together to discuss the request for the team to conduct the research project. This negotiation of the terms of the contract with the community takes place at the convenience of the elders and must occur before any further contact occurs. Conditions of the engagement must be met either that day or in the future. Even though the research study is approved by the elders of the community, the researcher must still solicit individual's consent. In many cultures in Africa individuals will decline to answer questions about their partners or other members of the family, preferring instead to invite them to speak for themselves. The collective ethics philosophy includes (Mkabela, 2005):

- An appreciation of the individual as part of a group
- An understanding that the research is a part of a community and a complex whole
- Respect for traditional authority
- The inclusion of elders and cultural committees in the research process
- The understanding of the interconnectedness or all things
- An understanding that researchers must act in an appropriate and respectful way to maintain harmony and balance of the community (Figure 2.16)

FIGURE 2.16. *Informed consent processes and practices.*

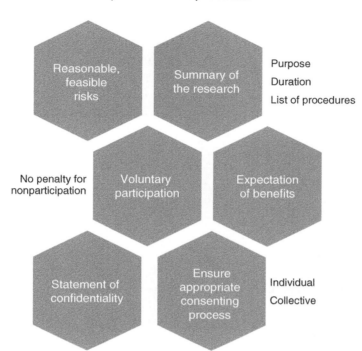

The Consent Form

The consent form and process specifically invite the individual who has been identified for the research study to participate in the research. The invitation is supported by descriptions of the purpose of the study, risks, and benefits associated with the study, payments, privacy, and confidentiality (Box 2.4). In addition, the form requires the researcher to provide contact information for those who are responsible for the research or who can be reached with concerns about the research or the researcher.

BOX 2.4 Obtaining Consent for Research

You are invited to take part in a research study because you _____. The study is being conducted under the direction of _____ (include investigator's degree) at [name the institution]

Provide information about the study as outlined in sections [a–e]
(a) Describe the nature and purpose of the study.
(b) Describe any tasks or procedures that will be performed on the participant (e.g., survey, interviews, document review) as appropriate.
(c) Describe any existing data (types and sources) about the participant that the investigators will access. Describe how long it should take the participant to complete any questionnaires or other procedures.
(d) Include total study length and session length and if participants will be audio or video recorded.
(e) Include a statement that the participant may decline to answer any questions that make them uncomfortable.

Potential Risks
Describe any risks the participant is likely to encounter during the study. These can be physical, psychological, or emotional.

Benefits
Describe any benefits the individual or community will get from participating in the study including any incentive payments. Compensation varies, but allowable incentive payments may cover participation costs. International research requires that the compensation is discussed and approved by collaborating researchers.

> **Confidentiality**
>
> Privacy can only be protected to the extent permitted by law. It must however be protected and the means of protection of the participant and the data must be described.
>
> Information from a research study may be shared while keeping the identity of respondents private.
> - List - sponsors, organizations, persons responsible for managing the project and processes, applicable government agencies and the office responsible for human research protections.

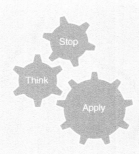

Develop an Informed Consent Form

Imagine you will administer the survey you designed earlier as part of a research study. Develop a consent form guided by the model in Box 2.4.

- The details of the study (items a–e)
- The risks associated with their participation
- Any individual or societal benefits that might come from their participation
- The voluntary nature of their participation
- Payments and incentives
- Protections for the individual and the data (anonymity and confidentiality including its limits)
- Contact individuals for the research team and other people who can be contacted if there are concerns about the study

STEP 2C: DESIGNING AND IMPLEMENTING THE RESEARCH STUDY

By the end of this step, learners will be able to:

- Discuss the mechanisms and ethical considerations in collecting quantitative data

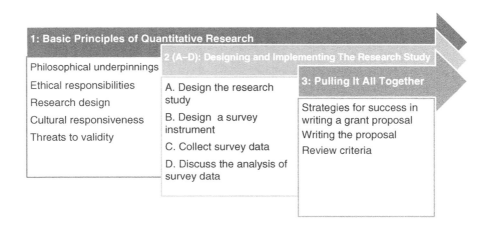

COLLECTING SURVEY DATA

Social Desirability

An important challenge in ensuring internal validity and reducing measurement error during the data collection process is respondents providing responses to survey questions that are influenced by socially desirability. When people respond to questions to be favorable to the research or the researcher and it does not necessarily reflect their real opinion, a social desirability bias occurs. It results in individuals' reporting both negative and positive behaviors in a more positive light than is accurate, an issue that influences all types of research for which self-reporting is the means of data collection. These exaggerations are likely a reflection of societal, community, cultural, and group norms and the respondent responds by bringing into congruence the many internalized norms and the ideal self in response to the survey question (Brenner and DeLamater, 2016), sometimes unconsciously. Social desirability bias was shown in a study by Latkin, Edwards et al., (2017) to be associated with key health measures; individuals who hide a health condition may fear being stigmatized or losing social status (Atre et al., 2011), and an individual who engages in illicit drug use may fear being arrested. In the study of drug use, questions about lifetime drug use produced more accurate self-reporting than drug use in the recent past (U.S. Department of Health and Human Services, 1997). Since responses are generally not consistent with what the individual would say on a repeat test, the instrument is likely to be unstable resulting in a bias that affects the conclusions the researcher draws about the participants in the study.

Training

Training the persons who collect the data in survey research is an important component to ensure research integrity. The National Institutes of Health (NIH) proposes ethics as the foundation for good science (Figure 2.17). Researchers must be trained and complete certification in Research Ethics before conducting any human subjects' research. NIH requires that researchers increase their knowledge of ethics and their sensitivity to the conduct of research, and learn the regulations, policies, statutes and guidelines as well as adopt a lifelong positive attitude to research ethics and the conduct of ethical and responsible research.

In addition to ethics and training for responsible research, training is required for the delivery of surveys to reduce error from instrumentation as a threat to validity due to the differences in how a survey or other research tool is deployed and the effect it has on the respondent. Training of interviewers has multiple components that include:

- Ethics training and the conduct of responsible research
- Training to understand the purpose of the study, the instrument, and how to ask the questions without modifying the intent of the question

FIGURE 2.17. *National Institutes of Health Responsible Conduct of Training Model*

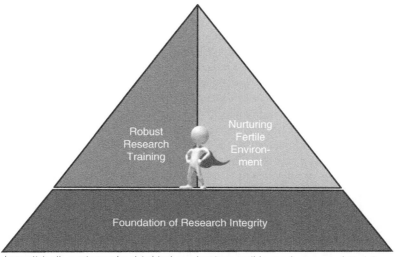

https://oir.nih.gov/sourcebook/ethical-conduct/responsible-conduct-research-training

TABLE 2.13. Action of the Interviewer and Possible Consequences for the Research

Action of the interviewer	Possible consequence
Overly positive feedback	■ Participants future responses fit a pattern that generates positive feedback ■ The respondent responds in a socially desirable way
Leading probes, prompts and explanations	■ Examples and explanations that clarify the question might skew a respondent's true opinion ■ Respondents may not respond in a way that would oppose the probe or prompt ■ Respondent learns something that makes them change their response ■ The respondent sees the interviewer as an expert

Adapted from Goodell et al. (2016, p. 579).

- Practice in conducting the interview as well as administering the consent form
- Orientation to the entire research study and protocols
- Practice in completing study instruments and forms required for management of the study and confidentiality of data

While the issues with delivery of questionnaires is limited to interviewer mediated surveys, which are more likely in cross-cultural research or in settings where the educational level of the participants does not lend itself to self-completion of the instrument, training in how to deliver the questions is critical. It is important that questions are delivered as presented in the survey and training enhances this feature but also provides opportunities for the trainees to discuss the alternative explanations that might be beneficial without skewing the question and biasing the respondent's response. The pretest and pilot-test phases of survey development provide opportunities for the researchers to learn how well the questions are written to facilitate understanding without the need for probes, prompts, and explanations. The consequences of bad interviewing are equally applicable and informative for training in quantitative research (Goodell, Stage, and Cooke, 2016) (Table 2.13).

DISTRIBUTING AND DELIVERING SURVEYS

The quality of the data from surveys is dependent on the expertise, ability, and creativity of the researcher and is reflected in the level of trust as well as the cultural connectedness of the respondent to the interviewer and to the data collection instrument. Other factors include the suitability of the respondent and their knowledge base as well as their receptivity to completing the survey. Cooper (2000) suggests that the order of questions and the visual display of a web questionnaire will affect its measurement. Technical problems in its delivery may be additional influences on completion directly affecting response rates and validity of the study findings.

The validity of the findings from a survey is dependent on the respondent, the extent to which that person has the knowledge appropriate for answering the question, and the approach that is used to collect the data. Surveys can be delivered to the respondent directly or indirectly. If delivered directly to the respondent, they can complete the survey in the privacy of their homes, school or workplace through a print version that may have been delivered individually in a face- to- face or telephone setting, or by mail. Indirectly, a survey can be delivered through an online/internet connection via email or a website. The primary limitation for internet mediated surveys is access to a computer for potential respondents. Even when they do computers, they still may not be able to complete the survey correctly due to their lack of computer skills (Elliott, 2002) and in some cases adequate access to the internet. In addition, sampling errors arise with computer-based surveys when the intent is to extrapolate the findings to the larger population.

Web based surveys have the advantage of being delivered quickly and do not suffer from the delays that are inherent in mailed surveys, however, the response rates range from 7% to 44% compared with a range of 6–68% for email surveys (Elliott, 2002). The formatting of the survey on the screen affects how responders experience the survey, and screen-by-screen survey designs take more than to complete compared to a scrolling type design that displays all the questions within one single web page although it may have the advantage of respondents skipping questions and reminding respondents to give consistent responses (Peytchev et al., 2006). Increasing the response rate requires changes in survey design and development as well as delivery factors that include respondents' access to computers and the internet. As in survey development for print surveys, pilot testing the instrument and the process in a web-based environment is critical. Prenotification of the survey by using letters or emails to individuals has improved responses (Elliott, 2002). Surveys may be delivered on the web through organizations like Ipsos, which host lists of users to whom surveys can be sent. Ipsos digital platform hosts the Knowledge Panel of 55,000 address-based potential respondents, including doctors and members of the public. Web-based resources like SurveyMonkey® allow the researcher to use an existing template or develop their own template and send emails to respondents. SurveyMonkey's pricing is based on the level of services. Features include gathering feedback via web link, email, mobile chat, and social media and then analyzing and exporting the results and data to the researcher.

Traditional Methods of Delivering Surveys

The cost of collecting survey data varies from one approach to the other, with the cost being calculated in terms of time associated with developing and analyzing the data, in addition to the time associated with collecting it. Standard means of data collection include one of two primary data collection approaches: interview-mediated or self-completion. Dillman (1978) proposed the use of telephone and mail, whereas in a later study comparing face-to-face, mail, and telephone delivery of a survey, De Leeuw et al. (1996) found that the delivery of the survey influenced the results producing different covariance and structural models when respondents were questioned about their general well-being and loneliness. Survey completion is influenced by gender, race, population type, survey content, and design and mode of delivery. Among respondents in a study of students, faculty, and staff, three influences of participation in self-administered surveys were societal factors, characteristics of the person, and attributes of the survey (Keusch, 2015). In the self-completion format of data collection, the respondent is given the survey to complete in a face-to-face setting, by telephone or mail or electronically, via email or web browser. The different approaches have advantages and disadvantages, but one feature in common is that they each rely on the respondent providing answers to questions within the survey with little opportunity for deviation from the validated and carefully pretested instrument. The limitation in survey research is compounded in cross cultural research with an undefined number of respondents possibly being unfamiliar with the terms used or the framing of the question.

The research mechanisms determine the quality of the report; the report reveals the quality of the research

Given the increased reluctance of members of the public to complete and return mail-in surveys, and the complications associated with diminishing telephone land line use as well as the mobility of the present populations, researchers are accepting the use of mobile phones for data collection as unavoidable. Unlike telephone landlines, there is less access to mobile phone lists. The expanded use of cell phones combined with the mobility of individuals makes it difficult to know where respondents are located at the time of the interview especially if the research is reliant on the exact geographical location of the respondent. In spite of these limitations the use of cell phones and text messaging has emerged as a viable approach to data collection, partly due to the high cost of internet data for individuals on low or fixed incomes. In a study conducted in Nepal, 450 respondents were randomized to three conditions, telephone interview, moderator-facilitated text messaging and an interview using text messages within a modular design framework. Researchers found that text messaging increased the likelihood of the respondent disclosing sensitive information (West et al., 2015).

Incentives have often been used to entice individuals to participate in surveys. These have ranged from cash, gift cards, and other promotional items per individual to participation in a raffle that carries significantly priced items. In one study I am aware of, individuals were entered into a drawing with a television as the raffle prize. In their systematic review of the evidence, Singer and Ye (2013) found that incentives vary depending on the motivation of the person asked to participate in the survey. The motivations were identified as altruistic, egoistic, or based on one or more survey characteristics. It appeared that increasing the level of the incentive did not necessarily increase response rates, which differed based on the study population. In a study of interview mediated surveys, differences were seen in the effectiveness of financial incentives that was based on interviewer behavior rather than the characteristics of the interviewer (Kibuchi et al., 2019).

The design of the study determines how likely it is to provide valid results!

Face-to-face interviews require travel to the individual to be interviewed, which has implications for time and cost in travel expenses. Imagine the indigenous population is hundreds of miles away and the researcher having to go multiple times in order to collect the data. The cost associated with this approach is often high, and respondents may be embarrassed having to answer sensitive questions face-to-face. However, an appropriate alternative could be the telephone. I recall occasions when individuals have not answered the doorbell or the telephone a previously scheduled interview. The Demographic and Health Surveys program incorporates Geographic Information Systems (GIS) technology in their data collection process to provide accurate coordinates associated with collecting household survey data. Eligible households and respondents are identified and interviewed by trained interview teams. The conditions associated with the spread of COVID-19 and the need for social distancing have left researchers with options that do not include any physical contact. In rural and marginalized communities and in low-resourced countries, access to a telephone or a cell phone may be a luxury when the phone may be shared among family members and an anonymous or confidential interview becomes an unrealistic expectation. In a recent study the author conducted, the cell phone was shared by neighbors, so when the research team called to schedule the appointment other families learned about the study and wanted to participate. Another factor in completing telephone surveys is the use of caller IDs to screen calls and for potential individuals in the sampling frame to not answer calls from numbers they do not recognize, often sending the call to voicemail or responding with a text message indicating their unavailability. However, in a facilitated interview each participant is asked the questions in the same order and with no changes to the structure or content of the questions. In one way or another, many of these issues affect the measurement capabilities of survey research and the training of interviewers is critical to reduce bias and systematic error.

Web-Based Surveys

As the use of web-based survey becomes more and more important in collecting survey data given the limitations of other mechanisms, researchers recognize specific features of the internet-based delivery that affect the response rates. Design features have been identified that have been shown to improve the response and completion of the surveys (Elliott, 2002).

- Include an invitation with a statement of the nature of the study similar to what would be provided in a consent form
- Ensure that respondent's privacy and perception or privacy
- List only a few questions per screen
- Group questions according to theme
- Use graphics sparingly to avoid unintended association of the graphics with the response
- Use matrix questions sparingly since they place an additional burden on the respondent
- Reduce errors by restricting response choices using radio buttons or drop boxes
- Provide some indication of progress through the survey (e.g., percent completed indicators at the bottom of the page)
- Allow respondents to come back to the survey at a later date
- Make sure to follow Americans with Disabilities Act (ADA) guidance and applicable guidelines to ensure access to individuals with disability

In an evaluation of online markets, 24% of workers in the sample appeared to have completed the survey at least twice, and 1% complete it more than five times, suggesting that individuals may not remember if they have previously completed an online survey and researchers need to consider restricting access to the survey once an individual has completed it the first time (Berinsky et al., 2012). Another important aspect of web-based data collection relates the ethical principle of respect for persons and therefore voluntary participation in the survey. When a researcher requires that the respondent completes each question before moving to the next one or prevents a submission of the survey due to the respondent not completing a question or a series of questions, this may actually be a violation of the promise of informed consent and must be considered in the light of survey delivery (Hammer, 2017). This varies from a text-based mail delivered survey, which by the nature of delivery allows for the option of individuals skipping questions (Buchanan and Hvizdak, 2009). The advantages and disadvantages of traditional and web-based surveys are summarized in Table 2.14.

TABLE 2.14. Advantages and Disadvantages of Survey Delivery Approaches

Survey delivery approach	Advantages	Disadvantages
Traditional approaches		
Mail surveys	<ul><li>Least expensive</li><li>A longer questionnaire is possible</li><li>Does not require any special equipment</li><li>Greater anonymity</li><li>Allows individuals to skip questions</li></ul>	<ul><li>Low response and completion rate</li><li>Self-selection bias</li><li>Requires the respondent to return the completed survey</li></ul>
Telephone	<ul><li>Random dialing allows for less self-selection</li><li>Can use highly trained data collectors on Computer Assisted Telephone Interviewing (CATI) software</li><li>Easier to reach "hard to reach" populations</li><li>Less likely to have nonresponse based on the design of the study</li></ul>	<ul><li>Fewer accessible telephone lines with the advent of cell phones</li><li>Could be costly if response rate is low</li><li>Place based research is more difficult since a phone can be registered in one state, yet the individual resides in another</li><li>Difficult to ask sensitive questions</li><li>Could result in a biased sample if the response rate is low</li><li>Use of caller-ids to screen calls</li><li>Cell phones can be shared with others making it difficult to conduct a confidential interview</li></ul>
Face-to-face	<ul><li>Questions can be asked in sequence</li><li>Completion rate is high</li><li>Interviewer can record responses</li></ul>	<ul><li>Requires travel and can be time consuming</li><li>Can be expensive</li><li>Training of interviewers is required to reduce bias</li><li>Individuals may be reluctant to share personal/sensitive information</li></ul>
Online surveys		
Web-based surveys	<ul><li>Ease of access leading to higher response and completion rates</li><li>Lower cost</li><li>Can be sent to respondents through multiple platforms (web, email, mobile phones)</li><li>Can be taken anywhere geographically</li><li>May include data analysis</li><li>Existing survey panels providing easy access to study populations</li><li>Privacy can be assured</li></ul>	<ul><li>Sample demographics may be skewed in favor of those who have computers/internet resulting in biased data</li><li>Limited to those who can read</li><li>Difficult to establish geographic restrictions</li><li>Impossible to ascertain who is actually completing the survey</li><li>Lack of randomization of the study sample</li><li>More difficult to skip questions</li></ul>

When an individual receives a request to complete a survey, they usually have not had advance notice of the study and therefore may be understandably hesitant to respond. Cover letters have been shown to improve the likelihood of a survey being completed. Cover letters are used to introduce the respondent to the study, the sponsors, and the protections of the individual personal information and data (Box 2.5).

> **BOX 2.5** Components of a Cover Letter to Improve Survey Completion
>
> - Description of the study
> - Identification of the sponsors
> - Reason for their inclusion in the study
> - How the results of the study will be used
> - Incentives
> - Confidentiality and anonymity policy

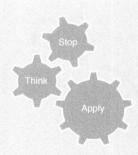

Reflections on Completing a Survey

Think about a time when you were asked to complete a survey, write a short half-page to one-page reflection about what contributed to your positive and negative feelings in your reaction to completing it. In your experience what is one thing you would do to increase data collection in conducting a survey research study?

STEP 2D: DESIGNING AND IMPLEMENTING THE RESEARCH STUDY

By the end of this step, learners will be able to:

- Discuss how to analyze survey data

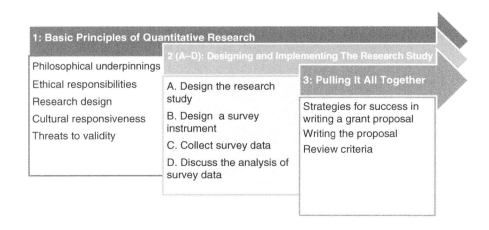

ANALYZING AND INTERPRETING THE SURVEY DATA

This section provides a brief overview of the analysis and reporting of survey data. The methods used for analysis of the data are generally described in detail in the methodology section of the paper. In writing the research study report for the final presentation and for publication, the researcher will usually include a descriptive analysis of the study sample, specific tests that show the association between the independent and dependent variables, global and specific tests that compare the population samples, and any specialized tests that dictated to answer the research question as well as the p-value that was used for testing significance (Kliewer, 2005).

In addition to the previously identified ethical considerations in the research process, ethical practice applies to the data analysis component. It calls on researchers to ensure

- Confidentiality of the respondent' information and data
- Accuracy in conducting the analysis and drawing conclusions
- Honesty in reporting the findings.

The American Statistical Association's Ethical Guidelines for Statistical Practice can be found on their website (American Statistical Association, 2022). The guiding principles outline the principles for good statistical practice, transparent assumptions, reproducible results and valid interpretations. It is organized into seven categories (A–H).

A. Professional integrity and accountability
B. Integrity of data and methods
C. Responsibilities to science, public, funder, and client
D. Responsibilities to research subject
E. Responsibilities to research team colleagues
F. Responsibilities to other statisticians and statistics practitioners
G. Responsibilities regarding allegation of misconduct
H. Responsibilities of employers, including organizations, individuals, attorneys, or other clients employing statistical practitioners

The ethical principle that best applies to this section of the module is (B) integrity of data and methods, and it is provided in Box 2.6. There are basically three goals for conducting statistical analysis: (1) to compare means or medians of the one or more samples; (2) to assess correlations between independent and dependent variables; and (3) to measure association between one or more independent variables and one of more dependent variables (Marusteri and Bacarea, 2010). While surveys may be used to collect the data to answer all or parts of the research question in a particular research study, the level and type of analysis required to answer the question will be very different. For example, in a cross-sectional study where descriptive data are analyzed to produce frequencies and percentages, the data analysis plan to assess the difference between the groups includes analysis of covariance (ANCOVAs) as well as regressions to determine associations between causal factors in the model (Rose et al., 2019). The level and type of analysis that can be conducted also depends largely on the response categories, how the data are collected, and whether the data lends itself to the type of data analysis required to answer the questions reinforcing the importance of ensuring when data are collected in a research study that a statistician is involved.

Analyzing quantitative data are a systematic process for examining the results of the survey data collected from the research project. As a reminder, it is important to think about the analysis at the very early stages of the research design, since the type of data collected is very closely aligned with the data analysis that is possible and appropriate. The analysis phase is a process of sorting and categorizing the survey data using available tools. Tools available for analyzing quantitative data include Excel©, SPSS©, R©, SAS©, and STATA©. Excel is the most readily available of these programs as part of the Microsoft Office Suite. It is a powerful data visualization and data analysis tool that lets the researcher create, view, edit, and share files like tables, charts, and budgets.

Data collected from the response items of a survey are categorized as nominal, ordinal, interval, and ratio. Categorical data consists of nominal variables, for example, gender and ethnicity. Nominal variables are the lowest level of measurement and include categories of people and things that are grouped by name. They are mutually exclusive, meaning individuals, places, or things are placed in only one category and hence the term *categorical* to represent the type of data. In interpreting this information for analysis, numbers can be assigned. So in a survey when the question about gender (male, female, or other) is asked, entering that data into the software (e.g., Excel) for analysis, the responses get represented as numbers. For example, male = 1, female = 2, other = 3.

> **BOX 2.6** **Integrity of Data and Methods**
>
> The ethical statistician practitioner seeks to understand and mitigate known and suspected limitations, defects, or biases in the data or methods and communicates potential impacts on the interpretation, conclusions, recommendations, decisions, or other results of statistical practices.
>
> The ethical statistician practitioner:
>
> 1. Communicates data sources and fitness for use, including data generation and collection processes and known biases. Discloses and manages any conflicts of interest relating to data sources. Communicates data processing and transformation procedures, including missing data handling.
> 2. Is transparent about assumptions made in the execution and interpretation of statistical practices, including methods used, limitations, possible sources of error and algorithmic biases. Conveys results or applications of statistical practices in ways that are honest and meaningful.
> 3. Communicates the stated purpose and the intended use of statistical practices. Is transparent regarding a priori versus post hoc objectives and planned versus unplanned statistical practices. Discloses when multiple comparisons are conducted and any relevant adjustments.
> 4. Meets obligations to share the data used in the statistical practices (e.g.) for peer review and replication as allowable. Respects expectations of data contributors when using or sharing data. Exercises due caution to protect proprietary and confidential data, including all data that might inappropriately harm data subjects.
> 5. Strives to promptly correct substantive errors discovered after publication or implementation. As appropriate, disseminates the correction publicly and/or to others relying on the results.
> 6. For models and algorithms designed to inform or implement decisions repeatedly, develops and/or implements plans to validate assumptions and assess performance over time, as needed. Considers criteria and mitigation plans for model or algorithm failure or retirement.
> 7. Explores and describes the effect of variation in human characteristics and groups on statistical practice when feasible and relevant.
>
> *Source:* American Statistical Association, 2022

Ordinal level data also allows the researcher to organize the data into categories that are mutually exclusive, but unlike nominal data this level of data can be organized into ranks such as in a Likert-type scale in a rank order of satisfaction. Respondents' satisfaction is specified at one of five possible levels from very dissatisfied to very satisfied with each level being assigned a number from 1 to 5. Interval-level data are continuous data that provide much more flexibility for how the data can be used in analyses. The distances between the categories or numbers are all assumed to be the same and can be measured; however, there is no zero. One example of an interval-level data with no zero is blood pressure. There is no such thing as a zero-blood pressure, similarly, height where is also no logical zero point. Ratio-level data are the highest data level among the measures, and it allows the researcher to organize the data in categories as in nominal and ordinal data as well as have the flexibility of interval data; however, ratio-level data does have a logical zero when the entity does not exist.

When only one variable is present, the analysis is referred to as univariate analysis. If the data are either ordinal or nominal, univariate analysis provides results of central tendency, frequencies, and dispersion measures. With interval data, in addition to the central tendency, frequencies, and dispersion measures, the researcher is able to obtain symmetry, peakedness, and normality statistics. In addition, statistical analysis available for interval data when there are two variables is bivariate analysis. Multivariate analysis is used for the analysis of more than two variables.

The initial step once survey data are collected is to code it so that any names used in the data to represent categories are converted into numbers so the quantitative data analysis can use it. The data are entered at least twice into two different files, and the data are compared to make sure data were entered accurately. A check of the data can also be done with at least 10% of the entries. The data are then cleaned to correct any errors in the data files to allow for accurate analysis of the data (Jacobson, 2012). Descriptive analysis describes the basic features of the data and provides a

FIGURE 2.18. *Types of data and associated descriptive data analysis.*

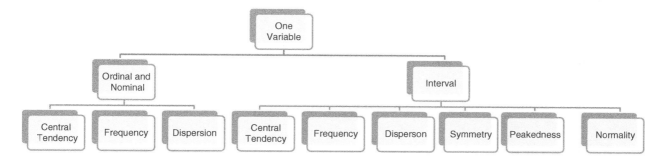

summary of the data. It provides a large amount of data are a simple more digestible format. Descriptive analysis is used to summarize the data initially with all public health research. It provides a profile of the group of individuals in the study is generally presented in graphs and charts showing the mean or average score, which is the most common indicator of central tendency; the mode, another measure of central tendency of the most frequently occurring value; and the median, the middle of a range of numbers.

In a distribution of the values, when two numbers occur at the same frequency, the distribution is referred to as bimodal. In a normal distribution of the data, the mean, median, and mode are all equal. Measures of spread refer to the difference in scores between the highest and the lowest score. Measures of spread include the range, the standard deviation, or variance and show how close the scores in the group are to one another. The bell curve (Gaussian curve) represents the normal distributions of the sample, and the data are shown as symmetrical around the mean (Figure 2.18). Most of the data are in the main body of the curve, with only a few of the data being in each tail (darker shaded areas). A normal distribution has the following characteristics:

- It is symmetrical around the mean.
- The mean, median, and mode are equal.
- The area under the curve is equal to 1.0.
- It is denser in the middle and less dense at the edges (tails).
- The area under the curve within 1 SD represents 68% of the data, while 95% is within 2 SD and >99% is within 3 SDs and 0 represents the sample mean.
- It is appropriate for parametric tests.
- It is assumed with large samples.

In a descriptive analysis the researcher summarizes the data to show how often each category of the survey is represented in the data. In addition to age, gender, and educational attainment, the data were analyzed to show the number and proportion of the sample who participated in community-based research activities (Table 2.15). In other kinds of data, the table might show how many individuals have a disease and how many do not or similar clinical date. This table provides a summary of the information to offer the reader a profile of the sample. There are likely to be multiple tables depending on how much data were collected. In addition to presenting data in tables, other formats may be used such as a pie chart or a bar graph (Figures 2.19, 2.20 and 2.21) to show the gender data and the education-level data to show the proportion of males and females who are represented at each level.

Similarly, inferential statistics for data that is nominal or ordinal utilizes nonparametric tests since the data cannot be assumed to be normally distributed. Nonparametric tests include chi-square, Mann–Whitney U test, Wilcoxon signed-rank test, and Spearman's ran-korder correlation. Interval and ratio data that are more likely to assume a normal distribution are analyzed using parametric tests. Parametric tests include t-tests, analysis of variance (ANOVA), and Pearson's correlation (McKenzie et al., 2017). Parametric tests require data that are normally distributed (Bell curve; Figure 2.13) and relies on ratio and interval data, whereas nonparametric tests use data that do not fulfill the requirement for normal distribution or make the assumption that the data are normally distributed. Categorical variables are usually tested using nonparametric tests. Parametric tests rely on large probability type samples, whereas nonparametric tests

TABLE 2.15. Table Showing Descriptive Analysis of Individuals Active in Research Activities

Characteristic	Value (%) N = 26
Mean age (SD)	38 (±6)
Gender	
Female	6 (23)[a]
Male	20 (77)
Education	
Less than high school	1 (4)
High school diploma	6 (23)
College	19 (73)
Participants in community-based research activities	
Yes	25 (96)
No	1 (4)

[a] Percentages rounded to the nearest whole number

FIGURE 2.19. Bell (Gaussian) curve showing a normal distribution.

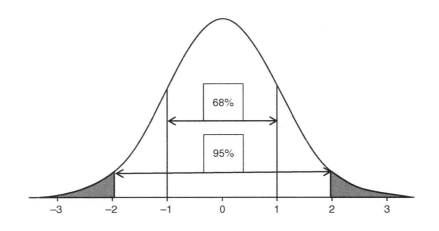

FIGURE 2.20. *Pie chart showing education levels of individuals active in research activities..*

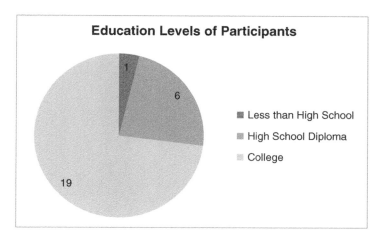

can handle much smaller samples, where the data are not normally distributed but usually have less power to detect significance in hypothesis testing and require larger sample sizes for the same degree of confidence in drawing conclusions. Samples that do not follow a Gaussian distribution may be transformed to create a Gaussian distribution by using logarithmic transformation (Marusteri and Bacarea, 2010).

BOX 2.7 When a Nonparametric Test Is Appropriate

- When the outcome variable is a rank or score with fewer than twelve categories
- When some values are either too high or too low, which would violate the assumptions of a parametric test
- When it is clear that the population is not normally distributed using the D'Agostino-Pearson normality test, the Kolmogorov-Smirnov test, or others, although not when the sample is small (<15)

Bivariate Analysis

Bivariate analysis is used to determine the relationship between two nominal variables simultaneously, and the chi square (X^2) test is used to test the relationship between categorical variables. It assesses the distribution of the variables using a 2 × 2 table showing the extent to which the variables are independent. The X^2 statistic represents the distribution of the total difference between the observed and expected frequencies (Suen and Ary, 1989). Similar to the X^2 test, the Fisher's exact test is useful for testing hypothesis and the independence of means when the sample size is small and the variables are nominal data (Jacobson, 2012).

The relationship between the two variables can be assessed for their direction and their strength through their covariance. A negative covariance indicates a negative relationship while a positive covariance indicates a positive relationship. There are also situations where there is no relationship. The magnitude of the relationship is assessed using the Pearson's r or correlation coefficient. Person's r assumes a linear relationship (Suen and Ary, 1989). A nonlinear relationship as for ordinal or ranked data are analyzed using Spearman's rho, whereas nominal data are analyzed using Kendall's tau.

The initial assessment of the relationship can be done using scatterplots, but the statistic measures how far away the points are to the line of best fit. Correlations are used to assess the extent to which two variables are related to each other but do not assign causation. In each of these relationships (Figure 2.21) the correlation runs from +1 to −1, +1 representing a positive correlation as in (a), −1 represents a negative correlation as in (b), and where there is no correlation between the variable, there is a straight (nearly straight line) as shown in (c) (Figure 2.22).

FIGURE 2.21. *Bar chart showing education levels of individuals active in research activities by gender.*

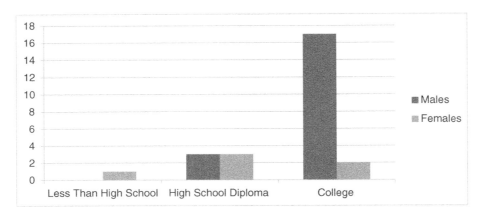

FIGURE 2.22. *The relationship between the variables in correlations (a) positive correlation. (b) Negative correlation. (c) No correlation.*

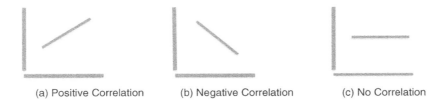

When the researcher wants to distinguish between the independent and the dependent variables and the relationship between the two variables is linear, the regression coefficient and the F test, may be feasible; however, if the relationship between the two variables is not linear, the researcher must select a different set of tests. When there is no distinction between the dependent and the independent variables and the test of the means on the two variables is equal, then a t-test for paired observations is appropriate, while if the answer to that question is no, but the researcher wants to treat the relationship as linear, then there are other specific statistical tests that are required. There are three versions of the t-test.

- Independent sample t-test that compares the means for two groups when the samples within the groups are independent
- Paired sample t-test that compares means for the same group at different times or the groups are related
- One sample t-test that tests the mean of a single group against a known mean

The ANOVA assesses the means of two or more groups and determines if they are different when the dependent variable is interval or ratio data when the distribution of the sample is normal (McKenzie et al., 2017). A complementary nonparametric test for testing the difference in means of two or more groups is the Krusal-Wallis test (Jacobson, 2012). The basic statistical tests for comparing one or more samples are summarized in Box 2.8 (Table 2.16).

BOX 2.8 When a Paired t-Test Is Appropriate

- When the variable is measured before and after and intervention
- When the samples are matched based on predefined criteria (e.g., age, race/ethnicity, disease severity)
- When there is an intervention and a control sample
- When samples are paired in the measurement of the outcome

TABLE 2.16. Basic Statistical Tests for Comparing One or More Samples

Number of samples	Paired or unpaired samples	Samples are normally distributed (yes/no)	Appropriate statistical test
1 sample	N/A	Yes	One sample t-test
		No	Wilcoxon rank sum test, one sample chi-square χ^2 test
2 samples	Paired	Yes	Paired t-test
		No	Wilcoxon matched pairs test
	Unpaired	Yes	Independent samples t-test
		Yes	Welch's corrected unpaired t-test
		No	Mann-Whitney U test
3 or more samples	Paired	Yes	Repeated measures one way ANOVA
		No	Friedman's test
	Unpaired	Yes	One-way ANOVA
		No	Kruskal-Wallis test

Adapted from Marusteri and Bacarea (2010).

Multivariate Analysis

The analysis of three or more variables simultaneously is known as a multivariate analysis.

Multiple regression models are useful for exploring relationships among variables or exploring the effects of multiple independent variables against the dependent variable. The model allows the independent variable's effect on the dependent variable to be explained while controlling for other variables using primarily two different approaches: (1) entering all the variables into the model; or (2) entering significant variables from the bivariate phase of the analysis one at a time. The fit of the model is assessed. In a backward stepwise approach, the variables are taken out one at a time to determine the best model fit. A logistic regression model is used when the outcome variable is dichotomous, and the independent variables can be either categorical or continuous variables. A linear regression model is used to assess if the relationship between the independent variable and the outcome variable is linear when the outcome variable is a ratio or interval variable. Discriminant analysis expressed as Linear discriminant function analysis, performs a multivariate test of differences between groups. The function is such that it can also be used to determine the minimum number of dimensions needed to describe these differences. Discriminant analysis is useful in determining whether the independent variables, which in this case are continuous variables, are effective in predicting an outcome that is a categorical variable.

Factor analysis used in scale development is a process in which the values of observed data are expressed as functions of a number of possible causes to find which are the most important. Factor analysis is a way to condense the data in many variables into a just a few variables. For this reason, it is also sometimes called *dimension reduction*. You can reduce the dimensions of your data into one or more super-variables. The most common technique is known as principal component analysis (PCA). It may help to deal with data sets where there are large numbers of observed variables that are thought to reflect a smaller number of underlying/latent variables.

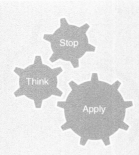

Reviewing Methods in Survey Data Analysis

Working in pairs, identify three to four peer-reviewed journals using survey research designs or survey data for answering the research question. Review the methodology section, and compare and contrast the different approaches used for analyzing the data. Draw a table showing the study design, the research question, and the planned data analysis. Describe the similarities and differences in the approaches used. Include the references for the articles that informed this assignment.

Reporting Quantitative Data

Reporting results of quantitative research occurs primarily in a narrative and a summary of findings followed by a table or chart. Data may also be reported as,

> *In a cross-sectional study of mentoring relationship formed by medical students, researchers performed descriptive analysis, X^2, Fisher's exact test and Mann-Whitney rank sum tests and bivariate analysis and used stepwise logistical regression to assess variables that were predictive of the mentoring relationship. Variables selected into the model were significant at the $p \leq 0.05$. (Aagaard and Hauer, 2003).*

In a study of consumption of fruits and vegetables, data were collected on a range of indices including perceived health, income, BMI, access to healthy foods, and prevalence of an obesity-related condition (Figure 2.23). In addition to providing the results for the study, researchers provide a clear analysis of the strengths and limitations of their study.

Study Strengths and Limitations

A well-designed study has many strengths, such as the size and appropriateness of the sample, methodology, and data analysis, followed by the limitations of the study, which are generally those that weaken the conclusions.

Limitations are usually noted in two primary categories of systematic bias as threats to internal or external validity. When a threat to internal validity occurs in a study design or in the measurement of the variables, the outcome is not accurately measured. If the research design or the instrument is free from bias, it is free from systematic error. Overall, the appropriate design and the implementation of the study are critical for reducing the threats of validity. Once a research study is complete, the researcher is required to report the threats to the validity within the discussion section. Reporting threats to validity is an obligation of the researcher and alerts the reader to what the researcher perceives are issues that limit interpretation of the findings. Some of the more likely threats are presented next.

Project Design

- Researcher did not design the study appropriately to answer the research question completely due to an inadequate literature review or conceptualization of the constructs
- Failure in the delivery of the survey due to technical difficulties either in the design of the survey for the delivery mechanism or a failure of the mechanism due to nonresearcher error such as computer/internet issues
- Use of an inappropriate method for example using a cross-sectional design to answer a cause-and-effect type research question
- Repeated testing that leads to instrumentation errors
- Interviewer demographics or style that changes the delivery of questions in a systematic way

FIGURE 2.23. *Table showing data from two groups on the consumption of fruits and vegetables.*

Variable (%)[c]	Consume three or more servings of Fruits and vegetables per day (%)[a]		P value[b]
	Yes (N = 594)	No (N = 700)	
Perceived General Health			0.004
Good or Better	80.0	65.9	
Fair or Poor	20.0	34.1	
Annual Household Income			0.001
Less then $35,000	36.0	53.5	
$35,000 or more	64.0	46.5	
Current Smoking status	20.0	21.4	0.79
Body Mass Index			<.001
Neither overweight nor obese	43.5	23.9	
Overweight	35.2	39.3	
Obese	21.3	36.9	
Physically Active	71.1	58.6	0.03
Easy to purchase healthy food in my neighborhood	83.7	82.4	0.83
Distance (< 1 mile) from home to grocery store	41.7	44.2	0.67
Access to healthy foods	37.8	33.3	0.41
Prevalent Medical Conditions Diabetes	10.8	14.1	0.29
Coronary Heart Disease	5.6	5.6	0.47

[a]Consumption of fruits and vegetables (1 = consume 3 or more times per day. 0 = less then 3 times per day)
[b]Rao-Scott Chi-Square p value
[c]All percentages are survey weighted
[d]Perceived safety of neighborhood (1 = Persons who answered 'quite safe' or 'extremely safe' to the question "How safe from crime do you consider your neighborhood to be?"   0 = otherwise   IDN: Initiative Designated Neighborhood

Sample Size Issues

- A small sample size due to inadequate or ineffective sampling
- Low survey returns or completion rates by any method
- Reduced sample size due to a loss of participants between the pretest and the posttest measurements—particularly important if there is a disproportionate loss from either the intervention or the control/comparison group

Measurement Issues

- Invalid or unreliable measurement instrument for the study population
- Respondents putting answers that are socially desirable, e.g., what they perceive is expected of them and not reflecting their true feelings—in some cases guessing what the question or the answer choices mean
- Self-reporting that might be influenced by recall, characteristics of condition or situation of the recall, the individual's characteristics, and the duration of the study
- Maturation bias when the participants age due to age or maturity

Data Analysis

- Statistical regression toward the mean from a high or low initial measurement
- Confounding variables that have not been accounted for in the study
- Prior sensitization of the study population to the outcomes of the study being observed before measurement

When the study is designed so its results apply only to similar limited populations, place, and time, the study is said to lack external validity. A study has to be internally valid to be externally valid, although it can be internally valid and not externally valid. Once the study and the researcher decide on the overall quality of the research, the final step is writing the report to share the findings. The basic structure for a report of a quantitative research contains a summary of the entire study. The researcher also notes any limitations of the study that would result in a bias in the findings or lack of internal or external validity. It provides the reader with information about the conditions or the challenges the research experienced, demonstrating an understanding of the research process. One that is often cited is a smaller than anticipated sample size. An example is provided in Box 2.9.

The outline of the structure of the report that incorporates the AIM(RaD)C (Cargill and O'Connor, 2009) model is shown in Box 2.10. The content for each of these sections is described in detail in Module 5 of this book. The NIH discusses the importance of ethics not just in the collection of data but also in writing the report. As a researcher considers how to present the findings from the research study, this becomes an important aspect of responsible research.

BOX 2.9 Study Limitation Example from the Literature

"Although beyond the scope of the current study, an additional limitation is a lack of a measure that examined the unique experiences that accompany being a non-White member of society in the United States. While Black and Hispanics were oversampled in NESARC, Asian, American Indian, and Alaskan Natives were not, leading to smaller sample sizes for interaction analyzes and a need to exclude these groups."

Glass et al. (2017, p.9)

BOX 2.10 Outline of the Final Report for a Quantitative Study

- The title page
- Abstract
- Acknowledgments
- Table of contents
- Abstract
- Introduction/literature review
- Aims and purpose of the study
- Research questions and hypotheses
- Study design and methodology
    - Study design
    - Setting
    - Participants
    - Sample size
    - Measurement
    - Variables
    - Statistical methods
- Data collection
- Results of the analysis
    - Participants
    - Descriptive data
    - Outcome data (where appropriate)
    - Main results
    - Other analyzes
- Discussion including limitations
    - Key results
    - Limitations
    - Interpretation of results
    - Generalizability
- Conclusion
- References
- Appendices

Deciding What Study Results to Publish and Transparency

Dr. Wyck is the lead investigator for a cohort-based case-control study of the genetic and environmental factors related to Parkinson's disease (PD) that compares 1,000 patients with 1,000 matched controls. Her team's analysis discovers that having a history of head trauma ($p = 0.005$), high blood pressure ($p = 0.01$), or exposure to agricultural pesticides ($p = 0.04$) is related to 25–60% higher risk of PD. Surprisingly, Dr. Wyck found that current cigarette smokers were at 40% lower risk of PD as compared to nonsmokers ($p = 0.02$). The analysis also indicated that nonsmokers exposed to secondhand smoke had 12% lower PD risk compared with nonsmokers without exposure to secondhand smoke, but this association was not formally statistically significant ($p = 0.07$). Dr. Wyck is concerned that the findings for smoking exposure may have a negative impact on public health by discouraging people from quitting (i.e., as a way to avoid developing PD). While preparing the study manuscript, she is considering whether or not to report the findings related to smoking (and if so, how to address those findings in the discussion).

Questions:

1. Should Dr. Wyck report all her findings, including those related to smoking? Why or why not? What if the result for smoking was opposite; that is, it was related to higher PD risk?
2. Should she report only findings with p-values?
3. Which findings should Dr. Wyck emphasize in title, abstract, and discussion?
4. How should she discuss the apparent protective association with smoking; for example, should she speculate on possible mechanisms, such as nicotine's role in increasing brain dopamine levels?
5. What, if anything, should the authors say about the secondhand smoke finding?
6. What aspects of the many health risks associated with smoking are relevant to the findings?

Source: National Institutes of Health, Office of Intramural Research (2017) Case #1

SUMMARY

Culturally and ethically responsive research includes residents of the community, colleagues across multiple professional areas, and staff of organizations, universities, and agencies. Ideally, stakeholders are involved in public health research throughout the process and have critical roles and responsibilities including giving voice to the study population.

A review of the literature provides the researcher with a clear justification for the study and situates it within the field as relevant and important. When the study is based on previous research and built from identified gaps in the literature, it is of greater value to the field.

Conceptualizing the framework of the research within the socioecological model allows the researcher to identify a more complete set of variables in the conceptual map as the basis for the study. Incorporating established and published theories increases the likelihood that concepts and constructs that are known to influence the behavior and drive the health and wellbeing outcomes are included in the research study.

The research question guides the study design and the methodology so make sure it is specific enough to give the researcher a road map for the study. If the aim of the study requires multiple questions, then each question must meet the same criteria.

When available, use an existing valid and reliable instrument rather than developing a new one given the time and effort required to an instrument. Determine the established psychometrics for an existing instrument and assess its applicability for the study population.

As far as possible, survey data collection should be based on probability sampling, where each person in the population has an equal chance to be selected into the sample for the study. The sampling design has implications for cost associated with the study.

When planning a research study, the sample size calculation may be different depending on the type of study. Calculating the sample size allows the researcher to obtain a smaller segment of the population for testing that is representative of the population.

Using an existing instrument often seems attractive until the researcher finds that the survey does not contain all the questions required for a particular study or that it was validated for a different population. First try to identify an appropriate instrument or questions that can be used in the design of a new questionnaire.

Social desirability is defined as a type of bias that has people responding in a way that would be favorable to the research or the researcher and not necessarily reflecting their true opinions.

Collecting primary data requires careful consideration of the survey methodology. Pretesting and pilot testing the tool is critical to ensure the survey is both culturally and linguistically appropriate.

Validity as it applies to measurement is the instrument's ability to measure what it is designed to measure, and it adequately reflects the real meaning of the concept under consideration. Reliability refers to the accuracy, stability, and predictability of the survey instrument.

The quality of the data from surveys is dependent on the expertise, ability and creativity of the researcher and is reflected in the level of trust as well as the cultural connectedness of the respondent to the interviewer and to the data collection instrument. Other factors include the suitability of the respondent and their knowledge base as well as their receptivity to completing the survey.

Each survey mechanism has advantages and disadvantages and requires addressing issues related to the respondent, the instrument, and research approach.

Ethical practice applies to the data analysis part of the research process as much as it does to earlier sections. Researchers must ensure confidentiality of the respondents' information and data, accuracy in conducting the analysis and drawing conclusions, and honesty in reporting the findings.

Analyzing quantitative data are a systematic process for examining the results of the survey data collection from the research project. It is important to think about the analysis at the very early stages of the research design, since the type of data that is collected is very closely aligned with the data analysis that is possible and appropriate.

Reporting results of quantitative research occurs primarily in a narrative and a summary of findings followed tables or charts. The researcher is required to report the limitations of the research that alert the reader to what the researcher perceives are issues that affect the interpretation of the findings.

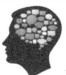

Now that I have reached the end this section, I am able to:

Course objective	Strongly agree	Somewhat agree	Neutral	Somewhat disagree	Strongly agree
Describe the process for conducting a research study					
Develop a problem statement and research question					
Outline the process for survey development					
Discuss the mechanisms and ethical considerations in collecting quantitative data					

STEP 3: PULLING IT ALL TOGETHER: AN OVERVIEW OF GRANT WRITING

By the end of this section, learners will be able to:

- Outline the steps for writing a grant
- Discuss the requirements for a successful grant submission
- Write a grant for submission for funding

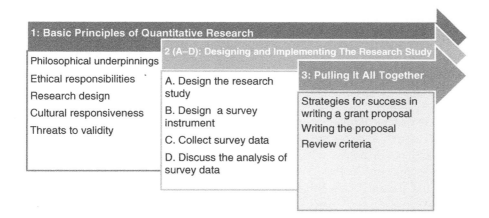

INTRODUCTION

Grant writing is often how public health researchers get funding to undertake research project. Grants may be funded by foundations, national research institutes, national, local, and state governments and local nonprofit and for-profit institutions and universities. Research is conducted at different levels and by different people and it can be funded or not. Not all research is funded, but often researchers request funding when the cost of the research is more than they can do without it being funded. Institutions are often able to fund small seed projects, if the researcher is developing a new idea or testing a new model or concept.

Some people are researchers in their professional roles, and others in academic institutions conduct research as one of their roles as researchers or as teachers at undergraduate, master's, and doctoral levels. At each of these levels, students may also be involved in writing grants to fund their research activities. One such opportunity is with more senior researchers, when for large funding institutions like the National Institute of Health in the United States; supplementary awards are made to researchers with established grants. There are two benefits to this, one the student gets to start their career with an established researcher, and secondly the student gets an opportunity to learn very early on how to write grants that are more likely to be successful. One of the markers of success in grant writing is having the experience to know what the reviewers are looking for, a skill that is built over time. In writing a winning grant, the reality that is created for the reader/grant evaluator is that the research study is worth conducting! A grant proposal is generally in response to a Request for Proposals (RFP) or sometimes called the call for proposals that provides clear guidelines for what the organization or agency will fund and how the response must be submitted. The turnaround time for the submission of a grant is often as short as six weeks although they can be shorter, so researchers have to have a well-developed idea often with an existing stakeholder advisory group set up and working on the project long before a call for proposals is published.

In an assessment of public and philanthropic organizations globally, the ten largest funders of health research based on 2013 data, spent $37.1 billion, the largest being the NIH in the United States followed by the European Commission and the UK Medical Research Council with WHO being the largest multilateral funder. Viergever and Hendricks (2016) also pointed out the need for greater transparency and evidence-based funding mechanisms. While spending by philanthropic organizations was significantly less, like public intuitions, their spending levels vary considerably. In the United States, the most common sources of funding are from the federal government, which is a mixture of formula and competitive grant programs. There is also funding available at the state, county, and city levels, although these amounts are considerably smaller. Unfortunately, not all grant proposals are funded the first time and grant writers must be persistent (Kwekkeboom, 2014). Proposals are scored by the peer evaluators based on specified criteria. The researcher that submits the grant will usually get a report on the peer review providing indications of the application's strengths and weaknesses. If a grant is not funded, the researcher has an opportunity to revise the submission and reapply in the future. Most researchers have some experience of having the opportunity to revise their submission and resubmit the following year.

Calls for proposals are put into the public domain in a number of ways, through print or electronic newsletters, websites, and special publications (Box 2.11). Grant writers and researchers searching for grants can request regular announcement bulletins from the organization that may be sent to a registered email address. Universities generally have offices responsible for grants management that will send out RFPs of interest to relevant departments in addition to helping researchers manage the grant application and monitoring process.

BOX 2.11 [Foundation] COVID-19 and Diabetes Research Award—Request for Proposals

The [foundation] is requesting applications for research focused on the impact of diabetes on COVID-19 and the impact of COVID-19 on diabetes and its complications.

Recent clinical results have shown that people with diabetes are at higher risk of death from COVID-19 and that COVID-19 drives an increased risk of hyperglycemia and other complications in those with and without diabetes. This is in addition to the risk due to advanced age and chronic disease. Both the biological mechanisms underlying this risk and how to minimize it remain poorly understood. There is an urgent need for research to understand the impact of diabetes on COVID-19 and vice versa. This is true at a basic and clinical level.

The main text of the application will be a **two-page application** to provide all necessary study components (aims, significance, preliminary data (if applicable), research plan, and expected actionable outcomes) with a one-page listing of critical references, PI biosketch, and budget form. The goal of this RFA is to use a rapid application and review process to identify **at least 10 grants of up to $100,000/each** in this area and of high scientific merit for immediate funding.

The expedited application deadline _____

Learn the Basics/Plan the Approach

Success in the process of grant writing is exciting for the researchers involved but the steps to being a successful grant writer lie in undertaking a thoughtful and deliberate process of presenting a proposal to a federal, national, or local agency or organization to fund their research or project implementation. Philanthropic organizations and foundations will also accept proposals to fund research and community-based interventions.

While the process differs somewhat from institution to institution the fundamentals of successful grant writing remain the same. A strong application should be easy to read, concise, and attractive. It must be clear and well-written and respond to the review criteria (Gholipour et al., 2014). Before considering writing a grant however, the team has a responsibility to:

- Identify the team leader, who will generally be referred to as the PI
- Develop a specific and meaningful research project idea
- Consider how the project idea is likely to fit the values and mission of the funding organization
- Review previous funded grants of that institution
- Engage other potential stakeholders
- Ensure there is likely to be appropriate supports and infrastructure for implementing the project (individuals with appropriate qualification or expertise, space, technology, financial management and other key resources)

The individual who writes the grant is often the researcher; however, there are skills associated with grant writing that can be developed, and many public health professionals have become successful consultants writing grants for other people and organizations, who may neither have the appropriate skills or the time to put together not just the content of the grant but all the accompanying documentation that is often required. Grant writing is a major financial investment in time and energy and successful grant writing requires sufficiently senior researchers to lead the team to assure the reviewers of the likelihood of the success of the research once it is funded. The use of review documents to check the quality of the approach, such as the CONSORT (Consolidated Standards of Reporting Trials) or STROBE (Strengthening the Reporting of Observational Studies in Epidemiology) statement, will enhance the quality of the application (Kwekkeboom, 2014). Additional tips for successful grant writing are listed in Box 2.12.

> **BOX 2.12** **Additional Tips for Successful Grant Writing**
> - Read the instructions in the RFP completely and thoroughly—each grant it different!
> - Make sure deadlines are met.
> - Be very detail-oriented as well as clear, logical, direct, and to the point.
> - Use the headings provided by the funding agency in the guidelines.
> - Be methodical, thorough, and persistent.
> - Have strong budgetary skills.
> - Meet tight deadlines.
> - Have strong professional ethics.
> - Have strong writing, grammar, and spelling skills.
> - Be proficient in word, PowerPoint, Excel, and other necessary software.
> - Ensure the document is properly formatted and references are adequately cited in the appropriate writing style (e.g., American Psychological Association [APA], American Medical Association [AMA])

While the basic structure of the grant is similar across public health disciplines, underlying research approaches may be specialized. For example, a community-based participatory research proposal will have the expectation for considerable and sustained community engagement and be undergirded by a transformative philosophy. The methodology will of course be guided by the research questions that will be answered and the expected outcomes of the research. However, a basic research grant or one that is seeking funding for a clinical trial will have additional criteria for scoring the merits of the grant. Many agencies and organizations now have web-based presentations of the grant submission process and give researchers and grant writers the opportunity to ask questions. Questions that are answered are generally limited to the process, administration, and technical issues as well as clarifying the grant requirements, although one-on-one calls may be entertained by the grants officer. Deadlines are an important feature of grant writing and funding agencies will close the portal for submission and late submissions will not be accepted. The two important deadlines are the due dates for the letter of intent (LOI) and the grant submission. Other information that must be considered in the grant's application process is the funding allocation. The funding agency (federal, national, local, or foundation) will specify how much is available and what their funding includes. For example, federal grants will generally have a rate that is negotiated for indirect costs associated with the project, but foundations will expect all indirect costs to be clearly stated. Proposal specific guidelines may also be included. In a Department of Justice grant application for example the expectation is that there is significant community support for the proposal as well as explicit commitments for its implementation from local agencies and public offices through letters of endorsement. They require that a Citizen Advisory Committee is formed, and the community is engaged in a needs assessment to justify the proposal. The process for writing and submitting grants as well as how the award and post award process may differ from agency to agency; however, the National Institutes of Health (NIH) provides an insight to the process (Figure 2.24).

The Letter of Intent

Funders will sometimes request a LOI in advance of requesting a full proposal. Visiting the organization's website and understanding their mission, vision, goals and objectives is critical to understanding what the organization is likely to fund. With a call for letters of intent the funder may offer opportunities for the researchers to get clarification and have their questions answered by a designated program manager or a frequently asked questions (FAQ) sheet is prepared and posted on the funder's website. Scheduled informational webinars may be available as well as a deadline for submission. A LOI includes the state of the field and the gap that the study will fill, the research question and the methodology as well as sufficient detail for the reviewer to judge the quality and feasibility of the study (Blanco et al., 2016) but is not limited to information such as the study purpose, goals and objectives and the budget (Box 2.13).

FIGURE 2.24. *National Institutes of Health central resource and grants funding overview.*

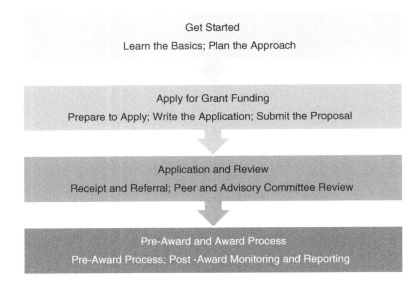

BOX 2.13 **Components of a Letter of Intent**

A summary statement about the intent of the LOI
- The [researcher/research institution] seeks funding to undertake research using an innovative approach to [purpose of the study]. Potential outcomes of this work include: [list potential outcomes]. We are requesting [amount] for a [propose length of study].
- A summary of why the project is needed (one to two paragraphs)
  - What is the issue to be addressed?
  - What makes it an important issue?
  - Who is likely to benefit from the results of the research?
  - Why would the funders care and be interested in funding this study?
- A description of what the research project will entail
  - Describe the research project in detail and why it is important/different/ expands the base of knowledge in the field/advances the science
  - Describe the research methodology
- State the specific outcomes the research project hopes to achieve
- Describe the credentials of the researchers, the organization, and its partners (one to two paragraphs)
- The budget describing the funding needs for the research and the total amount requested
- Closing paragraph
  - Interest in discussing the proposal with a member of staff
  - Offer to provide more information
  - Appreciation for the opportunity to apply
  - Contact information

Signature of appropriate organizations signatory—often a research compliance office of the institution

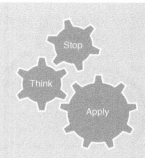

Draft a Letter of Intent

In groups of two to three, conduct a search of the internet and locate a call for proposals in any area of interest of your choice. Assume you have been asked to submit a LOI. Using the information above and any other guidance you may have, design letter intent to respond to the call for proposals. The goal of this exercise is to solicit funding for your idea that while not completely in line with any specific call for proposals, meets the overarching requirements for a grant submission to that agency. Make sure to include references.

Write the Application

- *Title page and abstract.* The title page and abstract provide an overview of the research project such that the funder knows the main idea associated with the application. The abstract is limited to 200–500 words. The abstract states the aims, research questions, and hypotheses as required and describes the research design and methods and the study's relevance to public health.

- *Study framework.* Planning the approach for a grant application mirrors the planning process for conducting a research study that was covered earlier in this chapter. The research study plan components include conducting the literature review; specifying study aim, the research questions, hypotheses, and the design of the study including the methodology for collecting and analyzing the data; and reporting the findings (Figure 2.25).

FIGURE 2.25. *Overview for designing a public health research study.*

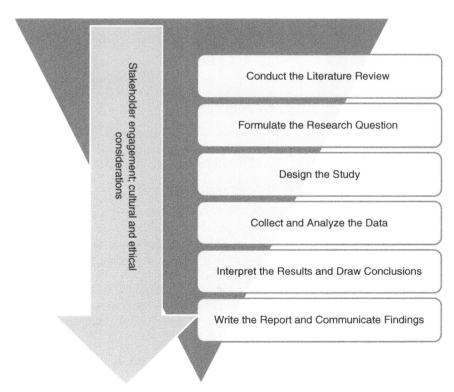

- *The literature review.* The literature review provides the philosophical and theoretical framework for the research study and the conceptual framework. Provide a clear indication of the existing state of knowledge of the problem the research will focus on. It leads to the development of the problem statement. It answers the question about the purpose for the study and what studies have been done in the past that support the present application. In addition to identifying specific publications that support the research, systematic reviews and meta-analyses that have already been conducted are especially helpful for (a) locating new peer reviewed publications that might have been missed, and (b) summarizing the existing research. Be sure to cite references appropriately both in the literature review and throughout the document as required. Style manuals offer standard guidelines for writing technical or scientific reports including guidelines related to formatting in-text citations and end-of text references, formatting headings and subheadings, structuring the manuscript, writing mechanics, and the display of tables and figures. While the American Psychological Association (APA) and the American Medical Association (AMA) styles are the most commonly used in public health research there are other styles that researchers may choose (see Module 5 for a list of common guides and manuals). See Module 1 for a complete description of how to search the literature and write a literature review.

- *Problem statement.* The problem statement serves as the needs assessment and provides the specific justification for the study. It provides a well-developed argument for why the research study is being conducted based on identifying what the gaps are that need to be filled. It is important to have a comprehensive yet concise section and include the potential impact and significance of the study. Tables, figures, and images should be clear, and the narrative should summarize the major points. The components of the problem statement are conceptualized in a summary statement that includes:
  - What is already known about the specific problem
    - What the problem is and why it matters
    - The risk factors associated with the problem at multiple levels of the socioecological model
  - The major gaps in knowledge in the literature
  - The proposed study and its relevance in addressing the gap, and
  - The benefits to understanding or resolving the problem, which should be significant enough to contribute to the existing body of research and lead to further research

The problem statement does not include any reference to the research question. It provides the justification for the study from the perspective of the literature. Once the problem is clearly stated, the researcher writes a statement that gives the reader an insight into how the problem that has been articulated through the literature review is leading to the research study.

- *Significance:* What scientific knowledge will be gained or what other significant outcome will accrue from the research; what will change in concepts, methods, technologies, and so forth. Use key components of the proposal to demonstrate the project's significance and feasibility.

- *Aims, research questions, and hypotheses:* The aims, research questions, and hypotheses are related to the problem statement and the gap in the literature that the study will address. Include hypotheses as appropriate for the study. This is one of the most important aspects of the study since they drive the research.

As always, the research aims, questions, and hypotheses drive the study!

- *Study design and description:* This section describes the research study design, the study population, sample size, the data collection design, and a detailed description of the methods, data analysis, and data management approaches. Describe any considerations that have to be included due to the cultural characteristics of the study population. Describe the engagement of the community and the role of stakeholders. Include specifics as they pertain to intervention or clinical studies. A diagram makes the researcher's thinking more visible and describes the project in visual terms. If the grant is for an intervention, a logic model works very well in providing a visual (Coley and Scheinberg, 2017). Training that must be carried out to facilitate ethical and credible research must also be described as well as how results from the study will be communicated. See earlier sections of this module for more details.

A timeline is helpful for the reviewers to see what the plan is for implementing the project. It includes project activities and dissemination of research findings (Blanco et al., 2016) (Table 2.17).

TABLE 2.17. **GANTT Chart of Project Timeline**

Activity	Quarter 1	Quarter 2	Quarter 3	Quarter 4
IRB/ethics review	■			
Hire and train staff	■			
Set up research study space		■		
Obtain study materials		■		
Recruit participants and confirm methodology		■		
Gather data			■	
Analyze data			■	
Prepare reports				■
Disseminate findings				■

- *Overall impact:* The likelihood that the project will have a strong and sustained impact on the field. Choose a novel high impact project.

- *Human Subject Protections:* Institutional Review Board (IRB) or Ethics Board clearance is required for all human subjects' research and must be carefully addressed in the application (Gholipour et al. 2014). The researcher provides information about how the study participants will be notified about the study, what they will be told and how they will be protected during the study, including the risks and benefits of their participation and who they can contact if they have any problems with the researcher or the research.

- *Study environment:* The study environment relates to the infrastructure that will be required for the study and their access. It includes the physical and budgetary infrastructure of the institution. It describes the laboratory, office and other project related spaces, computer, and library resources (Gholipour et al., 2014).

- A *reference list* of all materials reviewed and referenced within the grant is provided at the end of the narrative.

Additional materials and information may be required for inclusion with the application. It is important to review the instructions carefully and if in doubt call the program officer who is usually available to answer questions.

- *Researcher's credentials and experience:* The grant must include expertise commensurate with the requirements of the grant. The reviewers will expect to see that the person at the top of the ticket (the PI) has the appropriate credentials that support the work. The principal investigator is generally the most highly qualified full-time member of the team with expertise in the given subject. They are responsible for ensuring the implementation of the grant, and financial oversight associated with any monetary allocations to the grant. Others who are listed must also have credentials to justify their inclusion on the grant. Often submissions with less qualified individuals or new investigators who are listed as PIs will include more experienced and often known persons in the field as consultants or as Co-PI with at least 10% of their time paid for by the grant. Credentials of all lead players are provided as a curriculum vitae (CV) or biosketch (National Institutes of Health (NIH)/National Science Foundation (NSF) approved format for biographical information)

- *Letters of support:* These describe the support that other institutions will provide in the execution of the grant. Support could include providing space for implementation of the grant, laboratory testing if required, and referral sites. These letters of support are accompanied by memorandums of understanding (MOUs) that spell out very clearly what their commitment will be in implementing the grants. Letters of support may be obtained from any collaborating entity or individual who will play an integral role in the project and can include fiscal and/or material support.

- *Appendix:* The appendices contain supplementary materials that are pertinent to the study in addition to the Curriculum Vitae (CV) or biosketch, or Memorandum of Understanding (MOU) and letters of support. The appendix should not contain any material that is required reading for the reviewers as they review the grant. Any materials that support the understanding of the narrative must be included within the prescribed page limit.

Budget and Budget Justification

The budget is an important part of the research endeavor. The researchers must consider the cost of the project in the context of the funding that is being provided. The more funding is available, the more elaborate the research project can be. On a limited budget the researcher must consider the cost of a particular line item in the broader context of getting the project completed and achieving the goals of study. Often the budget that is allowed for a research study will influence the study approach. It is important that there is a clear alignment between the research design and the methodology and that the budget is developed concurrently with the research plan (Blanco et al., 2016).

The elements that determine the budget include the level of expertise and personnel related costs associated with the research team, the time available for the study, the sample size and logistics of data collection and data analysis, and any equipment and supplies required to meet the obligations of the research. These are considered to be *direct costs* of conducting the study. It is important that each item in the budget it is tied directly to the program design with a clear justification for the need for the expenditure (Gholipour et al., 2014).

When the research is conducted on behalf of an agency or organization or institution, there are often costs that are shared with others. For example, in a university, shared costs will include office space, electricity, administration, grants management, and technology. These costs are pooled into a category known as *indirect costs*. Indirect costs are generally calculated estimates that get passed on and included in the grant if outside funding is being sought. This rate may vary from <10% to >50% depending on the institution Universities tend to require higher indirect costs due to their higher overhead expenses. When a flat fee is not allowed for the indirect cost, the researcher itemizes their costs to ensure all expenses to be covered. Foundations and nonprofit organizations will require an itemization of the indirect expense that includes utilities and space that must be proportional to the project's needs. A line-item budget provides a line for each type of expenditure (Table 2.18). The directions in the announcement will include the budget format of the grant, the expected categories as well the time frame for the grant. The first year's expenses are generally the most important with an assumed limited or no increase in subsequent years unless there is clear indication in the narrative and the budget narrative justifying it. Any unspent amounts must be reported to the funder until the end of the grant period, at which point a no-cost extension may be approved if requested for completing the study/project. Once a grant is funded, the research may only move 10% of the budget across categories without permission from the funder.

TABLE 2.18. **Example Line Budget Format**

Personnel	Full time (FTE = 1)	Monthly range (FTE)	Monthly	Yearly (First Year)
	Research project title Date range			
Project director (PI)	0.1	$8,000–10,000	$900	$10,800
Project manager	1	$5000–$6,000	$5,000	$60,000
Data analyst				
Research asst. 1				
Research asst. 2				

TABLE 2.18. (Continued)

	Research project title Date range			
Personnel	Full time (FTE = 1)	Monthly range (FTE)	Monthly	Yearly (First Year)
Research asst. 3				
Administrative asst.				
Accountant				
Subtotal personnel				70,800
Benefits @ 25%				17,700
Total personnel				88,500
Equipment (laptops)				
Office and printing supplies				
Rental (photocopier)				
Incentives for participants				
Mileage @ 0.57 per mile				2,052
Survey distribution costs				
Travel for meetings out of state/ international				6,000
Total operating costs				96,552
Indirect costs @ 30% of the total budget				28,965
Grand Total				$125,517

In addition to the monies requested from funding agencies, in some grants, in-kind contributions are required as matching funds that are also indicated in the budget (Coley and Scheinberg, 2017). The amount of matching funds required may be specified as a percentage of the cost of the project, which could be contributed through fundraising activities of the organization or as a percentage of time donated by the executive director or volunteers' hours by members of the community.

Budget Justification

The budget justification describes how each dollar amount outlined in the budget will be spent. It breaks down individual costs. It explains how the funding will be expended and each item in the budget and the budget justification must be substantiated within the proposal through activities that are clearly outlined. Each budget item has a clear justification in job responsibilities, the amount of time that will be dedicated to the project and the salary.

Project manager: The project manager will work full time (100%) on this project providing day-to-day management for the implementation of the grant and will include staff supervision, coordination of the research assistants, overseeing the data collection, and report writing. The project manager has a master's degree in a social science with five years' experience managing similar projects. The salary is $60,000 per year.

Operating costs are also justified itemizing all the costs associated with implementing the project.

Travel expenses include mileage to research sites and meetings for an estimated 100 miles per month for three staff at 0.57 per mile for 12 months for a total of $2,052 per year. Also travel (transportation and per diem) for two staff members $1,500 per person for one major conference per year at $3,000 per year. Total travel is $6,000.

APPLICATION AND REVIEW

Once the application is complete and has been reviewed and signed off by the PI and other required staff at the institution, it is submitted to the funding agency as per their guidelines paying close attention to deadlines and other pertinent information. Once received the proposal is reviewed by a team of researchers. The grant review team might include subject as well as non-subject experts (Blanco et al., 2015). In addition, while the categories for the submission are similar, the level of review and the expectations as laid out in the RFP may look very different from one funder to the next with the foundation having a less formal and bureaucratic process that needs to be followed. While funding organizations have a "grants officer" that can be contacted to discuss specifics about the process, they are not usually part of the review and decision-making process and generally cannot make any promises of funding. That decision is usually up to the committee of reviewers who score the proposal and make recommendations and may even prioritize the applications in order of merit. Funding decisions are made in other "corridors of power." In the case of NIH, the second level of peer review is performed by an advisory council or board.

Review criteria: This is undoubtedly the most important aspect of the grant review and grant writers must keep these criteria in the forefront of their process as they compile the grant. Much of the information will be contained within the study design and description but keeping the criteria in mind will help in ensuring the best possible grant application is submitted for review. Be sure to spell out very clearly the overall impact of the study findings, the significance of the project, and the innovative nature of the proposal. Remember, it is important to think creatively and boldly, especially for an intervention research grant application, but it is also important to make sure innovative ideas are supported by the literature and the application is logical and cost sensitive.

There are generally two levels of review for large grants although it may differ for smaller organizations. The initial review of the application at the NIH is conducted by the Center for Scientific Review and focuses on the criteria against which the peer reviewers will score each application, based on the predefined criteria: (a) overall impact of the study findings and the likelihood for the project to have a sustained and powerful influence in the research field; (b) the project's significance; (c) innovation; (d) the approach; and (e) the environment. Additional criteria include the protection of human subjects, study timeline, inclusion of women, minorities and children, vertebrate animals, biohazards, and whether it is a resubmission, renewal, or a revision (National Institutes of Health, 2020). The review is based on a 9-point rating scale (1 = exceptional and 9 = poor), and 5 is considered a good-medium impact application and an average score.

The advisory council/board of the institute that awards the grant does the second level of review. The boards are comprised of scientists from the research community and members of the public. The applications are reviewed in addition to the overall impact scores, the percentile ranking, and the summary statements provided from the first round of reviews. The council considers the Institute's goals and their spending priorities and makes their recommendations to the director (National Institutes of Health, 2020).

BOX 2.14 Additional Considerations for Review of Grant Applications

- Study timeline
- Inclusion of females, minority populations, and children
- Vertebrate animals
- Biohazards
- Resubmission of a previous application

Preaward and Award Process

Once a decision has been made by the funding agency to award the funding, the next step is notifying the researcher and making any clarifications regarding the implementation of the grant. It could also include negotiating the scope of the grant or changing the timelines. During this period the funding agency may conduct a site visit to be sure that the conditions for undertaking the grant can be verified. The contact is generally made by the grants officer. The final award is communicated to the researcher and to the institution that will oversee the fiscal arrangements for the disbarment of funds. The financial arrangements will differ depending on the funding agency and the nature of the characteristics of the funded entity. For example, in 2020 the National Institute of Minority Health (2020) is providing $335,812,000 in funding for grants that take into consideration: In contrast, the National Institute of Diabetes and Digestive and Kidney Diseases (2020) will have available to award in grants, $2.114 billion. In a small grant award recently funded, 50% of the budgeted amount was provided for project implementation and the rest was paid on completion of the study and submission of the report. In other situations, the funder may reimburse the institution upon receipt of an invoice monthly or quarterly. Once the study is approved, IRB/ethics committee approval must be sought for a human subject's study before the study can proceed. The primary purposes for getting IRB approval include, the study seeks to collect data that is generalizable, the researcher seeks to publish the findings, and the study involves human subjects or protected health information (Table 2.19).

The review of grants and the funding opportunity will generally follow similar expectations that include:

- Scientific and technical merit of the proposed project
- Organizational recommendations
- Overall programmatic portfolio balance and specific needs of the agency
- Support for the next generations of underrepresented groups
- Potential for highly innovative scientific impact in advancing the science of public health and particular populations

In addition to monitoring the implementation of the grant, the institution is responsible to monitor the ethics protocols and the human subjects' protections. If there are any changes to the IRB/ethics committee approved protocols or instruments, those changes must be notified, and an updated letter of approval obtained from the IRB/ethics committee before the study can proceed. Large studies and clinical studies that are of more than minimal risk to the study participants are monitored more directly and more often, although the NIH laments the increasing evidence of poor ethical responsibility in research and proposed training for researchers and provides guidance through its publication, Guidelines and Policies for the Conduct of Research in the Intramural Research program at NIH (2019).

TABLE 2.19. Requirements for IRB Submission

Category	IRB review requirement
Purpose	If the study is to contribute to generalizable knowledge by being published in the scientific literature
Design	Generally, studies will have a larger sample size; may involve randomization of the study subjects; will be assessing the effects of a new technology or process; involves human subjects or their protected health information
Results	The intent is to publish or present the findings in research publications and forums to contribute to existing knowledge

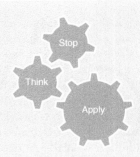

Develop a Strategy to Respond to a Call for Proposals

Imagine you are the head of a research organization that focuses on a public health issue of your choice. Using a recently published research grant RFP, and all the information you have at your disposal, develop a strategy for responding to a call for proposals including all the required components as specified by the call and the information provided in this section. Include draft letters of support and a budget that will support the research study/project.

 SUMMARY

The grant proposal is always written with the reviewer in mind. The reviewer needs to be able to understand what the study is all about as well as how the researcher intends to achieve the results. The budget must be closely tied to the proposed project.

Grant review focuses on the criteria against which the peer reviewers score each application, based on the predefined criteria that include (a) overall impact of the study findings and the likelihood for the project to have a sustained and powerful influence in the research field, (b) the project's significance, (c) innovation, (d) the approach, and (e) the environment. Resources for successful project implementation are important aspects of the review process.

Now that I have reached the end this section, I am able to:

Course objective	Strongly agree	Somewhat agree	Neutral	Somewhat disagree	Strongly agree
Outline the steps for writing a grant					
Discuss the requirements for a successful grant submission					
Write a grant for submission for funding					

REFERENCES

Aagaard, E. M., & Hauer, K. E. (2003). A cross-sectional descriptive study of mentoring relationships formed by medical students. *Journal of General Internal Medicine, 18*, 298–302.

Ambrose, S. A., Bridges, M. W., DiPietro, M., Lovett, M. C., & Noman, M. K. (2010). *How learning works, 7 research based principles for Smart Teaching*. Jossey Bass.

American Statistical Association. (2018). Ethical guidelines for statistical practice. Committee on Professional Ethics. https://www.amstat.org/asa/files/pdfs/EthicalGuidelines.pdf

American Statistical Association. (2022). Ethical guidelines for statistical practice. https://www.amstat.org/docs/default-source/amstat-documents/ethicalguidelines.pdf

Atre, S., Kudale, A., Morankar, S., Gosoniu, D., & Weiss, M. G. (2011). Gender and community views of stigma and tuberculosis in rural Maharashtra, India. *Global Public Health, 6*(1), 56–71. https://doi.org/10.1080/17441690903334240

Bandura, A. (1986). *Social foundations of thought and action: a social cognitive theory*. Prentice-Hall.

Beauchamp, T. L., & Childress, J. F. (2001). Principles of biomedical ethics. Oxford Press.

Becker, H., Cookston, J., & Kulberg, V. (2000). Mailed survey follow-up postcard reminders more cost effective than second questionnaires? *Western Journal of Nursing Research, 22*(5), 642–647.

Berinsky, A. J., Huber, G. A., & Lenz, G. S. (2012). Evaluating online labor markets for experimental research: Amazon.com's Mechanical Turk. *Political Analysis, 20*, 351–368.

Blanco, C., Jorge, M., Rodriguez-Fernandez, M., Baca-Garcia, Wang, S., & Olfson, M. (2015). Probability of predictors or treatment-seeking for substance abuse disorders in the U.S. Drug and Alcohol Dependence, 149, 136–144.

Blanco, M. A., Gruppen, L. D., Artino, A. R., Uijtdehaage, S., Szauter, K., & Durning, S. J. (2016). How to write and educational research grant: AMEE Guide no. 101. *Medical Teacher, 38*, 113–122.

Blaney, C. L., Robbins, M. L., Paiva, A. L., Redding, C. A., Rossi, J. S., Blissmer, B., Burditt, C., & Oatley, K. (2012). Validation of the measures of the transtheoretical model for exercise in an adult African-American sample. *American Journal of Health Promotion, 26*(5), 317–326.

Boateng, G. O., Neilands, T. B., Frongillo, E. A., Melgar-Quinonez, H. R., & Young, S. (2018). Best practices in developing and validating scales for health, social and behavioral research: A Primer. *Frontiers in Public Health, 6*, 149. https://doi.org/10.3389/fpubh.2018.00149

Boyton, P. M., & Greenhalgh, T. (2004). Selecting, designing, and developing your questionnaire. *BMJ, 328*.

Brenner, P. S., & DeLamater, J. (2016). Lies, dammed lies and survey self-reports? Identity as a cause of measurement bias. *Social Psychology Quarterly, 79*(4), 333–354.

Bronfenbrenner, U. (1977). Developmental research, public policy and the ecology of childhood. *Child Development, 45*(1), 1–5.

Brown, T. A. (2015). *Confirmatory factor analysis for applied research*. Guilford.

Buchanan, E. A., & Hvizdak, E. E. (2009). Online survey tools: Ethical and methodological concerns of human ethics committees. *Journal of Empirical Research on Human Research Ethics, 4*(2), 37–48.

Cargill, M., & O'Connor, P. (2009). Writing Scientific Research Articles. Wiley Blackwell, West Sussex, UK, 10.

Charan, J., & Biswas, T. (2013). How to calculate sample size for different study designs in medical research. *Indian Journal of Psychological Medicine, 35*(2), 121–126.

Chilisa, B. (2012). *Indigenous research methodologies*. Sage.

Effective grantmanship for fundingColey, S. M., & Scheinberg, C. A. (2017). Proposal writing. Sage.

Crenshaw, K. (1989). Demarginalizing the intersection of race and sex: A Black feminist critique of antidiscrimination doctrine, feminist theory and antiracist politics. University of Chicago Legal. *Forum, 1989*(1), Article 8

CSDH. (2008). Closing the gap in a generation: health equity through action on the social determinants of health. In *Final report on the commission on social determinants of health*. World Health Organization.

De Leeuw, E. D., Melenbergh, G. J., & Hox, J. J. (1996). The influence of data collection methods on structural models. *Sociological Methods & Research, 24*(4), 443–472.

DeVellis, R. F., & Thorpe, C. T. (2021). *Scale development. theory and applications*. Sage.

Dillman, D. A. (1978). *Mail and telephone surveys: The total design method*. Wiley.

Durhan, J., Brolan, C. E., & Mukandi, B. (2014). The convention on the rights of persons with disabilities: A foundation of ethical disability and health research in developing countries. *American Journal of Public Health, 104*, 2037–2043. https://doi.org/10.2105/AJPH.2014.302006

Egleston, B. L., Miller, S. M., & Meropol, N. J. (2011). The impact of misclassification due to survey response fatigue on estimation and identifiability of treatment effects. *Statistics in Medicine, 30*(30), 3560–3572. https://doi.org/10.1002/sim.4377

Elliott, M. (2002). *Conducting research surveys via e-mail and the web*. RAND.

Fawzy, A. F., & Salam, E. M. A. (2015). M-commerce adoption in Egypt: An extension to theory of reasoned action. *Business and Management Review, 6*(1).

Fishbein, M., & Ajzen, I. (1975). *Belief, attitude, intention and behavior: An introduction to theory and research*. Addison-Wesley.

Freeman, A. (2015). Blurred lines: Creating and crossing boundaries between interviewer and subject. In A. J. Jolivetté (Ed.), *Research justice methodologies for social change*. Policy Press.

Galama, T. J., & van Kippersluis, H. (2018). A theory of socio-economic disparities in health over the life cycle. *Economic Journal, 129*, 338–374.

Gholipour, A., Lee, E. Y., & Warfield, S. K. (2014). The anatomy and art of writing a successful grant application, a practical step-by-step approach. *Pediatric Radiology, 44*, 1512–1517.

Glass, J. E., Rathouz, P. J., Gattis, M., Joo, Y. S., Nelson, J. C., & Williams, E. C. (2017). Intersections of poverty, race/ethnicity, and sex: alcohol consumption and adverse outcomes in the United States. *Social Psychiatry and Psychiatric Epidemiology, 52*(5), 515–524.

Goodell, L. S., Stage, V. C., & Cooke, N. A. (2016). Practical qualitative research strategies: training interviewers and coders. *Journal of Nutrition Education and Behavior, 48*, 578–585. e1

Hammer, M. (2017). Ethical considerations for data collection using surveys. *Oncology Nursing Forum, 22*(2), 157–159.

Harris, M. J. (2010). *Evaluating public and community health programs*. Jossey-Bass.
Hochbaum, G. M. (1958). *Public participation in medical screening programs: A sociopsychological study*. PHS publication no. 572. U.S Government Printing Press.
Hoz, J. J., & Boeije, H. R. (2005). Encyclopedia of social measurement. *1*, 593–599.
Jacobson, K. (2012). *Health research methods: A practical guide*. Jones and Barlett Learning.
Johnson, A. G. (2001). *Privilege, power and difference*. Mayfield Publishing Company.
Jolivetté, A. J. (2015). In A. J. Jolivetté (Ed.), *Research justice methodologies for social change*. Policy Press.
Kadam, R. A. (2017). Informed consent process: A step further towards making it meaningful. *Perspectives in Clinical Research, 8*(3), 107–112.
Keusch, F. (2015). Why do people participate in Web surveys? Applying survey participation theory to internet survey data collection. *Management Review Quarterly, 65*, 183–216.
Kibuchi, E., Sturgis, P., Durrant, G. B., & Maslovskaya, O. (2019). Do interviewers moderate the effect of monetary incentives on response rates in household interview surveys? *Journal of Survey Statistics and Methodology., 8*(2), 264–284.
Kim, H., & Zakour, M. (2017). Disaster preparedness among older adults: Social support, community participation and demographic characteristics. *Journal of Social Service Research, 43*(4), 498–509.
Kinsman, J., de Bruijne, K., Jalloh, A. M., Harris, M., Abdullah, H., Boye-Thomson, T., Sankoh, O., Jalloh, A. K., & Jalloh-Vos, H. (2017). Development of a set of community informed Ebola messages for Sierra Leone. *PLoS Neglected Tropical Diseases, 11*(8), e0005742. https://doi.org/10.1371/journal.pntd.0005742
Kliewer, M. A. (2005). Writing it up: a step-by-step- guide to publication for beginning investigators. *American Journal of Roentgenology, 185*, 591–596.
Krieger, N. (2012). Methods for scientific study of discrimination and health: an ecosocial approach. *American Journal of Public Health, 102*, 396–345.
Kumar, R. (2014). *Research methodology, a step-by-step guide for beginners*. Sage.
Kwekkeboom, K. (2014). Overview and Tips for successful grant writing for infusion nurses. *Infusion Nurses Society, 37*(5).
Latkin, C. A., Edwards, C., Davey-Rothwell, M., & Tobin, K. E. (2017). The relationship between social desirability bias and self-reports of health, substance use, and social network factors among urban substance users in Baltimore Maryland. *Addictive Behaviors, 73*, 133–136.
Marin, G., & Marin, B. V. O. (1991). *Research with hispanic populations: applied social research series* (Vol. 23). Sage Publications.
Marusteri, M., & Bacarea, V. (2010). Comparing groups for statistical differences: how to choose the right statistical test? *Biochemia Medica, 20*(1), 15–32.
McGorry, S. (2000). Measurement in cross-cultural environment: survey translation issues. *Qualitative Market Research: An International Journal, 3*(2), 74–81.
McKenzie, J. F., Neiger, B. L., & Thackery, R. (2017). *Planning, implementing and evaluating health promotion programs*. Pearson.
Mkabela, Q. (2005). Using the Afrocentric methods in researching indigenous African culture. *Qualitative Report, 10*(1), 178–189.
Morton, R. B., & Williams, K. C. (2008). Experimentation in political science. In J. M. Box-Steffensmeier, H. E. Brady, & D. Collier (Eds.), *The Oxford handbook of political methodology*. Oxford University Press.
Murray, C. J., & Lopez, A. D. (1997). Alternative projections of mortality and disability by cause 1990–2020: Global burden of disease study. *Lancet, 349*, 1498–1504.
National Institute of Diabetes and Digestive and Kidney Diseases. (2020). 2020 Award Funding Policy. https://www.niddk.nih.gov/research-funding/process/award-funding-policy?dkrd=prspt0701 https://www.niddk.nih.gov/research-funding/process/award-funding-policy?dkrd=prspt0701
National Institute of Minority Health. (2020). NIMHD Financial Management Plan and Grant Awards. https://www.nimhd.nih.gov/funding/nimhd-funding/funding-strategy.html
National Institutes of Health. (2019). *Guidelines and policies for the conduct of research in the intramural research programs at NIH*. National Institutes of Health.
National Institutes of Health. (2020). Review Criteria at a Glance. National Institutes of Health. https://grants.nih.gov/grants/policy/review.htm
National Institutes of Health, Office of Intramural Research. (2017). Socially Responsible Science, Case #1. Research Cases for Use by the NIH Community. https://oir.nih.gov/sites/default/files/uploads/sourcebook/documents/ethical_conduct/case_studies-2017.pdf
O'Mahony, J. M., Donnelly, T. T., Bouchal, S. R., & Este, D. (2013). Cultural background and socioeconomic influence of immigrant and refugee women coping with postpartum depression. *Journal of Immigrant and Minority Health, 15*, 300–314.
Osypuk, T. L., Joshi, P., Geronimo, K., & Acevedo-Garcia, D. (2015). Do social and economic policies influence health? A revie. *Current Epidemiology Reports, 1*(3), 149–164.
Pepper, J. K., Squiers, L. B., Peinado, S. C., Bann, C. M., Dolina, S. D., Lynch, M. M., Nonnemaker, J. M., & McCormack, L. A. (2019). Impact of messages about scientific uncertainty on risk perceptions and intentions to use electronic vaping products. *Addictive Behaviors, 91*, 136–140. https://doi.org/10.1016/j.addbeh.2018.10.025
Peterson, R. A. (2000). *Constucting effective questionairres*. Sage.
Peytchev, A., Couper, M. P., McCabe, C., & S.D. (2006). Web survey design: Paging versus scrolling. *Public Opinion Quarterly, 70*, 596–607.
Polit, D. F. (2015). Assessing measurement in health: beyond reliability and validity. *International Journal of Nursing Studies, 52*(11), 1746–1753.
Price, L. R. (2016). *Psychometric methods: Theory into practice*. Guilford Publications.
Rolstad, S., Adler, J., & Rydén, A. (2011). Response burden and questionnaire length: is shorter better? A review and meta-analysis. *Value in Health, 14*, 1101–1108.
Rose, M. K., Costabile, K. A., Boland, S. E., Cohen, R. W., & Persky, S. (2019). Diabetes causal attributes among affected and unaffected individuals. *BMJ Open Diabetes Research & Care*, 7e000708. https://doi.org/10.1136/bmjdrc%202019-00708
Schweizer, M., Braun, B. I., & Milstone, A. M. (2016). Research methods in healthcare epidemiology and antimicrobial stewardship- quazi-experimental designs. *Research and Methologoy in Infection Control, 37*(10), 1135–1140.
Shadish, W. R., Cook, T. D., & Campbell, D. T. (2002). *Experimental and quasi-experimental designs for generalized causal inference*. Houghton Mifflin.
Singer, E., & Ye, C. (2013). The use and effects of incentives in surveys. *Annals of American Academy of Political and Social Sciences, 645*, 112–114.

Sudman, S., Bradburn, N. M., & Schwarz, N. (1996). *Thinking about answers: the application of cognitive processes to survey methodology.* Jossey-Bass.

Suen, H. K., & Ary, D. A. (1989). *Analyzing quantitative behavioral observation data.* Psychology Press.

Survey Research Center. (2016). Guidelines for best practice in cross-cultural surveys. Ann Arbor, MI: Survey Research Center, Institute for Social Research, University of Michigan. http://www.ccsg.ist.umich.edu

Terwee, C. B., Bot, S. D., Boar, M. R., van der Windt Knol, D. L., Dekker, J., et al. (2007). Quality criteria were proposed for measurement properties of health status questionnaires. *Journal of Clinical Epidemiology, 60*(1), 34–42.

Torraco, R. J. (2005). Writing integrative literature reviews: guidelines and examples. *Human Resource Development Review, 4*(3), 356–367.

United Nations. (2006). Convention on the Rights of Persons with Disabilities [A/RES/61/106]. https://www.un.org/esa/socdev/enable/rights/convtexte.htm

US Department of Health and Human Services. (1997). *NIDA research monograph 167.* National Institutes on Drug Abuse.

Valentine, M., Nembhard, I. M., & Edmondson, A. C. (2015). Measuring teamwork in health care settings. A review of survey instruments. *Medical Care, 53,* e16–e30.

van de Mortal, T. F. (2008). Faking it: social desirability response bias in self-report research. *Australian Journal of Advanced Nursing, 25*(4), 40–48.

Viergever, R. F., & Hendricks, T. C. C. (2016). The 10 largest public and philanthropic funders of health research in the world: what they fund and how they distribute their funds. *Health Research Policy and Systems, 14*(12), 1–15.

West, B. T., Ghimire, D., & Azinn, W. (2015). Evaluating a modular design approach to collecting survey data using text messages. *Survey Research Methods, 9*(2), 111–123.

MODULE 2: RESOURCES

INTRODUCTION

This section of the book provides a set of resources for use by faculty teaching the course and their students. Resources include the outline of the research process; IRB regulations and model forms and student resources to support a semester-long course project including working in groups and giving feedback.

Number	Title of resource
1	Outline and design of a research study
2	Institutional Review Board (IRB) Regulations
3	A Model Informed Consent form
4	Preamble consent form
5	Assent form
6	Short-form consent suitable for translation
Student resources for a semester-long-project course design and giving feedback	
7	Working in groups
8	Semester-long project model
9	Giving feedback

Integrated Research Methods In Public Health, First Edition. Muriel Jean Harris and Baraka Muvuka.
© 2023 John Wiley & Sons, Inc. Published 2023 by John Wiley & Sons, Inc.
Companion website: www.wiley.com/go/harris/integratedresearchmethods

Resource 1

Outline and Notes for the Design of a Research Project

Step	Actions
1.	Write down the topic you are interested in researching. Develop a research question that will help guide the literature review. What were the gaps in the literature or limitations of previous studies that you identified?
2.	Write a problem statement that clearly identifies the gap (s) in the literature that this study will address. What emerges as the focus of the study? Write an aim/purpose statement for your project.
3.	**Using the aim/purpose of the study as a guide** ▪ Without looking at any resources yet, draw a concept map to help shape your thinking about the topic and the relationships of the variables to the dependent variable and to each other as identified in the literature. The variables that are included in this map may also be variables that are conceptualized as important for this study, but not having previously been tested as part of a public health related study. However, these variables may exist in other fields of study and have been included in research in different ways than you intend for your study. For example, trust may not have been previously included in studies related to work in program and policy development in public health, but it had proven to be an important variable in the business literature. This hypothesized relationship could lead to its inclusion in your study. ▪ Review your literature review and update it as necessary to show the linkages between the variables and create a central theme/topic of your study and the relationships of the independent variables to the dependent variable ▪ Draw a table that shows the constructs and the references and the theory that provides a foundation for the assumptions of the relationships. Make notes that you can come back to later. ▪ Draw a new concept map when you are sure about the relationship of the variables.
4.	**Formulate the research question** ▪ Write down the research question that will guide the study. ▪ Confirm the constructs for the study. ▪ Develop hypotheses to be tested (if required).
5.	**Design the research study to answer the research question** ▪ Discuss the philosophy that undergirds the research study and how the philosophy guides the rest of the study (e.g., postpositivist, constructivist, pragmatic). ▪ Describe the design of the research study (e.g., experimental, nonexperimental, cross-sectional, longitudinal, mixed methods). ▪ Identify study population and note inclusion and exclusion criteria. ▪ Describe the sampling approaches and sample size for the study. ▪ Design data collection method (quantitative, qualitative, mixed). ▪ Develop/adopt/adapt data collection tools as appropriate. ▪ Pilot-test the instruments. ▪ Validate instruments.
6.	**Collect the data** ▪ Describe recruitment strategies. ▪ Distribute the data collection tool and collect the data.
7.	**Analyze the data** ▪ Select methods that are appropriate for answering the research question or testing the hypothesis. Choose the significance level and conduct the relevant statistical test. For example, if the purpose of the study is to compare two population sample means, then it is important to follow the protocols for inferential statistics.
8.	**Disseminate findings of the research study** ▪ Describe how the findings from the study will be shared with stakeholders and the greater population.

Resource 2

IRB REGULATIONS

Research regulations in the United States are provided in Section 46.109 of the 2018 requirements (2018 Common Rule) that outlines the IRB Regulation for the Review of Research. See Box 2.14.

BOX 2.14 IRB Regulations

(a). An IRB shall review and have authority to approve, require modifications in (to secure approval), or disapprove all research activities covered by this policy, including exempt research activities under §46.104 for which limited IRB review is a condition of exemption (under §46.104(d)(2)(iii), (d)(3)(i)(C), and (d)(7), and (8)).

(b) An IRB shall require that information given to subjects (or legally authorized representatives, when appropriate) as part of informed consent is in accordance with §46.116. The IRB may require that information, in addition to that specifically mentioned in §46.116, be given to the subjects when in the IRB's judgment the information would meaningfully add to the protection of the rights and welfare of subjects.

(c) An IRB shall require documentation of informed consent or may waive documentation in accordance with §46.117.

(d) An IRB shall notify investigators and the institution in writing of its decision to approve or disapprove the proposed research activity, or of modifications required to secure IRB approval of the research activity. If the IRB decides to disapprove a research activity, it shall include in its written notification a statement of the reasons for its decision and give the investigator an opportunity to respond in person or in writing.

(e) An IRB shall conduct continuing review of research requiring review by the convened IRB at intervals appropriate to the degree of risk, not less than once per year, except as described in §46.109(f).

(f) Unless an IRB determines otherwise, continuing review of research is not required in the following circumstances:
  (i). Research eligible for expedited review in accordance with §46.110;
  (ii). Research reviewed by the IRB in accordance with the limited IRB review described in §46.104(d)(2)(iii), (d)(3)(i)(C), or (d)(7) or (8);
  (iii). Research that has progressed to the point that it involves only one or both of the following, which are part of the IRB-approved study:
    (A) Data analysis, including analysis of identifiable private information or identifiable biospecimens, or
    (B) Accessing follow-up clinical data from procedures that subjects would undergo as part of clinical care.
      (1) [Reserved]

(g) An IRB shall have authority to observe or have a third party observe the consent process and the research

Ref: https://www.hhs.gov/ohrp/regulations-and-policy/regulations/revised-common-rule-regulatory-text/index.html

Resource 3

Informed Consent

Title of Research Study (Required) _____

Introduction and Background Information

You are invited to take part in a research study because you _____. The study is being conducted under the direction of _____ (list investigators degree) at the [Name of Institution].

Purpose

The purpose of this study is _____

Procedures In this study, you will be asked to –

a. Describe any tasks the participants will be asked to perform (e.g., view video, walk on treadmill). Describe any procedures that will be performed on the participant (e.g., blood pressure measurement, cheek swab for saliva).

b. Describe the nature and purpose of any questionnaires, surveys or other instruments the participant will be asked to complete.

c. Describe any existing data (types and sources) about the participant that the investigators will access.

d. Include information in this paragraph about how long it should take the participant to complete any questionnaires or other procedures performed by or on the participant.

e. Include total study length and session length.

f. Include a statement that the participant may decline to answer any questions that may make them uncomfortable. Include how long their participation in the study will last If participants will be audio or video recorded, indicate it here.

Required if applicable: Your research test results (will or will not—choose one) be shared with you. Results of the overall research study (will or will not—choose one) be shared with you. (If so, describe when and under what conditions).

Choose option 1 or 2 depending on whether or not the data/specimen will be stored for future research.

- Option 1: Your [*data and/or specimen*] will be stored and shared for future research without additional informed consent if identifiable private information, such as your name are removed. If identifying information is removed from your [*data and/or specimen*], the [*data and/or specimen*] may be used for future research studies or given to another investigator for future research studies without additional consent from you.

- Option 2: Your [data and/or specimen] will not be stored and shared for future research even if identifiable private information, such as your name and medical record number, are removed.

Potential Risks

There are risks associated with *(study procedure)*. Those risk(s) is/are *(Describe any risk(s) that may occur in the study. Possible risks to participants you may address are: physical, psychological, social, economic, and/or legal risks if they are a part of the research)*. There may be unforeseen risks. *If there are no foreseeable risks, say* "There are no foreseeable risks other than possible discomfort in answering personal questions. There may also be unforeseen risks." *If the investigators cannot identify any foreseeable risks, say,* "There are no foreseeable risks, although there may be unforeseen risks."

Benefits

The possible benefits of this study include *(present personal or societal benefits. Do not list any financial payments. There is a separate section to discuss payment)*.

Payment

Payment for participating and type and level of payment to be received [describe format of payment]

Confidentiality

Privacy statement. If the results from this study are published, your name will not be made public. Once your information leaves our institution, we cannot promise that others will keep it private.
Your information may be shared with the following:

- The sponsor and others hired by the sponsor to oversee the research
- Organizations that provide funding at any time for the conduct of the research.
- The University's Institutional Review Board, Human Subjects Protection Program Office, Privacy Office, others involved in research administration and research and legal compliance at the University, and others contracted by the University for ensuring human participants safety or research and legal compliance
- The local research team
- Researchers at other sites participating in the study
- People who are responsible for research, compliance and HIPAA/privacy oversight at the institutions where the research is conducted
- People responsible for billing, sending and receiving payments related to your participation in the study
- Applicable government agencies, such as:
    - Office for Human Research Protections
- Others

OR – IF INFORMATION WILL NOT BE KEPT PRIVATE: Your identity as a participant in this study and the information you provide may be released and *published (only to be used if the participant has been fully informed of potential for information to be made public, and has still consented to participate)*

Security

The data collected about you will be kept private and secure by *(e.g., locked cabinet, encrypted, password protected computer or secured server, limited access, locked area)*

Voluntary Participation

Taking part in this study is completely voluntary. You may choose not to take part at all. If you decide not to be in this study, you won't be penalized or lose any benefits for which you qualify. If you decide to be in this study, you may change your mind and stop taking part at any time. If you decide to stop taking part, you won't be penalized or lose any benefits for which you qualify. You will be told about any new information learned during the study that could affect your decision to continue in the study.

Research Participant's Rights

If you have any questions about your rights as a research participant, you may call the Human Subjects Protection Program Office at [phone number]. You may discuss any questions about your rights as a research participant, in private, with a member of the [Institutional Ethics Board]. You may also call this number if you have other questions about the research, and you cannot reach the study doctor, or want to talk to someone else. The IRB is an independent committee made up of people from the University community, staff of the institutions, as well as people from the community not connected with these institutions. The IRB has approved the participation of human participants in this research study.

Questions, Concerns and Complaints

If you have any questions about the research study, please contact (add PI name and phone number)
If you have concerns or complaints about the research or research staff and you do not wish to give your name, you may call the toll free number [number].

Acknowledgment and Signatures

This document tells you what will happen during the study if you choose to take part. Your signature and date indicates that this study has been explained to you, that your questions have been answered, and that you agree to take part in the study. You are not giving up any legal rights to which you are entitled by signing this informed consent document though you are providing your authorization as outlined in this informed consent document. You will be given a copy of this consent form to keep for your records.

Signatures and dates for the participant, PI, Sub-I or Co-I
Grant number; contact information for the study investigator who will answer questions about the study and Site of the study
Adapted from the University of Louisville.

Resource 4

Sample Preamble Consent Form

TITLE OF RESEARCH STUDY: _____
Dear _____ :   Date

You are being invited to participate in a research study. The purpose of the study is _____. This study is conducted by _____ of _____ (list any collaborators).
Your participation in the study will involve _____. The study will take approximately (*give time*) to complete. There are no known risk for your participation in this research study. The information you provide will (*explain what the information is being used for*). Your information will be stored (*state site of physical and or electronic data storage*). The information collected may not benefit you directly. The information learned in this study may be helpful to others. Individuals from the Department of (*give name of the sponsoring department*), the Institutional Ethics Board, the Human Subjects Protection Program Office (HSPPO), and other regulatory agencies may inspect these records. In all other respects, however, the data will be held in confidence to the extent permitted by law. Should the data be published, your identity will not be disclosed.

[There may be additional paragraphs when collecting identifiable data or protected health information]
Taking part in this study is voluntary. By answering survey questions you agree to take part in this research study. You do not have to answer any questions that make you uncomfortable (*or prosecutable by law; if appropriate*). You may choose not to take part at all. If you decide to be in this study you may stop taking part at any time. If you decide not to be in this study or if you stop taking part at any time, you will not lose any benefits for which you may qualify.
If you have any questions, concerns, or complaints about the research study, please contact: (*Name and phone number of the researcher*)

If you have any questions about your rights as a research subject, you may call the Human Subjects Protection Program Office at [telephone number]. You can discuss any questions about your rights as a research subject, in private, with a member of the Institutional Review Board (IRB). The IRB is an independent committee made up of people from the University community, staff of the institutions, as well as people from the community not connected with these institutions. The IRB has reviewed this research study.

If you have concerns or complaints about the research or research staff and you do not wish to give your name, you may call [telephone number]. This is a 24 hour hot line answered by people who do not work at the [Institution overseeing the research].

Signatures and dates for the PI, Sub-I or Co-I
Adapted: University of Louisville

Resource 5

Sample Participant Assent

Study Title _____

You are invited to be in a research study being done by (*state investigator name*). When a person is in a research study, they are called a "subject" or "participant". Research studies are done when people want to find new ways to do things. You are invited because (*explain the condition that renders the child eligible to take part, in very simple terms*). In this study, we want to find out more about (*describe the study*). If it is okay with you and you agree to join this study, you will be asked to (*describe what they will be asked to do*). Your participation in this research will last (*specify how long their participation will last*). Describe which part of the study is experimental.

Explain any possible risks to the child, in simple terms. If something might be painful, state this in the assent. Explain that the child should inform his/her parents if they are sick or in pain as a result of being in the study.

Describe known benefits for participating in this study (*give the list of benefits, if any*). You may include possible future benefits to others. If there are no known benefits, state so.

State any alternative procedures that might be available to the child other than this study.

Your family, the researcher and the research team will know that you are in the study. If anyone else is given information about you, they will not know your name. A number or initials will be used instead of your name.

Describe that the child's parents/legal guardians have been given information on what to do if the child is injured during the study.

If I have any questions about the study or any problems to do with the study, you can contact the study investigator (*insert telephone number*). You do not have to be in the study if you do not want to. It is up to you. You can also ask all the questions you want before you decide. If you want to quit after you are already in this study, you can tell the study investigator and they will discuss with your parents.

You have been told about the study and know why it is being done and what you have to do. Your parent(s) have agreed to let you be in the study. If you have any questions, you can ask the research investigator and research team at any time.

Signatures and dates for the Study participant, parent/guardian, PI, Sub-I or Co-I
Ref: University of Louisville.

Resource 6

Sample English Short Form for Translation

[THIS DOCUMENT MUST BE WRITTEN IN A LANGUAGE UNDERSTANDABLE TO THE SUBJECT]
Consent to Participate in Research

You are being asked to participate in a research study.

Before you agree, the investigator must tell you about (a) the purposes, procedures, and duration of the research; (b) any experimental procedures; (c) any reasonably foreseeable risks, discomforts, and benefits of the research; (d) any potentially beneficial alternative procedures or treatments; and (e) how confidentiality will be maintained.

Where applicable, the investigator must also tell you about (a) any available compensation or medical treatment if injury occurs; (b) the possibility of unforeseeable risks; (c) circumstances when the investigator may halt your participation; (d) any added costs to you; (e) what happens if you decide to stop participating; (f) when you will be told about new findings that may affect your willingness to participate; and (g) how many people will be in the study.

If you agree to participate, you must be given a signed copy of this document and a written summary of the research.

You may contact [**name**] at [**phone number**] any time you have questions about the research.

You may contact [**name**] at [**phone number**] if you have questions about your rights as a research subject or what to do if you are injured.

Your participation in this research is voluntary, and you will not be penalized or lose benefits if you refuse to participate or decide to stop.

Signing this document means that the research study, including the above information, has been described to you orally, and that you voluntarily agree to participate.

Signatures and dates for the Study participant, witness, PI, Sub-I or Co-I
Ref: University of Louisville

Resource 7

Working in Groups

Group work is stimulating and rewarding, but it can be both frustrating and exhilarating. The important thing is to recognize the value of group work. If everybody gives it their best, the group will be proud of its achievement! Public health requires group work. There is almost no research project that does not require working with others. In order to maximize the benefits of teamwork, the members of the group must work effectively. This includes thinking about group work and the achievement of the outcome as occurring in a step wise manner. Groups sometimes run into trouble! Regular meetings and honest and open conversations will help get the group back on track.

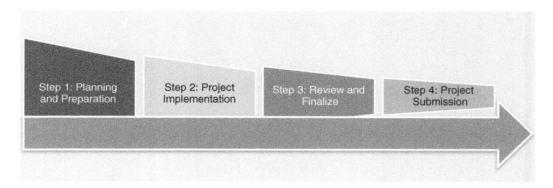

Step 1: *Planning and Preparation:* This is the stage when the individual members of the group get to know each other and begin to understand the task they need to undertake. During this early phase understand each other's strengths and weaknesses and commit to resolve how individual weaknesses can be addressed. A couple of topics to get you started

- The task: what is it and what it takes to get it done
- The timelines: how much time is allocated for the project and how does the time get divided up to get to deadlines?
- The ground rules: what are the group's operating guidelines? What are members' roles and responsibilities? It is helpful to have folks in specific roles that can be rotated although at the very minimum identify a coordinator who will take notes and keep the group on task. Decide on what constitutes a violation of the ground rules and how it will be handled by the group.
- The contract: develop a group contract that commits members to the timelines and the work
- Plan *the work*!

Step 2: *Project Implementation:* The step is the longest and the most important. It is the step where *the work* is done. Maintaining the momentum through this step and meeting individual obligations is crucial to achieving the goals. If things start slipping, review the guidelines and hold each other accountable.

- Check in with each other; set up specific meeting times but allow for flexibility if the time needs to change
- Meet deadlines that have been set; missing deadlines results in frustration and can cause delays in the final submission
- Stay on task and do the work!

Step 3: *Review and Finalize:* This is probably the most difficult step since it means pulling all the pieces of "*the work*" together into one coherent piece. At this point, the project could potentially have multiple parts (final report, PowerPoint presentation; publication or other deliverables), if so, identify different members of the team to work on the different deliverables.

- Submit all the pieces according to the established deadlines
- Compile the final document(s) based on the specified guidelines
- Decide on who does what for closing out the project

- Distribute the work to each member through a shared portal like OneDrive or Google Docs
- Review *the work*; edit as appropriate
- Read over the final product(s), check spelling, grammar, organization, style, references, and so forth. Ensure the final product(s) meets acceptable standards for submission.

Step 4: *Project Submission*: This is the last and final stage of *"the work."*

- Submit it as per the guidelines
- Review feedback and incorporate it in the final submission
- Resubmit

Resource 8

Semester-Long Activity

This semester long activity provides the students with experience in completing multiple steps in the research process. In addition, learners have the opportunity to present their findings.

Part 1: Write a research proposal following the guidance outlined in Appendix 6
Part 2: Peer review of the research proposal with structured feedback

Part 1

- Form groups to form an even number of groups.
- As a group, identify a research question.
- Identify six to eight research articles that support answering the research.
- Review the articles and develop a summary of the articles using a thematic approach. Review the methodologies of each article and identify the strengths and weaknesses/limitations of each.
- Design a five-page research proposal with a methodology that seeks to address the limitations of the studies as it answers the research question

Part 2

- Submit the proposal.
- Distribute each proposal to other groups to review and provide feedback.
- Each person reviews the assigned proposal and gives feedback including helpful comments to improve the proposal to answer the research question.
- The original group reviews the feedback and submits the final proposal accompanied by the peer review feedback for grading. "Targeted feedback gives students prioritized information about how their performance does or does not meet the criteria so they can understand how to improve their future performance".

Resource 9

Giving Feedback

Purpose: The purpose of the feedback is to provide the other group information that will be useful for them to improve the quality of the research proposal. Giving specific feedback allows the individual to engage in a more targeted response and gives the recipient of the feedback and opportunity to develop their knowledge and skills. Provide both positive and negative feedback to facilitate the learning through elaboration (Ambrose, Bridges, DiPietro, Lovett, and Norman 2010).

- Positive feedback indicates areas of the grant that are good and should be retained. It should be given first to help build self-efficacy and enhance motivation.
- Negative feedback on the other hand is intended to provide guidance for what needs to be reviewed and changed/edited.
- Provide feedback on one dimension at a time and aimed to improve the final product

Attribute	Component needs addressing	Component covered and adequate
Research question(s)	<ul><li>The research question(s) are poorly defined</li><li>Weak or missing rationale for the research question(s)</li><li>Unclear how the planned study will answer the stated research question(s)</li></ul>	<ul><li>The research question(s) are clearly defined</li><li>Clear rationale for the research question(s) grounded in existing research</li><li>Planned study logically and adequately answers stated research question(s)</li></ul>
Literature review	<ul><li>Weaknesses in depth of knowledge in subject matter</li><li>Insufficiently focused regarding the research topic</li></ul>	<ul><li>Demonstrates adequate knowledge in subject matter</li><li>Sufficiently focused regarding the research topic</li></ul>
Quality of the science	<ul><li>Arguments are illogical, incoherent, or have no basis in existing literature</li><li>Objectives/hypotheses are poorly defined with a poorly articulated problem statement</li><li>Demonstrates no originality</li><li>Demonstrates poor understanding of theoretical/conceptual concepts</li><li>Methodology not adequately supported by the literature</li><li>The methodology is not appropriate for the theoretical/conceptual framework of the study</li><li>Data analysis is not consistent with the research questions or hypothesis</li></ul>	<ul><li>Arguments are logical, coherent, and supported with existing literature</li><li>Objectives/hypotheses are clear and support the problem statement</li><li>Demonstrates originality</li><li>Demonstrates understanding of theoretical/conceptual concepts</li><li>Methodology is adequately supported by the literature</li><li>Methodology is consistent with the research questions/hypotheses</li><li>Data analysis is adequate for answering the research questions or hypothesis</li></ul>
Study limitations	<ul><li>Proposal fails to acknowledge limitations of the study</li></ul>	<ul><li>Proposal acknowledges limitations of the study</li></ul>
Contribution to the discipline	<ul><li>Limited publication potential</li></ul>	<ul><li>Clear publication potential</li></ul>
Comments that would improve the publication in a bulleted format		

CHAPTER 3

MODULE 3: QUALITATIVE RESEARCH METHODS

This module provides an overview of the philosophical underpinning of qualitative research and presents practical steps for designing and conducting a qualitative research study, building on the fundamental research concepts and frameworks discussed in Module 1. The concepts of stakeholder engagement, ethical and cultural considerations, and reflexivity are integrated throughout the module. In addition, this module also incorporates exercises and examples from the literature and the authors' research and teaching experiences. This module is divided into three sections: (a) Introduction to Qualitative Research, (b) Conceptualizing a Qualitative Research Study, and (c) Applying Qualitative Research Methods.

By the end of the module, learners will be able to:

- Explain the philosophical underpinnings and attributes of qualitative research
- Describe the qualitative research process
- Formulate qualitative research questions
- Develop a qualitative data collection tool
- Apply qualitative data analysis methods
- Discuss the ethical and cultural considerations in qualitative research

Integrated Research Methods In Public Health, First Edition. Muriel Jean Harris and Baraka Muvuka.
© 2023 John Wiley & Sons, Inc. Published 2023 by John Wiley & Sons, Inc.
Companion website: www.wiley.com/go/harris/integratedresearchmethods

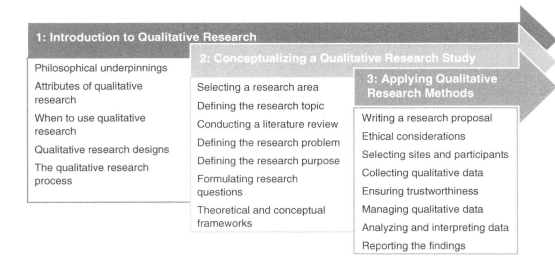

SECTION 1: INTRODUCTION TO QUALITATIVE RESEARCH

By the end of this section, learners will be able to:

- Explain the philosophical underpinnings of qualitative research
- Describe the attributes of qualitative research
- Describe the common qualitative research designs
- Describe the qualitative research process

INTRODUCTION

This section challenges the learners to critically reflect on qualitative research method as a distinct, independent, and rigorous research method. It introduces the philosophical paradigms associated with qualitative research and describes the distinctive features of qualitative research that are rooted in these paradigms. This section provides an overview of qualitative research designs and the qualitative research process.

PHILOSOPHICAL UNDERPINNINGS

Our philosophical paradigms or assumptions about the world, reality, and knowledge shape how we formulate research questions and how we seek to answer these questions (Ataro, 2020; Creswell, 2013). Module 1 discussed some philosophical paradigms that shape our approaches to research. Qualitative and quantitative research both seek to understand social issues using rigorous data collection, analysis, and interpretation approaches. However, they are fundamentally different in their underlying philosophical paradigms.

More specifically, quantitative and qualitative research differ in their ontological, epistemological, and axiological assumptions. *Ontology* refers to the nature of reality. While quantitative research assumes an objective truth or reality as discussed in Module 2, qualitative research considers multiple subjective realities. *Epistemology* refers to the nature of knowledge and how we know what we know. The quantitative research method is underpinned by the positivist paradigm, which posits a truth that can be systematically and objectively observed, verified, and measured. It primarily tests hypotheses or theories by measuring the relationships between variables while controlling for confounders (alternative explanations) and researcher bias. Conversely, qualitative research is primarily grounded in the *interpretivist/constructivist* worldviews, which are premised on the notion that reality is socially, culturally, and historically constructed as individuals interact with the world and among themselves (Creswell, 2013). *Axiology* is concerned with the nature of values. Quantitative research assumes a value-free (i.e., objective) research, where the researcher is considered independent from the study. However, qualitative research is value-laden or value bound (i.e., subjective) since it stipulates that the researcher cannot be separated from the study given their role as the research instrument and co-constructor of knowledge. Rather than detaching themselves from the study, qualitative researchers continuously and explicitly reflect on their values and biases to better represent their participants' voices. While qualitative research itself is underpinned by the interpretivist/constructivist paradigms, it should be noted that not all qualitative researchers strictly fit within these paradigms. There are qualitative researchers and scholars espousing elements of other paradigms such as positivism, pragmatism, or realism, thus resulting in variations in methodologies even within specific qualitative research designs. Overall, the philosophical differences between quantitative and qualitative research account for their methodological variations.

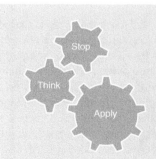

Reflecting on your Research Philosophy

Which philosophical paradigm(s) do you identify with (see Module 1)?
What are your assumptions about qualitative research?
Discuss how your philosophical orientation influences your assumptions about qualitative research.

ATTRIBUTES OF QUALITATIVE RESEARCH

The philosophical underpinnings of qualitative research give rise to the distinctive attributes of qualitative research that are depicted in Figure 3.1 and discussed subsequently.

Multiple realities: The interpretivist/constructivist paradigm suggests the notion of multiple realities and interpretations rather than a single, observable reality. In other words, this worldview posits that individuals perceive, understand, experience, and attribute meanings differently. Qualitative research is therefore focused on generating a deeper understanding of complex phenomena through participants' experiences and the meanings they ascribe to these experiences.

Transactional, naturalistic/contextual, holistic: Interpretivism/constructivism stipulates that researchers do not "find" or discover knowledge but rather co-construct it with their participants (Merriam, 2009, pp. 8–9). This view

FIGURE 3.1. *Key attributes of qualitative research.*

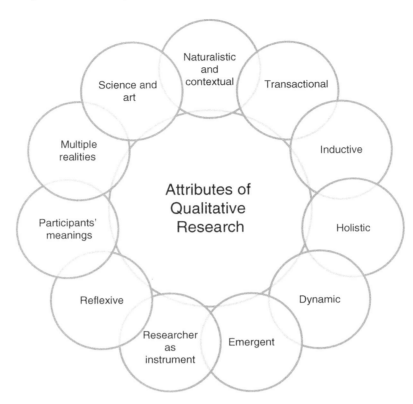

supports a *transactional and naturalistic* method of inquiry, in which the researcher and participants co-construct knowledge through direct interactions within their *natural setting*. As such, qualitative researchers ask *open-ended questions* related to the topic, listen carefully, observe closely, and interpret the findings based on *participants' meanings and experiences* (Creswell, 2013). A qualitative research design paints a *holistic* picture of the phenomenon under investigation by situating the participants and the researcher within the natural social, cultural, and political *context*.

Researcher as the instrument: One of several distinctive features of qualitative research is the researcher's unique role as a co-constructor of knowledge and primary research instrument for data collection and analysis. This role is useful for investigating complex and dynamic processes because the researcher as an instrument is best positioned to achieve an in-depth understanding of an issue given the following abilities described by Merriam (2009, p. 15):

- Respond and adapt immediately
- Capture both verbal and nonverbal communication
- Process information immediately
- Clarify and summarize materials
- Check with respondents for accuracy of interpretation, and
- Explore unusual or unanticipated responses

Reflexive research method: In any type of research, researchers come with their personal and philosophical assumptions and experiences. In qualitative research, there is an understanding that the researcher's background, assumptions, and experiences may shape (Charmaz, 2014):

- What they see, how, when, and to what extent
- What they do not see
- How they interpret what they see or do not see

The researcher's role as the primary research instrument and co-constructor of knowledge comes with an obligation to take a critical and reflective stance toward their position relative to the study (i.e., topic, research processes, and outputs), the participants, and the research context. Qualitative researchers engage in an ongoing process of critical self-reflection on their personal backgrounds, values, biases, and experiences, as well as their potential impact on the study (reflexivity). Ongoing reflexivity enables researchers to determine their position in relation to the study, which in turn opens them up to capturing the understanding and meanings of their participants (Creswell, 2013; Holmes, 2014). This often culminates in a reflexivity or positionality statement in which they bring these personal biases to consciousness and articulate how their background potentially influenced their research. Reflexivity and positionality are imperative to ensure ethical and culturally appropriate research (Sultana, 2007). Reflexivity and positionality are dynamic and context dependent rather than fixed (Holmes, 2014; Sultana, 2007). That said, the researcher must self-reflect and reexamine their position as the study progresses.

Inductive: Qualitative research often uses an inductive (bottom up) approach that seeks to identify recurrent patterns or themes across the data, which can be used to construct a theory that is grounded in the data. This contrasts with a deductive (top-down) approach that begins with and tests a prespecified theory or hypothesis as in quantitative research.

Inductive process: Specific observations ➡ recurrent patterns ➡ theory

Deductive process: Theory/generalization ➡ hypothesis ➡ observation ➡ specific conclusions

Some qualitative studies employ deductive approaches or combine both inductive and deductive approaches. For instance, deductive qualitative studies test the applicability of a theory or framework to specific situations and contexts or use a preexisting theoretical framework to direct data collection and analysis. Deductive–inductive qualitative studies begin with preexisting frameworks or categories but also incorporate the new categories that are identified from the data.

Dynamic and emergent: As with other types of research, a qualitative research study starts with a research plan in the form of a proposal. The qualitative research plan is not rigid but rather structured yet flexible enough to adapt to changing contexts and new findings or ideas to deepen the understanding of the phenomenon as the study progresses. These adaptations should be transparent and purposeful. The researcher leaves an audit trail that documents the major decisions and adaptations made throughout the research process, including their rationale.

A science and an art: As a science, qualitative research requires rigorous data collection and analysis methods with varying levels of complexity depending on the study and design. Furthermore, it requires that the researchers explicitly discuss their presuppositions or personal assumptions and how they influence the interpretation of the findings. As an art, qualitative research incorporates elements of esthetics in its design. It enables the use of all senses to achieve a holistic understanding of the issue being studied. It also embraces both conventional and novel forms of data collection, presentation, and dissemination, recognizing the complexity of communities and social issues. Being both an art and a science positions qualitative research to explore and uncover complex patterns or processes occurring in the natural context.

WHEN TO USE QUALITATIVE RESEARCH

Considering the plurality of research methods, one may wonder on what basis to select an appropriate research method for their study. Ideally, the research method depends on the nature of the research topic or problem, the research purpose (i.e., exploratory, explanatory, descriptive), and more importantly the research questions. Qualitative research is focused on understanding what is happening, how, and why, whereas a quantitative design is most appropriate to answer questions related to relationships between measurable variables (e.g., how many or how much). For instance, a qualitative study may ask: How do family members of victims of maternal deaths perceive maternal death

Qualitative research is appropriate:

- To answer what, how, and why
- When behaviors or settings cannot be manipulated
- To understand subjective experiences, perceptions, and meanings
- To explore contextual factors influencing a phenomenon
- To understand complex and dynamic issues that are not easily measurable

reviews? By asking open-ended questions, qualitative research enables an in-depth understanding of complex and dynamic concepts and contextual factors that are not easily measurable. Qualitative research is focused on understanding subjective experiences, perceptions, ascribed meanings, and their influences on behaviors, processes, or outcomes. This mode of inquiry is also appropriate when participants' behaviors and/or settings cannot be manipulated or controlled by the researcher as in experimental studies.

In terms of purpose, qualitative research is designed to explore, describe, or explain complex phenomena.

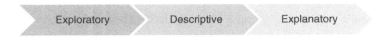

An *exploratory* qualitative study is undertaken when little or nothing is known about a topic. It asks general, open-ended questions seeking to uncover experiences, perceptions, meanings, patterns, discourses, and processes. It lays the groundwork for future studies as it generates new insights, more specific questions, and hypotheses that can be further investigated through qualitative, quantitative, or mixed methods studies. For instance, the authors conducted a qualitative study exploring women's perceptions of gold mining activities on their health in a small mining community in Ghana since much of the literature had focused on assessing the health of mine workers and mining communities (Muvuka and Harris, 2019), with little attention to women's health.

A *descriptive* qualitative study describes the nature, profile, characteristics, or aspects of the people, behaviors, events, situations, systems, or organizations being studied. It provides more detailed information on selected aspects of the phenomenon than an exploratory study. For example, Muvuka's (2019) doctoral dissertation employed a qualitative case study to generate a rich and thick description of the structures, processes, and outcomes of Maternal death surveillance and response (MDSR) in an urban health district in eastern Democratic Republic of Congo (DRC).

Finally, an *explanatory* study goes beyond exploration and description to explain the reasons (i.e., why?) behind a particular phenomenon. Distinctions can be made between a quantitative and qualitative explanatory study. While a quantitative explanatory study sets out to explain the relationships between variables, an explanatory qualitative inquiry is intended to explain the patterns and meanings of participants' experiences and the mechanisms by which they influence the phenomenon of interest. This is the hallmark of the grounded theory method (GTM) which develops a data-driven theoretical explanation or interpretation of the phenomenon. For instance, an explanatory qualitative study may seek to understand how masculine norms influence men's decisions to seek an HIV test within a specific cultural context.

QUALITATIVE RESEARCH DESIGNS

There are several designs in qualitative research and several variants within these designs. The key elements driving the selection of an appropriate qualitative research design are the researcher's philosophical orientation, theoretical framework, and more importantly, the research questions. The following are the most common qualitative research designs: case study research, ethnography, GTM, phenomenology, narrative research, and qualitative participatory research (e.g., photovoice).

Case Study Research

A qualitative case study involves an in-depth investigation of a bounded system (a case) or multiple bounded systems (cases) using multiple data collection methods (Creswell, 2013). The *case or* unit of analysis in a case study can be an individual, group, organization, community, event, program, policy, or process that is bounded by time, geographic area, person or population, or organization. The boundary of the case represents its scope (Crowe et al., 2011). The case is selected for its unique or interesting features and its ability to generate rich insights into the phenomenon being investigated. A case study enables a thorough investigation of complex issues within their natural contexts by specifically asking how, why, and what questions and capturing dynamic interactions between the case(s) and contextual factors. This approach therefore generates powerful and contextually rich information on public health issues, programs, theories, policies, and interventions. There are varying paradigms underpinning case study research. For instance, some prominent seminal authors such as Yin (2003) and Flyvbjerg (2006) have been viewed as espousing postpositivist worldviews while others such as Merriam (2009) and Stake (1995) express constructivist or interpretivist paradigms.

Yin (2003) suggests that case study research is appropriate when the following conditions are met:

- The study's focus is to answer how and why research questions.
- Participants' behaviors cannot be manipulated or controlled by the researcher.
- The study seeks to explore contextual factors influencing the case.
- The boundaries between the phenomenon and the context are not clear.

Case studies can be used for exploratory, descriptive, explanatory, or a combination of purposes (Yin, 2003). Regardless of the purpose, case study research should provide a detailed description of the case, an account of the key themes identified during the investigation, and the conclusions or lessons learned from the study that can be applied to similar cases (Creswell, 2013). Muvuka's (2019) doctoral dissertation adopted both descriptive and exploratory case study approaches as it sought to provide a detailed description of current MDSR processes while gaining deeper insights into internal and external factors influencing MDSR implementation. Additionally, case studies can involve a single case or multiple cases. Stake (1995) identified three types of case studies: instrumental, intrinsic, and collective. Intrinsic and instrumental case studies involve single cases, while collective case studies involve multiple cases. In an intrinsic case study, the case itself is of primary interest to the investigation given its unique or unusual features while an instrumental case study examines a specific case to shed light on a broader issue of interest (Stake, 1995). A collective case study examines multiple cases sequentially or simultaneously to gain insights into a broader issue.

A key strength of case study research lies in its ability to generate an in-depth and holistic understanding of a phenomenon by converging evidence from multiple sources, also known as data triangulation. Yin (2003) identified the following data sources for case study research: documents, archival records, interviews, physical artifacts, and observation. Converging evidence from multiple sources enables a coherent understanding of the case and its context. Baxter and Jack (2008, p. 554) describe each data source as a piece of the "puzzle" that contributes to the researcher's understanding of the whole phenomenon. In addition, data triangulation enhances the accuracy and credibility of the study findings.

Case study research, as with any research design, is not without limitations and challenges. While case studies are best known for their ability to provide in-depth description of complex phenomena, they can produce overwhelmingly large amounts of information and can be labor and resource-intensive (Baxter and Jack, 2008; Crowe et al., 2011). To mitigate this, Creswell (2013) suggests clearly defining the boundaries of a case (i.e., time, events, processes) and developing a data collection matrix to estimate the amount of information to be collected. Given the varying paradigms underpinning case study research, some critiques of case study research reflect an evaluation of qualitative case study research against positivist criteria designed for quantitative research rather than actual limitations of a qualitative case study. It is important to distinguish the limitations of case studies from such misunderstandings. Flyvbjerg (2006) addresses the most common misunderstandings of case studies and provides alternative statements to correct each of them. For instance, one common misunderstanding is that a single-case study cannot substantially contribute to scientific development because findings from a single case are not generalizable. Flyvberg's counterargument to this critique points out that "formal generalization is overvalued as a source of scientific development, whereas "the force of example" is underestimated" (Flyvbjerg, 2006, p. 228).

Ethnography

Ethnography is rooted in anthropology. It is focused on understanding the shared meanings, values, and belief systems underlying sociocultural structures, interactions, symbols, practices, and norms of a distinct group, community, or organization. This approach involves the prolonged and deep immersion of the researcher into the day-to-day lives of participants within their natural setting, during which they participate in activities and engage in various formal or informal research-oriented interactions. This approach posits that cultural phenomena are complex and multifactorial, thus prolonged immersion is expected to generate rich, deep, and holistic insights into sometimes hidden phenomena that other designs cannot adequately uncover. More importantly, the goal is to understand the phenomenon being studied from an insider or local perspective (i.e., emic). As in a case study, data triangulation is also important in ethnography as it converges evidence from observations, formal and informal interviews, and extensive field notes alongside other data collection methods (e.g., document reviews) to understand the phenomenon from the lens of the cultural group. It involves the co-construction of knowledge between the immersed researcher and the participants. For instance, an ethnographic study examined how young people envisioned getting out of an inner-city drug scene in Vancouver, Canada, as well as the factors that shaped their experiences as they attempted to exit this setting (Knight et al., 2017). In the researchers' own words, this ethnographic study involved "hundreds of hours in the places where young people were living, working, sleeping, socializing, and accessing services and systems, documented through written field notes, audio recordings, and photographs" (Knight et al., 2017, p. 2). Reflexivity is central to ethnographic studies, given the researcher's immersion and prolonged interactions with participants. It is common to find reflexivity or positionality statements in an ethnographic research report as it enables readers to assess the potential influence of the researcher on the findings.

While ethnography enables the researcher to acquire first-hand experience and, in some cases, an emic (i.e., insider) understanding of the cultural phenomenon, its inherent features can pose several challenges or limitations. For instance, the prolonged immersion, repeated contact, and need to establish trust makes it time-consuming and unpredictable, thus requiring flexibility on the part of the researcher. This may pose a challenge in meeting strict deadlines for projects such as dissertations or theses. A traditional ethnographic study often extends over a year or several years, although contemporary ethnographic studies are undertaken for shorter durations given resource limitations and the increasing use of an ethnographic design in applied research (Guest et al., 2013). Another challenge associated with ethnography is related to achieving an emic perspective of an issue. This is difficult to achieve because it depends on several factors including the nature of the phenomenon being studied—whether it can be experienced, reexperienced, or observed the same way; the participants; the duration and extent of the immersion; as well the researcher's initial position when undertaking the study. Having an "insider" status does not automatically translate into shared experiences and understanding of participants' meaning and experiences. In addition, the insider-outsider status is a dynamic process that is negotiated between participants and the researcher. The researcher's assumptions of an insider position can still be challenged by some participants as it is processed through their lenses. However, as the study progresses and the dynamics evolve, the insider–outsider boundary can begin to blur (Sultana, 2007). There are more novel forms of ethnography such as auto-ethnography, in which the researchers document their own perspectives and understandings of their social interactions with participants while investigating the sociocultural phenomenon.

Finally, there are potential ethical issues associated with ethnographic studies that examine sensitive or hidden cultural practices or utilize incomplete disclosure and deceptive practices such as informal conversations and covert observations. Such features have been reported to challenge the ethical approval of a study. Deception involves intentionally misleading participants by omitting or giving false information about key aspects of the study, such as the researcher's role or relationship and real purpose of the research, so as not to bias or compromise the quality of the study findings. It is not unique to ethnographic or qualitative research; it is also used in some experimental studies. Research studies involving deceptive methodologies or incomplete disclosure have lower chances of being approved by Institutional Review Boards or ethics committees. In unique circumstances where such studies are required, additional demands and responsibilities are placed on researchers to ensure that they do no harm to participants. The following are common conditions for approving studies with deceptive methodologies:

- Provide a scientific justification for the use of deception.
- Demonstrate that there is no equally effective nondeceptive alternative.
- Demonstrate that the study poses no more than minimal risk to participants.
- Demonstrate that the benefits of the study outweigh the risks.
- Depending on the level of deception, debrief participants after the study. Debriefing involves disclosing and justifying the use of deception and answering participants' questions after the study.

Despite these challenges and limitations, ethnographic research has generated rich evidence into sociocultural phenomena that were otherwise hidden or less understood. In addition, the data collection and analysis methods used in ethnography have inspired other qualitative approaches such as GTM, narrative inquiry, and Community Based Participatory Research (Morse, 2016).

Grounded Theory Method

The GTM aims to generate a theoretical explanation of a phenomenon that is grounded in participants' perceptions and experiences through an inductive analysis of the data. Grounded theory is both a qualitative research design and a product of the research process, thus the use of the term GTM in this module to distinguish the research design from its product (i.e., the grounded theory). The GTM was initially developed by Glaser and Strauss (1967) to establish a rigorous basis for qualitative research, challenging the predominant positivist view of quantitative research as superior (Bryant 2017).

There are several iterations of the original GTM varying in philosophical and methodological orientations. We briefly discuss three common iterations of GTM. The *classic GTM* was first introduced and articulated in the work of Glaser and Strauss (1967) who are considered the founders of GTM. This approach has some positivist underpinnings, as evidenced by an emphasis on an external, objective reality and the centrality of developing theory to predict phenomena (Bryant, 2017; Timonen et al., 2018). It asserts that the theory is inductively generated from the data by a researcher who maintains an objective stance by "bracketing" their personal biases. Some of its prescribed procedures conflict with current institutional requirements related to research (Timonen et al., 2018). For instance, the classic GTM views the researcher as a blank slate and advises against conducting a literature review prior to data collection, while more recent iterations (e.g., constructivist GTM) encourage literature reviews early in the research process provided that researchers maintain reflexivity and do not force the data into preexisting theories or frameworks. Similarly, this approach also encourages the formulation of specific research questions after data collection as discussed in the subsequent section.

The *Straussian GTM*, introduced by Strauss and Corbin, started with positivist and postpositivist underpinnings which assumed an external, objective reality that can be systematically investigated while also acknowledging that reality cannot be fully apprehended by the researcher (Corbin and Strauss, 2008; Strauss and Corbin, 1990). The Straussian GTM evolved over time to embrace symbolic interactionism, pragmatism, and constructivism. The more recent versions emphasize the construction of social reality through human interactions, the interpretive role of the researcher in generating the theory, the importance of reflexivity throughout the process, and endorse less prescriptive analytical techniques (Creswell, 2013; Timonen et al., 2018). Unlike the classic GTM, this version of GTM supports a literature review and formulation of research questions prior to data collection to orient the study but advices against starting with a theoretical framework (Corbin and Strauss, 2015; Rieger, 2019).

Finally, the *constructivist grounded theory* originates from the work of Charmaz (2006, 2014). This approach endorses the notion of multiple socially constructed realities rather than an external, objective reality and views the researcher and participants as active co-constructors of knowledge to generate the grounded theory. This approach encourages the use of the literature and the formulation of research questions prior to conducting the study. It also accepts the use of theoretical concepts to guide the study provided that the researcher is reflexive and does not impose these preexisting theories on the data.

Despite their philosophical and methodological differences, these iterations of GT adhere to the following fundamental concepts or principles of grounded theory. Their interpretation of these concepts and the degree of adherence may vary:

- *Process-orientation:* GTM aims to capture, understand, and explain the processes, interactions, or actions emerging from the data. When examining the data, the researcher essentially asks: What is going on here? Why?

- *Induction:* GTM emphasizes the importance of remaining open to new themes rather than imposing any preexisting frameworks or theories on the data. The theory that is generated should be grounded in the data collected, not in the literature. Part of the inductive process involves remaining open to generating new research questions or modifying existing research questions as data are collected (Sbaraini et al., 2011; Timonen et al., 2018).

- *Concurrent data collection and analysis:* data collection and analysis occur simultaneously. In other words, data analysis begins with the first interview, focus group, observation, or document review and is ongoing throughout data collection (Merriam, 2009). This is further explained in subsequent sections of this module.

- *Constant comparison:* a data analysis method that involves comparing the data against each other to identify recurrent patterns across the data. This is further explained when discussing data analysis in Section 3 of this module.

- *Theoretical sampling and saturation:* Theoretical sampling involves purposively selecting participants as data collection and analysis unfolds. This is done to fill the gaps in certain categories and reach theoretical saturation, where all concepts of the grounded theory are well understood.

- *Development of a grounded theory:* The intended outcome of the GTM is a grounded theory, and in some versions, a conceptual framework, model, or schema, that describes, explains, predict, and interprets structures and processes related to the phenomenon being investigated (Sbaraini et al., 2011). This theory is not final or infallible and can continue to be developed in subsequent studies.

Several published studies are labeled as GTM without fully or correctly adhering to the core principles of GTM. This is in part due to the time-consuming and complex nature of GTM, the disputes or contradictions between variations, and the conflict between some GTM principles with current institutional requirements (Timonen et al., 2018). For instance, the practice of delaying the literature review and research questions until after data collection may not align with requirements of dissertation committees and Institutional Review Boards or ethics committees. However, given its rigorous procedures, there is a proliferation of grounded-theory oriented studies that incorporate certain aspects of GTM into their designs (e.g., data analysis) without aiming to generate a grounded theory (Bryant, 2017; Timonen et al., 2018).

Phenomenology

Phenomenology seeks to understand the nature and essence or meaning of a phenomenon through the shared experiences and perspectives of individuals who experienced it. The researcher collects data from several individuals about *what* they experienced, *how* they experienced it, and what this experience *means* to them, and generates themes reflecting their collective experiences and meanings (Moustakas, 1994; Teherani et al., 2015). Phenomenology has been used to provide rich and thick descriptions of common or shared experiences related to various public health and social phenomena such as experiences of loss, grief, stress, and stigma. For instance, a phenomenological study by Smith et al. (2018) explored young people's experiences of thyroid cancer diagnosis and treatment as well as the meaning they ascribed to these experiences. While phenomenological data are primarily collected through in-depth interviews and focus groups, other data collection methods such as physical or electronic documents can be used to generate rich insights into participants' experiences of a phenomenon.

There are several types of phenomenological studies varying in philosophical paradigms and in their conceptions of lived experiences (Creswell, 2013; Neubauer et al., 2019). The most common variations of phenomenology are transcendental phenomenology and hermeneutic phenomenology. *Transcendental phenomenology* seeks a descriptive understanding of the essence of a phenomenon. This approach requires that the researcher take an objective stance by "bracketing" or separating their personal assumptions and biases in an effort to describe the essence of the phenomenon from participants' perspectives. It is most appropriate when little or nothing is known about the phenomenon being investigated. Contrastingly, *hermeneutic phenomenology* goes beyond the description of the essence of a phenomenon and seeks an interpretation of the meaning of participants' lived experiences related to the phenomenon. This interpretive process takes into account the influence of participants' backgrounds on their experiences of a phenomenon. Rather than assuming that researchers are a blank slate, hermeneutic phenomenology acknowledges that researchers come with their personal background and biases, which they bring to consciousness and report transparently through ongoing reflexivity (Creswell, 2013; Neubauer et al., 2019).

A major critique of transcendental phenomenology pertains to bracketing, which requires the researcher to become a blank slate (Creswell, 2013). This practice of bracketing one's personal background and biases in transcendental phenomenology is rooted in a positivist tradition. Proponents of hermeneutic phenomenology believe that this form of bracketing is not achievable and rather recommend various measures for enhancing the trustworthiness of the study such as reflexivity, respondent validation of preliminary findings, data triangulation, and peer review.

Narrative Research

Narrative research involves the development of a written and chronological narrative of an individual's life story, experience, and attached meanings related to a phenomenon of interest. It originates in social sciences, where it was first used by Connelly and Clandinin (1990) to describe the personal stories of teachers. It is inspired by oral storytelling traditions and is based on the premise that human beings construct narratives to make sense of their lived experiences and convey their meanings or interpretations of these experiences by telling their stories. Connelly and Clandinin (2006) assert that a story "is a portal through which a person enters the world and by which their experience of the world is interpreted and made personally meaningful" (Connelly and Clandinin, 2006, p. 375).

Narrative research emphasizes the co-construction and shared understanding of the participant's real-life story through an active collaborative relationship between the researcher and the participant. It employs a variety of data collection methods including semistructured or unstructured interviews, document reviews, photo-elicitation, and observations to generate powerful insights into the complexity of the participant's identity and experience related to a phenomenon within its social, historical, and cultural context. Narrative research tends to focus on the story of a single individual and, in some cases, the cohesive story of a small group of participants that have lived through a similar situation or phenomenon. When involving a small group of individuals, a narrative inquiry may be similar to a case study, an ethnography, or a phenomenology. The key difference between these approaches and narrative research lies in the consideration of stories as raw data and in the storytelling presentation of the data collected in narrative inquiry.

Some of the limitations associated with ethnography and phenomenology also apply to narrative inquiry. For instance, one important criticism of narrative inquiry concerns the accuracy of the researcher's interpretation and representation of the participant's lived experience and ascribed meaning. Since the narrative is a product of the interaction between the researcher and the participant, the researcher must reflect on their position and influence on the participant's narrative and must utilize additional measures to ensure the trustworthiness of the study findings as discussed in Section 3 of this module. Some argue that experiential meanings are complex, layered, and sometimes subconscious concepts that cannot be completely understood or articulated through language (Polkinghorne, 2007). This concern can be partly addressed by using various interviewing techniques such as probing or asking reflexive questions that enable participants to dig deeper. In addition, using other forms of communication or data collection methods such as symbols, artifacts, and photographs can supplement the oral narration of a participant's story. Finally, there are ethical concerns surrounding sensitive or traumatic events since interactions around such events may trigger flashbacks that could be psychologically harmful to participants.

Participatory Qualitative Research: Photovoice

Photovoice is a qualitative research approach within the category of participatory action research (Module 1), which primarily explores social justice-oriented issues and gives voice to historically marginalized or vulnerable groups. The term *Photovoice* was originally proposed by Wang and Burris (1994, 1997) in their work assessing the health and socioeconomic needs of women in rural villages in Yunnan Province, China. This approach builds on the evidence that photographs are powerful tools with the capacity to prompt conscious and subconscious thoughts, memories, emotions, and ascribed meanings in ways that text, words, or narratives cannot (Harper 2002). The *voice* in Photovoice stands for *voicing our individual and collective voice* because Photovoice promotes critical dialogue on community strengths and concerns through group discussions around photographs that are taken by participants themselves (Wang and Burris 1994, 1997). The goal is to stimulate collective action for social change. Photovoice promotes the active co-construction of knowledge between participants and researchers and enables researchers to view social and health issues from the lens of community members. Having participants produce their own photos reduces the power distance between the researcher and participants and acknowledges their roles as co-constructors of knowledge. This also empowers participants to be self-reflective and to control their own voice and narrative, which in turn paves the way for more productive discussions and action. The Photovoice approach generally follows the following steps:

1. The team and community partners collaboratively select the research topic and participate in a Photovoice training.

2. Guided by broad instructions, participants take photographs reflecting their experiences related to the phenomenon.

3. In small groups, participants select photographs that will form the basis for small group discussions based on their significance and representation of their lived experiences.

4. Participants and researchers collectively interpret the photographs through critical and reflective discussions on their context, lived experiences, and meanings. These focus group discussions are structured around the SHOWeD acronym (Shaffer, 1983):

    S: What do you **S**ee here?

    H: What is really **H**appening here?

    O: How does this relate to **O**ur lives?

    W: **W**hy does this concern, situation, or strength exist?

    e: How can we be **E**mpowered through our new understanding?

    D: What can we **D**o about it?

5. Participants and researchers codify and identify themes from the discussions.

6. Participants and researchers strategically and creatively disseminate the findings to diverse stakeholders.

7. Appropriate action is taken at multiple levels.

There are several types of qualitative visual methodologies that reflect some Photovoice features but do not adhere to the principles of participatory action research. One such approach is photo-elicitation. Photovoice and photo-elicitation both utilize photographs to explore a phenomenon of interest. However, unlike Photovoice, photo-elicitation is not necessarily a participatory approach because it is often designed, implemented, and disseminated by the researcher or research team (Liebenberg, 2018). In addition, photo-elicitation employs interviews or focus groups as the primary data collection methods, with photographs serving a secondary or supportive role to prompt conversations in interviews or focus groups (Liebenberg, 2018). While Photovoice participants produce their own photos, photo-elicitation photos can be produced by the participants or the researchers. More specifically, photo-elicitation participants can take their own photos, they can bring old photos that were not necessarily taken by them (e.g., family photos, images retrieved online), or the researcher can bring preexisting photos. While Photovoice occurs in small or large groups, photo-elicitation can be conducted on an individual basis or in groups.

Both Photovoice and photo-elicitation have been extensively employed to explore a variety of health and social issues affecting minority or underserved groups. As part of a faculty-led summer educational trip to Ghana in 2017, the authors conducted a collaborative mixed methods research study exploring the perceived impacts of gold mining activities on health and quality of life among residents of a small mining community in Ghana. This study was designed, implemented, and disseminated by a research team comprising students and faculty from the University of Louisville in the United States and the Kwame Nkrumah University of Science and Technology in Ghana. The qualitative arm of the study consisted of semistructured interviews with photo-elicitation. The participants were asked to produce photographs representing the factors within their community that influence their health and quality of life. The following were the semistructured interview prompts to guide the discussion around the photographs:

- What was your reason for taking the picture?
- What does the picture show? Describe the picture.
- How does the picture represent something about the health of individuals in your community?
- How do you think you or members of your community can address this issue/problem? What do you think people should do?
- Is there anything you would like to add about the picture?

Figures 3.2 and 3.3 are among the photographs produced by participants. Figure 3.2 depicts water contamination by discharges from mining activities in the community and represents water insecurity resulting from mining-related

FIGURE 3.2. *A photo-elicitation image of water pollution in a mining community.*

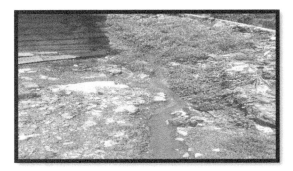

FIGURE 3.3. *A photo-elicitation image of deforestation in a mining community.*

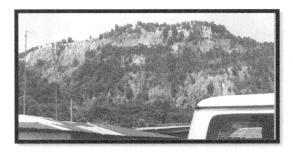

water pollution. Figure 3.3 represents the deforestation associated with mining activities, which the participant linked with food insecurity and the loss of traditional sources of livelihood (i.e., agriculture) to gold mining. Participants' narratives around both photographs alone exposed deep-seated issues of environmental injustice, power imbalances, helplessness, women's low social status, and a heavy reliance on an unstable mining industry.

While Photovoice provides a platform for addressing social and public health issues, there are potential ethical, legal, and cultural issues that must be carefully taken into account when designing, conducting, and disseminating a Photovoice study. Photovoice participants receive a short training or introductory session on research, photography techniques and etiquette as well as the ethical, legal, and cultural considerations of Photovoice (Wang and Burris, 1997). Privacy is an important ethical consideration in Photovoice. Participants must refrain from taking photographs that can potentially identify individuals and private spaces without obtaining consent or permission. They are trained to obtain written or signed informed consent from individuals who agree to be photographed for research purposes. In addition, Photovoice should be conducted with sensitivity to the sociocultural and religious norms concerning research and photography (Hannes and Parylo, 2014). Photovoice often culminates in the wide physical and electronic dissemination of the photographs and their narratives (Creighton et al., 2018). As such, the ownership and copyright of participant-produced photographs should be determined and discussed in the planning phase. In Photovoice, participants own or retain the copyright to their photographs but are asked to sign release or consent forms that give permission for researchers to use the photographs for dissemination purposes (e.g., research report, conferences, scientific publications, etc.) specified by participants (Creighton et al., 2018). Creighton et al. (2018) propose that participants must be made aware of the potential risk that the terms of use of the photographs may be violated by others, especially when disseminated online where they can be easily copied and reused beyond the control of the researcher. In summary, Wang and Redwood-Jones (2001) identified three types of consent needed in a Photovoice study: (a) a consent form for participation in the Photovoice study, (b) a consent form for individuals who agree to be photographed by Photovoice participants, and (c) a consent form signed by Photovoice participants permitting the dissemination of participant-produced photographs.

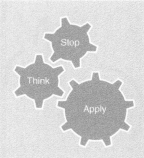

Practicing Photovoice

Take one photograph around your classroom, building, or workplace that represents health or public health. Share your photograph with a peer, colleague, or small group and discuss your responses to the following questions:
- What was your reason for taking the photograph?
- What does the photograph show?
- How does the photograph relate to health or public health?
- How does the photograph relate to your life?
- Is there anything else you would like to add about the photograph?

THE QUALITATIVE RESEARCH PROCESS

The qualitative research process is not linear, rigid, or static, but rather iterative, emergent, and evolving as the study progresses. Qualitative research generally involves the following major phases (Figure 3.4), each comprising specific tasks: (a) conceptualize and design the study, (b) conduct the study, and (c) report the research findings. Throughout each phase, the researcher engages various stakeholders, maintains reflexivity, and observes the necessary ethical and cultural considerations. The qualitative research process is discussed in detail in the subsequent sections of this module.

FIGURE 3.4. *The qualitative research process.*

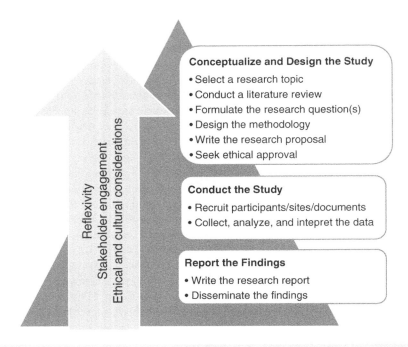

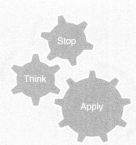

Reexamining your Assumptions About Qualitative Research

After reading this section, have your initial assumptions about qualitative research (see previous stop-think-apply) changed? If yes, in what ways have they changed?

List three pertinent facts or takeaways about qualitative research.

 SUMMARY

Qualitative research is grounded in the interpretivist/constructivist worldview, which is premised on the notion of multiple subjective realities that are socially constructed. In qualitative research, the researcher cannot be separated from the study given their role as the research instrument and co-constructor of knowledge. However, the researcher reflects on and reports their position in relation to the study. The interpretivist/constructivist paradigms underpinning qualitative research explain its distinctive features, including its transactional, naturalistic/contextual, holistic, reflexive, dynamic, emergent, scientific, artistic, and inductive nature.

Qualitative research is appropriate for answering what, how, and why research questions and can be used to explore, describe, and explain phenomena within their natural context, drawing from participants' experiences, perceptions, and meanings. There are several qualitative research designs, including case study research, ethnography, GTM, phenomenology, narrative research, and photovoice. The qualitative research process is iterative, emergent, and evolving.

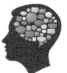

Course objective	Strongly agree	Somewhat agree	Neutral	Somewhat disagree	Strongly agree
Explain the philosophical underpinnings of qualitative research					
Describe the attributes of qualitative research					
Describe the common qualitative research designs					
Describe the qualitative research process					

Now that I have reached the end of this section, I am able to:

SECTION 2: CONCEPTUALIZING A QUALITATIVE RESEARCH STUDY

By the end of this step, learners will be able to:

- Select a research topic for a qualitative research study
- Explain the elements of a problem statement
- Develop a purpose statement for a qualitative research study
- Formulate qualitative research questions
- Explain the use of theoretical and conceptual frameworks in qualitative research

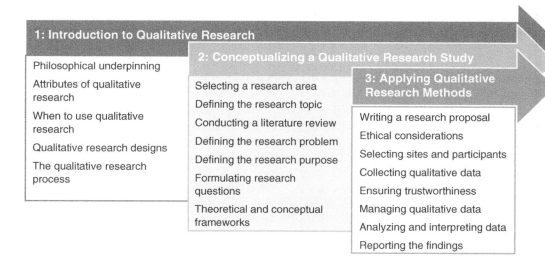

INTRODUCTION

Conceptualizing the research study is a challenging but critical step of the research process as it defines the focus of the entire study and directs the subsequent steps of the process. Researchers begin the research process at different starting points, with diverse backgrounds, levels of knowledge, and experiences in their field. Some begin with a specific topic or research question that stems from their personal and professional experience (i.e., research, teaching, or practice). However, many, especially students and early career researchers, start the research process with a broad research area or subject matter of interest that sparks their passion or intellectual curiosity. This broad research area is then gradually refined into a specific research topic, research problem, research purpose, and focused research

FIGURE 3.5. *From broad research ideas to focused research questions.*

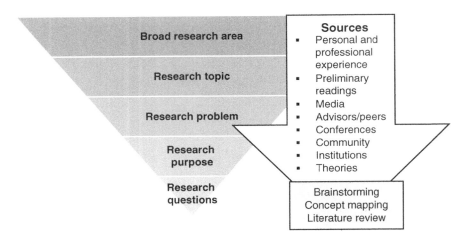

questions through an iterative process that involves the review of related literature, brainstorming with advisors and peers, and concept mapping. The process of conceptualizing the qualitative research study follows an inverted pyramid pattern, flowing from a broad or general research area to narrow, focused, and specific research questions (Figure 3.5).

SELECTING A BROAD RESEARCH AREA

Selecting a broad research area of interest is a starting point for those without predetermined research topics or questions. The broad area of study can be identified by reflecting and brainstorming on public health issues, populations, processes, activities, settings, systems, or phenomena of interest to the researcher and of significance to the institution, the discipline, or the community. The following questions can guide the identification of research areas of interest:

- Which public health areas, topics, or issues are you most interested in, passionate about, or concerned about? Why?
- Which of these areas of interest represents current priorities in your field, organization, or community?
- Which of these areas warrants further research and why?

The broadness of the research area depends on the researcher's particular interests, knowledge, exposure, and experience. Some examples of research areas include HIV prevention, the social determinants of health, health literacy, minority health, refugee and internally displaced populations, domestic violence, health insurance, maternal and child health, female genital mutilation, chronic diseases, reproductive health, or emerging infectious diseases. Research interests arise from multiple sources (Figure 3.5) including personal and professional experience, the literature, the media, advisors, peers, other scholars in the field, the community, and existing theories.

Personal and professional experience as sources of research ideas. Our daily personal and professional experiences or anecdotal observations of health and social needs, behaviors, discourses, communities, systems, practices, processes, policies, and outcomes can stimulate intellectual curiosity and inspire new research ideas. For instance, a researcher who has uninsured family members with mental health issues may develop an interest in systematically exploring the mental health-seeking behaviors, experiences, and attitudes of uninsured individuals. On a professional level, a front liner in the 2018–2019 Ebola outbreak in eastern DRC may be interested in examining healthcare workers' and community members' perceptions of the Ebola vaccine in this setting, with the goal of informing Ebola prevention and control efforts.

The literature as a source of research ideas. The literature is a valuable source of research ideas or questions. More specifically, preliminary exploratory readings of published and unpublished public health or nonpublic health literature, such as peer-reviewed articles, organizational reports, books, and dissertations/theses can highlight gaps, point to directions for future research, and inspire new research questions that can be further refined through a structured literature review.

Media as a source of research ideas. Traditional media and social media platforms such as television, radio, newspapers, Facebook, Twitter, Instagram, and newsletters feature current events, health and social issues, and controversial debates or dialogs that warrant further research. Many professional organizations circulate electronic and print newsletters to subscribers or members, with an overview of the existing evidence on priority issues, new developments in the field, as well as the gaps and calls for research proposals. It is important to subscribe to such newsletters in order to stay up to date on research priorities within one's field. For instance, during the COVID-19 pandemic, several organizations circulated calls for research proposals on COVID-19 among minority and vulnerable populations including homeless individuals, residents of nursing homes, and residents of refugee camps.

Peers, advisors, experts, and other professionals as sources of research ideas. Interactions with faculty, mentors, advisors, and peers within and beyond the researcher's institutions are important sources of research ideas. More specifically, local, national, or international scientific conferences, research presentations, lectures, community forums, workshops, and webinars have a great potential for inspiring new research ideas and creating research collaborations because such platforms convene professionals, subject matter experts, and other stakeholders with vast knowledge and experience in the field. For instance, the American Public Health Association's Annual Meeting and Exposition is the largest conference for public health professionals that hosts oral, roundtable, and poster sessions presenting the current evidence and research priorities in various public health areas of concentration.

Community as a source of research ideas. Research ideas can originate from communities in response to the community's perceived needs or the researcher's observations of the community's needs. Community Based Participatory Research studies are often conceptualized around community-initiated research ideas addressing priority issues within their communities.

Theory as a source of research ideas. By proposing relationships between various constructs, theories and models can generate new research questions while also providing a guiding framework for conducting research. For instance, Herrmann et al. (2018) utilized the Health Belief Model to explore the factors influencing women's decisions for or against the removal of their ovaries for cancer prevention purposes.

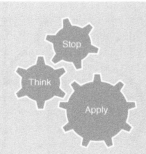

Selecting a Broad Research Area

Answer the questions below regarding your research area of interest and share your responses with a peer or colleague.

1. How did you learn about your research area of interest?
2. Does this area of interest represent current priorities in your field, setting, or organization?
3. Why does this area warrant further research?

Selecting the research area is a step forward toward developing the research topic. However, the research area is too broad to investigate in a single research study. Once a broad research area has been determined, the next step is to identify and define a specific research topic within the research area of interest.

DEFINING THE RESEARCH TOPIC

The research topic refers to the central idea or specific focus within the broad research area, from which the research problem and questions are derived. This topic can take the form of a health or social condition, behavior, health determinant, event, experience, activity/process/practice, system, institution, intervention/program, among several others. Since the research topic guides the formulation of the research problem and questions, selecting an appropriate research topic requires time and careful consideration. The research topic should be clearly defined by specifying its characteristics, scope, or boundaries, essentially the who, what, when, and where related to the topic. The parameters used in defining the topic include but are not limited to any or a combination of the following:

- Population: defined by sociodemographic characteristics such as race/ethnicity, culture, age, education, income, occupation, or health insurance status.

  Example: food insecurity among older adults

- Place or geographic setting (e.g., country, region, community, institution)

- Time period (e.g., century, era/period, decade, year)

- Components: involves breaking down the topic into multiple facets and focusing on one facet. One example is focusing on HIV-related stigma as one of several barriers to HIV pre-exposure prophylaxis (PrEP) uptake

- Relationships: how concepts compare, contrast, or relate with one another

  Example: perceived versus technical quality of care

- Unit/level: includes the levels of the socioecological model (Figure 3.6). Example: male partner's involvement in antenatal care services (i.e., interpersonal level)

The process of defining the research topic is iterative, reflective, interactive, and interrogative. It can span over several weeks to months, during which the researcher engages in preliminary readings of the literature, brainstorming, and concept mapping with advisors, mentors, or research team members to narrow the focus. These activities are ongoing and conducted concurrently until the formulation of the research questions.

Background or preliminary readings of relevant literature in the broad area of interest are a critical starting point for identifying the research topic. Note that these preliminary readings are different from the structured literature review that is carried out once a preliminary research topic has been determined. Some authors refer to these preliminary readings as the initial (Walliman, 2005) or preresearch literature review because it provides a snapshot or overview of the evidence, gaps, debates, or controversies within the broad research area for the purpose of identifying a specific research topic. Conversely, the structured literature review provides a more detailed and critical synthesis of the evidence and gaps surrounding the research topic for the purpose of defining the problem, the research questions, and positioning one's research study within the context of the broader literature. To avoid confusion, we refer to the preliminary review of the literature as background or preliminary readings. While not as structured as a literature review, these preliminary readings should be intentional and strategic such that the researcher identifies and generates a list of interesting or significant topics within the research area and captures the controversies, debates, questions, or knowledge gaps. The researcher can choose to focus the study on a topic with unresolved conflicts or knowledge gaps, alternatively, they can choose to challenge or expand a well-established topic within the broad research area (Walliman, 2005).

FIGURE 3.6. *The socioecological model.*

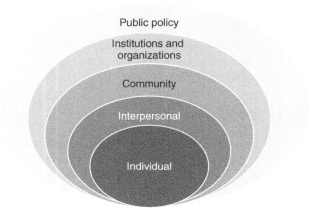

Brainstorming with advisors, peers, and key stakeholders is another useful, practical, and interactive approach for defining or narrowing down the research topic. Brainstorming generally involves asking and answering a series of questions about a topic to identify important aspects of the topic. Using any brainstorming technique, the research team discusses the preliminary findings from the readings, identifies interesting subtopics and related concepts, and discusses the specific aspects of the topic that they are interested in investigating. Purposeful and organized brainstorming sessions are productive, often generating outlines, diagrams, or concept maps. For example, a research team that started with a broad interest in HIV prevention may develop an interest in HIV PrEP after preliminary readings, which they can further narrow down through brainstorming around the following prompts: Which aspects or components of HIV PrEP are we interested in investigating (e.g., attitudes, experiences, beliefs, perceptions, knowledge, quality, accessibility, stigma)? In whom (e.g., women, older adults, health care providers)? Why? Where (if applicable)? Concept maps can be produced from the brainstorming sessions on the topic.

Concept-mapping is the visualization of key concepts and relationships between these concepts using traditional methods (e.g., board, paper, and colored markers) or digital tools. A concept map is often produced from preliminary readings and brainstorming. The main concepts related to the topic are listed at the top of the map and the sub-concepts are organized under each main concept, with lines indicating relationships between concepts and subconcepts (Figures 3.7 and 3.8). This organization and visualization of the key concepts and interrelationships stimulates productive discussions between research team members or stakeholders and facilitates the formulation of the research topic, problem, and questions.

FIGURE 3.7. *Example #1 of a concept map.* **FIGURE 3.8.** *Example #2 of a concept map.*

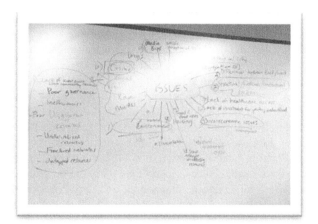
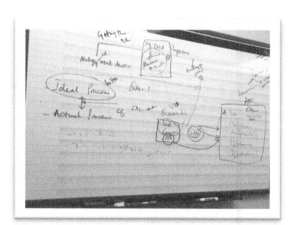

Box 3.1 presents a mini case study illustrating the process of selecting a research topic from a broad area of interest using some techniques presented in this section.

BOX 3.1 Selecting a Research Topic Within a Research Area

Danielle, a public health student, develops a general interest in noncommunicable diseases (NCDs) after reading global and local reports that they have persistently accounted for the majority of deaths over the years. She meets with her advisor who asks a series of questions about her research interests. During this initial brainstorming session, they conclude that *noncommunicable diseases* is a broad topic that can be further narrowed down by: (a) disease category such as cardiovascular diseases, cancer, chronic respiratory diseases, and diabetes; (b) metabolic risks including obesity, elevated blood pressure, blood glucose, and abnormal lung function; (c) behavioral risk factors including physical inactivity, unhealthy diet, tobacco use, and harmful use of alcohol; (d) social determinants such as social inequalities, housing and built environment, agriculture and food supply, health system, cultural factors, and policies;

(Continued)

> *(Continued)*
>
> or (e) demographic characteristics of the priority population (e.g., age, gender, race/ethnicity, socioeconomic status, geographic setting). Based on this initial meeting, Danielle has to decide whether any or a combination of these subtopics presents a problem of interest to her investigation as she continues to engage in preliminary readings, brainstorming, and concept-mapping with her advisor.
>
> As Danielle learns more about NCDs in her preliminary readings, she finds that the global burden of type 2 diabetes mellitus (T2DM) has nearly quadrupled since 1980 (Roglic and World Health Organization, 2016). The burden of T2DM is equally on the rise within the United States, with the highest prevalence of diagnosed diabetes reported among American Indians/Alaska Natives (Centers for Disease Control and Prevention, 2020). In addition, Danielle finds that previous studies and public health efforts related to T2DM have focused on behavioral factors such as physical activity and healthy diet but have not produced population-level results. Based on the knowledge gaps identified through the preliminary readings, she decides to focus on sociocultural factors influencing diabetes prevention and control among American Indians. She will work on refining this topic as she conducts a more thorough and critical review of related literature. Overall, she hopes that her study will expand the current evidence base and inform public health prevention efforts.

The following are important considerations when selecting a research topic:

Interesting: The research topic should be of deep interest to the researcher, stakeholders, and the organization to enhance the relevance and utility of the research study. In addition, since research can be a challenging, labor-intensive, and frustrating endeavor, this passion or deep interest in the topic can help sustain one's motivation and commitment to the process. It is especially important that students undertaking a dissertation or thesis find it enjoyable since such projects are conducted over long periods of time, during which they may experience moments of frustration, isolation, or fatigue in addition to investing substantial amounts of resources. A topic of deep interest to the researcher goes a long way in sustaining their motivation throughout the research process. However, the interest in a topic should be balanced with other critical considerations such as feasibility, relevance to the community, and significance to the field.

Original/novel: That a topic be novel or original is a common statement in academic and research circles. Novelty or originality in research does not mean that the research is completely new. Rather it means that it makes a significant contribution to the scholarly literature or discourse on the topic or sheds new light on the topic. This contribution can entail expanding what is known about the topic, disproving/challenging what is known, or contributing new knowledge to an identified research gap. For instance, a study may examine a similar issue as a previous study but in different populations, settings, or using different approaches. Researchers often select a topic that addresses a gap identified in the literature review. Researchers should critically reflect on their proposed topic and articulate what is unique or different about it and what potential contribution it makes to the literature or the field.

Significant and relevant: It is important to select a topic that will further the understanding of an issue and make a significant empirical, conceptual, theoretical, or methodological contribution to research, practice, policy, and/or teaching. The significance and relevance of a topic can be determined by answering the following question: Why is it important to research this topic? As much as possible, the topic should be timely and relevant to the current needs and priorities of one's discipline and community of interest. Staying up to date on current priorities in the field and engaging stakeholders in selecting a research topic are ways of ensuring its relevance and significance.

Ethical: Ensuring the ethical soundness of a research study is a proactive process that begins as early as selecting the research topic. Since the research topic defines the focus of the study and informs the formulation of the research questions, the researcher should select a topic that can be investigated in an ethically sound manner without violating any ethical codes or causing potential harm to the participants and the researcher. While not all ethical issues can be fully predicted, it is important to critically examine the potential ethical issues or unintended consequences of investigating the topic in order to mitigate their occurrence, reformulate the topic, or find alternative topics. For instance, one may ask: Would researching this topic put the researcher or participants at risk for physical, psychological, social, financial, or legal harm? Would confidentiality be an issue in researching a reportable or illegal behavior? Would research around traumatic events cause psychological harm to participants?

Feasible: Ensuring the feasibility of a topic earlier in the research process minimizes roadblocks throughout the remainder of the process. There are several aspects of feasibility that must be accounted for when selecting a topic. One aspect is whether the topic is researchable or do-able given its scope and nature. Previous literature can shed light on whether and how a similar topic has been researched in the past and can also aid in formulating a researchable topic.

Other important aspects of feasibility include the resources (human, material, financial), time frame, and competency/skills required to investigate the topic. For instance, some qualitative research designs such as ethnography require prolonged immersion in the study setting and multiple interactions with participants, thus may not be feasible for projects with tight deadlines and limited resources. Funding is a particularly critical consideration when selecting a topic since the nature and scope of the topic determines the potential expenses associated with the project. For instance, students proposing a dissertation or thesis that requires international travel may need to acquire external funds to support their travel and data collection. In some settings, an ethics committee review alone can cost as much as 1000 USD for foreign researchers who are not affiliated with the local institution. In addition, researchers should also reflect on the accessibility of the study setting and potential participants. Engaging various stakeholders throughout the research process and identifying local gatekeepers or connections facilitates access to study sites and participants for recruitment and data collection purposes. Additional feasibility considerations include the technical, linguistic, or interpersonal expertise of the researcher or the research team. For instance, a cross-cultural researcher who is not proficient in the local language may require professional translation and interpretation services that present additional expenses.

Culturally appropriate: The formulation of the research topic should be appropriate and relevant to the cultural context of the participants. Some topics may be considered sensitive or taboo within a particular cultural context, thus posing significant issues when implementing the study. This not only compromises the feasibility of the study but also poses an ethical concern as it may potentially harm or stigmatize the participants or community. Consulting, involving, or engaging key stakeholders from the cultural group in developing research topics and questions can help ensure their cultural appropriateness. Another important cultural consideration when selecting the research topic is the researcher's position in relation to the cultural context of the study (i.e., insider–outsider), whether and how they will gain access to the participants considering their position, as well as their cultural humility, technical, and interpersonal skills to carry out the research.

Selecting a Research Topic

Identify a broad research area of interest within your discipline. You can use your responses from the previous stop, think, and apply.

Next, list one topic within the research area you identified. Then answer the following questions:

1. Why are you interested in this topic?
2. Why is it important to research this topic?
3. What are the potential risks or harms (e.g., physical, psychological, social) to participants when researching this topic?
4. In two to three sentences, discuss the feasibility of researching this topic considering the required resources, technical skills, and the accessibility of the setting and potential participants.

This section has established that the research topic is often an area of personal or professional interest to the researcher, indicating that they have prior knowledge, experience, and assumptions about the chosen topic. The self-reflective process should therefore begin in the conceptualization phase of the research process, where the researcher acknowledges and articulates their philosophical assumptions, motivations for selecting the topic, assumptions or preconceptions about the topic, prior knowledge and experience with the topic, expectations from the research study, and potential influence on the study. Reflexivity is carried out with the goal of understanding the researcher's position in relation to the study, thus enabling them to remain open and grounded in participants' meanings and construction of the phenomenon as the study progresses. Box 3.2 presents an excerpt of a positionality statement, focusing on the section that articulates the researcher's position in relation to the research topic.

> **BOX 3.2** **Excerpt of a Researcher's Reflection on the Research Topic**
>
> *. . . I begin by positioning myself in relation to the research subject/topic. Having lived and worked in the Democratic Republic of Congo (DRC), I have witnessed the toll of fragile sociopolitical contexts on women and children, who are often the most vulnerable and neglected in such contexts. This led to my passion for Maternal and Child Health as I felt compelled to pursue endeavors that improve women and children's health, quality of life, and well-being amid competing sociopolitical priorities. My particular interest in investigating MDSR was prompted by the persistently high maternal mortality rate in the DRC and the dearth of research on MDSR in the DRC despite its high maternal mortality burden. My motivation for pursuing this study was driven by the evidence-informed value I place on MDSR as a promising high impact and cost-effective quality improvement tool for reducing preventable maternal deaths. I initiated this study with expectations that the findings will make important contributions to understanding and strengthening MDSR in the DRC, which will ultimately improve practice, policy, and maternal health. . . . While I entered into this study with no direct experience with MDSR, I had been immersed in the literature on MDSR in developing countries throughout the conceptualization and development of this study. Recognizing the potential influence of these preconceived ideas acquired from the literature, I remained open and grounded in my participants' unique experiences, perceptions, and context so as not to impose any preconceived codes and patterns on my data. . . . (Muvuka, 2019, pp. 125–126)*

The process of developing the research topic is iterative. At this early stage, the researcher is not expected to come up with a definitive or very detailed research topic because it is further developed or refined as they engage in a more structured critical analysis and synthesis of the literature. However, at this stage, the research topic should be focused enough to enable a focused review of related literature, during and after which it can be refined as needed.

CONDUCTING A LITERATURE REVIEW FOR A QUALITATIVE RESEARCH STUDY

After identifying the research topic, a more structured review of related literature can be conducted around a specific review question(s) related to the topic. As discussed in Module 1, a literature review provides a critical synthesis of the evidence on the topic, highlights the conflicts, gaps, and debates in the literature, and justifies the need and potential contribution of the proposed study to the existing body of knowledge. Essentially, it helps frame and focus the proposed study because it guides the formulation of the problem and research questions. In addition, the literature review provides the basis for comparing or relating the research findings with existing studies and theories in the discussion section of the research report. The three-phased literature review road map (Figure 3.9) discussed in Module 1 applies to literature reviews conducted as part of a qualitative, quantitative, or mixed methods study.

While qualitative research recognizes the value of a literature review, when to conduct it and to what extent it should be used is still debated and variable across the qualitative research designs (Tummers and Karsten, 2012). There are two main positions related to the use of a literature review in qualitative research. One position supports a review of related literature earlier in the research process (i.e., prior to data collection) to focus the study and inform the formulation of the research questions. Strauss and Corbin (1990), proponents of the evolved GTM, argue that a literature review conducted at the onset of the research process can stimulate questions and sensitivity to theoretical concepts from the data. A contrasting position that originates from the traditional GTM recommends delaying the review of related literature until after data collection and analysis, where it can be used to compare the study findings to the previous literature (Creswell, 2013; Glaser and Strauss, 1967). This position posits that a comprehensive review of related literature at the beginning of the study increases the researcher's likelihood of imposing preconceived notions or preexisting frameworks on the data and may suppress their openness to new themes or theories in the data (Glaser and Strauss, 1967). In addition, this position asserts that a literature review conducted after data collection and analysis is more likely to be focused and relevant as it covers the themes or categories that are identified from the data collected. Overall, both positions recognize the value of a literature review and share the common concern of protecting the researcher from imposing existing knowledge, patterns, or concepts on the data unless using a deductive analytic approach.

FIGURE 3.9. *The literature review process.*

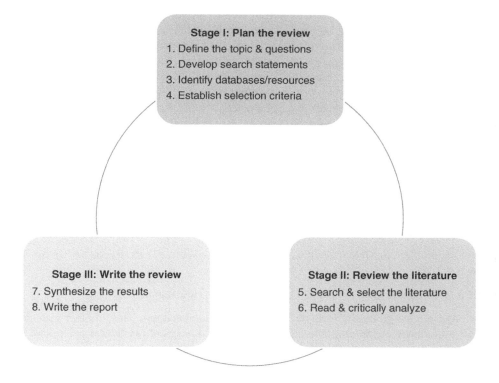

In practice, the recommendation of delaying a literature review until the end of the research process conflicts with most institutional requirements. Ethics committees, research committees, and funding agencies require a literature review to situate the proposed study in the context of the broader scholarly debate on the topic. As such, we present several options that take into consideration these institutional requirements and the variability of qualitative research designs, while staying true to the inductive qualitative research process. Researchers proposing a traditional grounded theory study can provide a strong rationale or justification for delaying the literature review in the research proposal submitted to their institution (Tummers and Karsten, 2012). Alternatively, a mini or preliminary literature review can be conducted when conceptualizing the study, just enough to justify the significance of the research problem and of the proposed study, while a more thorough literature review can be conducted in the later stage of the research process once the data are collected and analyzed (Creswell, 2013; Tummers and Karsten, 2012). Third, we recommend a formal and thorough literature review at the beginning of the research process to focus, justify, and position the study, provided that special measures are taken to remain grounded in the data rather than imposing concepts or theories from the literature. Whether a literature review is conducted earlier or later in the research process, we specifically recommend reflexivity during the literature review process, where the researcher questions and critically reflects on the preconceived notions acquired from the literature, the potential role of the literature in shaping the study or findings, and the measures to maintain the trustworthiness of the research findings (see Section 3) (Tummers and Karsten, 2012).

Given the emergent nature of qualitative research, the literature review can be expanded after data collection and analysis to accommodate and support the new themes or categories identified in the analysis. The literature review generates additional information needed to refine the topic, define the research problem, and formulate the research questions.

DEFINING THE RESEARCH PROBLEM

The research problem refers to a knowledge or practice gap, unresolved conflict or debate, issue, controversy, question, challenge, or need within the chosen research topic that calls for systematic investigation or resolution. In other words, the problem is the issue at the heart of the research process and the main reason for conducting the research study. The evidence and justification for the research problem can originate from the literature review, theory, or practice. Rather than starting with a broad research area or topic, some researchers begin the process with a specific research problem stemming from their prior knowledge and experience. For example, the limited participation of pregnant women living with HIV in an elimination of mother-to-child transmission of HIV (EMTCT) program can lead the researcher to design a qualitative study exploring the factors influencing EMTCT uptake among women in a specific setting. The literature review can highlight several problems but the researcher's decision to focus on a particular research problem should be based on: (a) the scientific and practical significance of the problem to the field/discipline, society/community, and organization; (b) the feasibility of the research study around the problem considering the context and resources; and (c) the researcher's interest and skills. Overall, the research problem should reflect the current priorities in the field and the society, and should be selected with the goal of making a significant and unique contribution to the field. The attributes of a good research topic discussed earlier in this section also apply to the research problem. The following questions can help the researcher in identifying a problem and in evaluating its potential as a research problem:

- What is the problem (e.g., issue, gap, controversy) that leads to the need for your proposed study?
- Who is affected? When? Where? How?
- Is the problem significant enough to merit investigation?
- Will your research make a significant contribution to the field or body of knowledge?
- Is research on the problem feasible given the current context, resources, time frame, and competency or technical requirements?
- Is the problem researchable in an ethical and culturally appropriate manner?

These questions can also guide the formulation of a problem statement. The *problem statement* describes the nature, scope, and importance of the problem using scholarly evidence and provides a persuasive argument for the necessity of the proposed research study. This statement should be carefully crafted to draw interest in and attention to the research problem and consequently, the study itself. The problem statement is often found in the introduction section of a research article or a thesis/dissertation report, where it varies in length from a few sentences in a research article to one or more pages in a thesis or dissertation report. While there is no specific formula for writing a problem statement, an effective problem statement contains the following elements (Table 3.1; Box 3.3): (a) a description of the ideal or desired situation; (b) a description of the general and specific problem or deviation; (c) a description of the impacts or significance of the problem; and (d) the proposed solution and role of the proposed research study.

TABLE 3.1. Elements of a Problem Statement

Description of the ideal or desired situation
- Brief description of the normal/desired/ideal/acceptable situation related to the specific topic

Description of the general and specific problem or deviation
- Description of the general and specific problem or deviation from the ideal, including its nature, scope, and context—the who, what, when, where, how of the problem
- Summary of previous research on the specific problem
- The gaps or limitations in the literature on the specific problem

Description of the impacts or significance of the problem
- Description of the impacts of the problem on society and on the priority population
- Description of the potential consequences of not addressing the problem
- Description of the potential benefits of resolving the problem—So what?

Proposed solution and role of the proposed research
- Statement of the necessity of research into the problem and how research may support or inform solutions to the problem.
- Description of the role of the proposed research in understanding or addressing the problem

BOX 3.3 A Dissection of a Problem Statement from a Peer-Reviewed Article

Jeffrey et al. Diabetol Metab Syndr (2019) 11:84
https://doi.org/10.1186/s13098-019-0480-4

Diabetology & Metabolic Syndrome

RESEARCH **Open Access**

Mobile phone applications and their use in the self-management of Type 2 Diabetes Mellitus: a qualitative study among app users and non-app users

Bronte Jeffrey[1], Melina Bagala[1†], Ashley Creighton[1†], Tayla Leavey[1†], Sarah Nicholls[1†], Crystal Wood[1†], Jo Longman[2], Jane Barker[2] and Sabrina Pit[3,4*]

Background

In Australia, people living in regional or remote areas have higher rates of diabetes and experience worse health related outcomes than people living in urban areas [1]. Type 2 Diabetes Mellitus (T2DM) is a major contributor to higher death rates outside major cities and accounts for 6% of excess deaths in all age groups [1, 2]. This is attributed to several factors, including decreased accessibility to health services (fewer health professionals and financial accessibility), decreased testing and possibly less effective management [2]. self-management strategies may help to e issues.

Self-management is considered the most important factor in ensuring well-controlled blood glucose levels (BGL) and, thereby, preventing diabetes complications [3, 4]. It has the potential to ease the burden on the healthcare system by encouraging patient autonomy and allowing disease monitoring outside clinical settings [5–8]. Self-management strategies include tracking blood glucose trends, adhering to medication or insulin therapy, monitoring nutrition and increasing physical activity [9]. Current research has established that apps are feasible tools to improve self-management of diabetes [4, 6, 10]. App use has been demonstrated to result in positive self-management behaviours, such as improved diets and attitudes towards diabetes self-management, increased physical activity and BGL monitoring [4, 11]. ecent meta-analysis has demonstrated e with T2DM, the use of diabetes apps standard self-management results in a nt reduction in HBA1C, a long-term marker of BGL control [6, 9].

Despite these positive outcomes, in Australia, only 8% of people with T2DM are reported to use apps to support diabetes self-management [12]. This poor uptake is multifactorial, with limitations including a lack of education integration into app technology, generic and impersonal information, perceived difficulty of use and an inability to export data or integrate with health professionals' records [4, 7, 9, 13]. Additionally, there is concern about the feasibility of sustained use of apps [14–16] with minimal data exploring long term app usage outside of short randomised control trials. From the patient perspective, studies have identified that people with T2DM do not believe apps will be useful, resulting in low uptake [12, 16–18]. Recent data from an Australian qualitative study demonstrated that people with T2DM would prefer an app to address the practical aspects of diabetes self-management and to improve, and reduce the cognitive burden of self-management [17]. Further s focus groups for app development have hi importance of blood glucose monitoring, d ing, education, interactive content, peer realistic goal setting [19–22]. Despite this, the uptake of apps usage to support diabetes self-management remains low, [12]. Additionally, current research has concluded that there is a paucity of qualitative data on current user app experience and factors influencing consumer engagement [5, 11, 12, 18].

The lack of qualitative evidence surrounding health app usage was addressed by Anderson et al. [5] who conducted the first study combining three theoretical frameworks to qualitatively explore users' experience of apps in relation to chronic conditions; The Technology Acceptance Model (TAM) measures how users accept technology and is based on the Theory of Reasoned Action [23]. The Health Information Technology Acceptance Model (HITAM) furthers the concepts in TAM to focus on health by incorporating the Health Belief Model [24]. The Mobile Application Rating Scale (MARS) includes theoretical constructs of engagement, functionality, aesthetics and information quality [25]. The integration of these frameworks provides robust theoretical grounding for research into the consumer experience of mobile phone apps [5].

The present study uses the interview guide developed by Anderson et al. [5], based on the three frameworks, in relation to T2DM. To our knowledge, there are no studies that have focused on app use in an Australian rural population where issues of healthcare access may increase the importance of self-management strategies.

Overall, further qualitative evidence is required to obtain an accurate summary of consumer experiences and preferences to shape targeted app innovation and development. User-centred diabetes apps have the potential to improve health outcomes, particularly in rural areas where access to formal health services is relatively restricted. Therefore, this study aims to acquire a greater understanding of the perceived useful features, facilitators and barriers to app usage for the self-management of T2DM in a rural population.

Source: Adapted from "Mobile Phone Applications and Their Use in the Self-management of Type 2 Diabetes Mellitus: A Qualitative Study among App Users and Non-app Users," by Jeffrey, B. et al., 2019, *Diabetology & Metabolic Syndrome*, 11, 84. Copyright 2019 by the Authors. Creative Commons Attribution 4.0 International License (http://creativecommons.org/licenses/by/4.0).

Dissecting the Problem Statement

Select a research article and identify the problem statement. Dissect the problem statement and highlight or annotate the following elements of the problem statement:

- Description of the ideal or desired situation
- Description of the problem or deviation from the desired situation
- Description of the impacts or significance of the problem
- Proposed solution and role of the proposed research study

Overall, there are two main positions related to the process of deriving the research problem and questions in qualitative research. The traditional or classic grounded theory endorsed by Glaser and Strauss (1967) argues that the specific research problem and questions emerge from the research process, during data collection and analysis. In this approach, a detailed problem statement is developed or finalized when writing up the research report. This contrasts with Strauss and Corbin's (1990) stance that aligns with current institutional requirements of developing the research problem and questions prior to undertaking the study. We recommend specifying the research problem, purpose, and questions when conceptualizing the study with the expectation that more specific research problems and questions can arise from the predefined problem and questions over the course of the study, given the emergent and dynamic nature of qualitative research.

DEFINING THE PURPOSE OF THE STUDY

The purpose statement often follows and complements the problem statement. In some cases, it is an extension of the problem statement as it partially fits into the aforementioned "proposed solution and role of the proposed research" section of the problem statement. The purpose statement communicates the general goal or intent, direction, and focus of the study in response to the identified research problem. Note that the purpose statement does not communicate a solution to address the problem but rather highlights the focus or direction of the research study itself, whether it is to explore, describe, explain, evaluate, or assess the phenomenon of interest. In addition, it indicates the method of inquiry, the sample or unit of analysis, and the setting. The purpose statement can be a sentence in the introduction section of a research article or a few paragraphs in the introduction chapter of a thesis or dissertation. An effective purpose statement contains all or most of the following elements (Creswell, 2013):

- The purpose of this **[insert qualitative design:** e.g., case study, grounded theory, phenomenological, ethnographical, or narrative] study is to **[insert appropriate qualitative verb**: e.g., explore, identify, describe, explain, assess, evaluate, investigate] the **[insert the central phenomenon being investigated]** in/among/for **[insert participants or unit of analysis**: individual, group, organization/institution, system] in/at **[insert study setting]**.

- This **[insert qualitative design**: e.g., case study, grounded theory, phenomenology, ethnography, or narrative study] study aims to **[insert appropriate qualitative verb**: e.g., explore, identify, describe, explain, assess, evaluate, investigate] the **[insert the phenomenon being investigated]** in/among **[insert participants or unit of analysis**: individual, group, organization, system] in/at **[insert study setting]**.

Note that the verbs used in the purpose statement should be consistent with the general purpose of qualitative inquiry. For instance, exploring, describing, explaining, and evaluating are more indicative of qualitative research while measuring, quantifying, or testing are more appropriate for quantitative studies. Box 3.4 provides specific examples of purpose statements for different qualitative research designs.

BOX 3.4 **Examples of Purpose Statements**

- **Example of a purpose statement in a case study**
  "We used a qualitative case study approach to explore the various features of the NHRC's [Navrongo Health Research Center] CE [Community Engagement] process and how it has been perceived by a range of stakeholders such as researchers, community leaders, and research participants." (Tindana et al., 2011, p. 1858).

- **Example of a purpose statement in a grounded theory study**
  "This study aimed to generate a theory of shared resilience using a constructivist grounded theory approach. This study therefore aimed to explore what resilience means in the context of couplehood in dementia, how dyads experience a shared sense of resilience, how they develop and maintain resilience and how this impacts upon their relationship." (Conway et al., 2020, p. 219).

- **Example of a purpose statement in an ethnographic study**
  "We used community-based ethnography and public health risk assessment to assess beliefs about pesticide exposure risks among farmworkers in the Lower Yakima Valley of Washington State" (Snipes et al., 2009, p. S616).

- **Example of a purpose statement in a phenomenological study**
  "Our study aims to understand the subjective experience of nurses participating in nursing COVID-19 patients through semistructured interviews and to analyze the data using phenomenological methods, providing fundamental data for the psychological experience of nurses." (Sun et al., 2020, p. 593)

- **Example of a purpose statement in a narrative study**
  "Our aim is to explore how mental health recovery unfolds through individuals' engagement in everyday activities." (Reed et al., 2020, p. 2)

FORMULATING THE RESEARCH QUESTIONS

Once the purpose of the study has been formulated, the research questions can be crafted. Given its exploratory nature, qualitative research does not test a hypothesis but is rather guided by one or more research questions. Research questions are the overarching or central questions about the problem or phenomenon that the research study sets out to answer. The research questions are an extension and breakdown of the purpose statement, formulated in an interrogative or question format. They drive and focus the study, directing the methodological decisions pertaining to the research design, data collection, sample, data analysis and interpretation, and the reporting of findings. Given their fundamental role, the research questions should be properly formulated because poorly conceptualized research questions can affect the feasibility and quality of the study. Research questions should not be confused with interview or focus group questions that are specific questions asked of participants during data collection in attempt to respond to the research questions. A well conducted literature review often culminates in focused research questions for the proposed study, although these questions can also be derived from practice.

Some qualitative research designs (e.g., traditional grounded theory) recommend the formulation of the research questions during data collection and analysis on the grounds that the preliminary data and findings can inspire more relevant and specific research questions about the problem or phenomenon. However, for practical and ethical reasons, we recommend formulating the research questions when conceptualizing the study to focus the inquiry and enable a proactive evaluation of the study's ethical and practical feasibility. In addition, including well-crafted research questions in the research proposal facilitates its review and approval by research committees, funding agencies, and ethics committees because these questions communicate the direction of the study. Unlike quantitative research questions, qualitative research questions can evolve throughout the research process. As the study progresses and generates preliminary findings, new questions can be generated, or old questions refined to deepen the understanding of the phenomenon being investigated. At the minimum, the initial research questions should be focused but general and open-ended to accommodate new themes, concepts, theories, and sub-questions as needed over the course of the data collection and analysis.

The process of formulating focused research questions is iterative, reflexive, and interactive (Agee, 2009). It is an iterative process because formulating focused research questions requires several rounds of writing, feedback, and revisions. This process begins with brainstorming on what the researchers would like to know about the research problem, including how, and why. Brainstorming sessions generate a list of potential research questions related to the problem, from which the researchers selects one or more priority or central research questions to guide the inquiry. The process of formulating qualitative research questions is also reflexive because it requires the researcher to proactively reflect on the ethical, cultural, methodological, and practical implications of asking and answering the research questions. More specifically, when formulating the research questions, the researcher should reflect on their own assumptions and presuppositions, how these questions position them relative to their potential participants (i.e., insider–outsider, power dynamics), as well as the potential effects of answering the research questions on participants' lives (Agee, 2009). In addition, the researcher should anticipate the participants, data collection methods, and data analysis methods that will be required to answer the research questions. Practicing reflexivity when formulating the research questions protects the researcher from asking leading research questions with embedded assumptions and ensures the feasibility of the study given the ethical, cultural, and practical/logistical considerations. If the initial research questions are deemed problematic, there may be alternative questions or alternative ways of formulating the questions. Finally, the formulation of research questions is interactive and collaborative. To ensure the ethical and cultural appropriateness of the research questions, researchers should consult or engage advisors, peers, and stakeholders in formulating appropriate research questions. Those conducting qualitative research as part of a community-based participatory research (Module 1) are particularly expected to involve their community partners in formulating appropriate research questions.

The following are the attributes of qualitative research questions:

Open-ended. Qualitative research questions do not have a simple yes/no answer but are formulated using how, what, or why questions to enable an in-depth exploration of perspectives, meanings, and experiences related to the phenomenon of interest. In addition, qualitative research questions should not be leading but should be formulated in a way that is open to discovering new themes.

Evolving. As the study progresses and generates preliminary findings, new research questions can be generated, or old research questions can be refined to deepen the understanding of the phenomenon being investigated.

Focused or specific. The research questions should be formulated in a way that delineates the scope of the inquiry. The research questions should specify the phenomenon or situation being investigated and the particular population of focus. For example, the research question, "What are the health insurance-related experiences of residents of West Louisville, Kentucky?" clearly indicates that the study was interested in exploring health insurance experiences (the phenomenon) in a sample of residents of West Louisville, a geographical location defined by specific zip codes (Ali et al., 2018). While specific, this research question was also broad enough to capture diverse experiences related to health insurance such as applying or signing up for health insurance, utilizing health insurance, and changing or discontinuing health insurance.

Answerable/researchable. The research questions should be answerable given the resources and time available to the researchers and participants, as well as the context in which the research is being conducted.

Ethical and culturally appropriate. Research questions should be answerable or researchable without violating the ethical codes for conducting research and the cultural norms of a community. In other words, the research questions should be designed in compliance with the ethical principles discussed in Section 3 and should be sensitive to the cultural context of the investigation.

Clear. The research questions should be clear, explicit, and stand-alone statements of what the research attempts to answer, leaving no room for misunderstanding or additional explanations by the researcher.

Concise. The research questions should be brief, with each question expressing a single idea or focus. Double barreled or embedded questions should be broken down into separate research questions or sub-questions. The number of research questions depends on the complexity and scope of the proposed research study. Some studies have a single research question while others have more than one research question with sub-questions. It is important to limit the number of research questions for feasibility purposes and to keep the study focused. One to three well-crafted research questions may be sufficient as a starting point, knowing that additional questions may be generated during the inquiry.

BOX 3.5 Examples of Research Questions by Study Designs

Example 1: Case study
A qualitative case study exploring the perceptions of the health implications of climate change and the links between these perceptions and mitigative behaviors among residents of the Canadian Golden Horseshoe region asked the following research question: "What are the knowledge, attitudes, and practices related to global environmental change and health of residents of the greater Hamilton area of the Canadian Golden Horseshoe region?" (Cardwell and Elliott, 2013, p. 2)

Example 2: Ethnographic study
An ethnographic study exploring the community's reception of community health workers (CHWs) posed the following research questions: "How are CHWs professional roles enacted? Do professional roles interact with other CHWs roles? If so, which ones and how?" (Rafiq et al., 2019)

Example 3: Grounded theory
Khisa et al. (2017) conducted a grounded theory study exploring the heath seeking behaviors of women with obstetric fistula, guided by the following research question: "What patterns of health seeking do women with obstetric fistula display in their quest for healing?"

Example 4: Phenomenological study
A phenomenological study by Lännerström et al. (2013, p. 2) describing the lived experiences of individuals with long-term sickness who had been sick-listed or placed on prolonged sick leave posed the following research questions: "What does it mean to be sick-listed? What does it mean to not be able to work because of illness? What are the aftermaths of life as a sick-listed person? How is one's life-world changed?"

Example 5: Narrative study
A constructivist, feminist, narrative study describing the trauma recovery process among women who survived childhood maltreatment (CM) posed the following research question: "What does thriving look like in women surviving CM [childhood maltreatment]?" (Hall, 2011, p. 3)

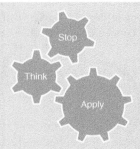

Formulating Research Questions

1. Identify a broad research area of interest and a specific topic within this research area. You can use your responses from the previous stop, think, and apply.
2. State the purpose of your research.
3. Generate three research questions about your research topic.
4. Ask your instructor or peer to provide feedback on your research questions based on the following criteria:

	Yes	No
Open-ended	☐	☐
Focused or specific	☐	☐
Answerable/researchable	☐	☐
Ethical and culturally appropriate	☐	☐
Clear	☐	☐
Concise	☐	☐

USING THEORETICAL AND CONCEPTUAL FRAMEWORKS IN QUALITATIVE RESEARCH

Apart from the philosophical paradigms that offer a broader lens through which the researcher views the world, the theoretical framework shapes the researcher's perspectives and methodological decisions. The literature review, theoretical framework, and conceptual framework are interlinked and collectively serve as the foundation for conceptualizing the research study. The empirical and theoretical findings derived from the literature form the basis for developing the theoretical and conceptual frameworks guiding the study. Currently, the use of theoretical and conceptual frameworks in qualitative research is still debated given its largely inductive nature. Quantitative studies apply theories deductively (i.e., from the beginning of the study) to test and verify these theories (Creswell and Creswell, 2018). While some qualitative studies utilize a deductive approach to examine the applicability of preexisting theories to specific circumstances, qualitative research is primarily designed to inductively build theory from the data rather than testing or verifying preexisting theories. An inductive qualitative approach therefore offers a new conceptualization of the topic or expands the existing conceptualization of the topic. Some qualitative designs, such as grounded theory, discourage the utilization or application of a theoretical framework so that the researcher does not impose any theoretical frameworks on the data but rather allows the theory to be built from the data.

Overall, the use of theory in qualitative research is highly variable. There are four main applications and placements of theory in qualitative research (Collins and Stockton, 2018):

1. Theory can be used as a guiding framework for conceptualizing the study and informing the methodological decisions.

2. Theory can be applied in data analysis (i.e., deductive analytic approach), where the data are coded using predetermined codes derived from theory.

3. A theory can be built from the data as the final outcome or product of the research study through an inductive analytic approach (e.g., grounded theory).

4. Theory can be used to interpret and contextualize the findings.

Many qualitative research reports do not explicitly articulate the theoretical framework guiding their study. However, this does not mean that they are not theory driven. Like other qualitative researchers and authors (Guba and Lincoln, 1994; Merriam, 2009), we acknowledge that all research is implicitly or explicitly driven by deep seated philosophical paradigms and theoretical frameworks that shape the researcher's worldview, thus their research priorities or problems they perceive to be important, the research questions, the methodological decisions to investigate these questions, as well as their interpretation of the findings. This is also true for researchers using an inductive qualitative approach (Merriam, 2009). Collins and Stockton (2018, p. 2) argue that

"a researcher who cannot articulate a theoretical framework may not have done the difficult and essential work to unearth their deepest operating principles and preconceptions about their study. The belief that preconceived notions do not exist or impact a study is, in fact, a theoretical disposition."

Since our theoretical frameworks operate implicitly or explicitly to shape the study, the main concern with using theory in qualitative research is the over-reliance on theory or the imposition of theoretical frameworks on the data. Theoretical frameworks direct what we see and ask but can also influence what we do not see and ask in our research (Merriam, 2009). A key question in qualitative research is therefore how to use theories appropriately such that they guide the research rather than dictating, obstructing, restricting, or limiting it. Collins and Stockton (2018) argue that when correctly used and acknowledged, theories can help researchers in identifying and questioning their theoretical assumptions and in remaining open to new findings that either confirm or negate these assumptions. While some propose the process of bracketing or extracting the researcher's view from the data, we agree with Collins and Stockton (2018) that this operationalization of bracketing is impossible to achieve. We rather view bracketing as an act of reflexivity that allows the researcher to reflect on and report their biases and interpretations, thus enabling them to remain open to new theories despite being guided by preexisting ones.

While the terms theoretical and conceptual frameworks are often used interchangeably, they are two distinct terms. The theoretical framework is an intersection of theories; it incorporates constructs from multiple theories, forming a coherent theoretical lens through which knowledge related to the phenomenon is processed. It is a road map that guides the formulation of the research questions and informs decisions related to the research design, data collection and analysis, and ultimately the interpretation of the research findings (Calba et al., 2015). The theories forming part of the theoretical framework are derived from the following sources:

- *Discipline/field*: individuals are introduced to multiple theories within their respective disciplines throughout their studies and practice (Merriam, 2009)

- *Literature*: a review of related literature reveals concepts, theories, or models that have been applied by previous studies on the topic as well as their strengths and limitations

- *Philosophical paradigms*: the researcher's philosophical paradigms influence their theoretical orientations and perspectives

Conversely, a conceptual framework is more specific and concrete than a theoretical framework. It is a logical narrative or visual representation of the main ideas, concepts, and relationships that the study aims to explore (Miles and Huberman, 1994; Reichel and Ramey, 1987). It is a concept map that displays the main concepts of the study and a tentative theory of their interrelationships. For instance, Figure 3.10 depicts a conceptual framework for a qualitative research proposal to assess women's perceptions and experiences of the quality of health facility–based childbirth services. This conceptual framework was adapted from Donabedian's (1966) model of quality of care and Hulton et al.'s (2000) framework for the evaluation of quality of care in maternity services.

In qualitative research, the conceptual framework can be refined to reflect new findings as data are collected, analyzed, and interpreted. Unlike the theoretical framework, which is formed from multiple theories, a conceptual framework is constructed from the concepts and relationships derived from multiple sources in addition to theories. Maxwell (2009) asserts that a conceptual framework is built by incorporating elements from the following major sources: theory and research, experiential knowledge, thought experiments, and pilot/exploratory studies. Overall, the conceptual framework is shaped by the empirical literature and theoretical framework. This means that the research study and its conceptual framework are situated within the theoretical framework, which is in turn situated within the philosophical paradigms.

FIGURE 3.10. *A conceptual framework for the quality of health facility-based childbirth services.*

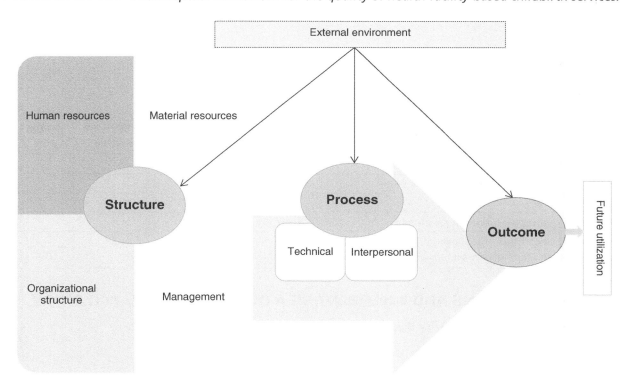

SUMMARY

The conceptualization phase of the research study follows an inverted pyramid pattern, starting with a broad research area that is gradually refined into a specific research topic, research problem, research purpose, and research questions through the literature review, brainstorming, and concept mapping.

While a literature review is typically conducted in the conceptualization phase, some qualitative designs (e.g., traditional grounded theory) recommend delaying the literature review until after data collection and analysis so as not to impose preconceived notions on the study. In qualitative research, the literature review can be expanded after data collection and analysis to address new themes or categories identified in the analysis.

The problem statement describes the nature, scope, and importance of the problem at the heart of the study and justifies the need for the proposed study. The purpose statement articulates the goal or intent of the study in response to the identified research problem and often indicates the method of inquiry, the sample or unit of analysis, and the setting.

Qualitative research does not test a hypothesis but is rather guided by one or more open-ended research questions. While formulated during the conceptualization phase, qualitative research questions can evolve as the study generates preliminary data and findings, to deepen the understanding of the phenomenon.

The theoretical framework incorporates constructs from multiple theories and provides a road map that informs methodological decisions. Conversely, a conceptual framework is a narrative or visual representation of the main concepts and relationships that the study aims to investigate. It is constructed using evidence from theory, experiential knowledge, thought experiments, and research. In qualitative research, the conceptual framework can be refined to reflect new findings as data are collected, analyzed, and interpreted.

Reflexivity and positionality begin in the conceptualization phase, where the researcher acknowledges and articulates their philosophical assumptions, motivations for selecting the topic, preconceptions about the topic, expectations from the research study, how these factors potentially influence the study, and measures to remain grounded in the data.

Now that I have reached the end of this section, I am able to:

Course objective	Strongly agree	Somewhat agree	Neutral	Somewhat disagree	Strongly Agree
Select a research topic for a qualitative study					
Explain the elements of a problem statement					
Develop a purpose statement					
Formulate qualitative research questions					
Explain the use of theoretical and conceptual frameworks in qualitative research					

SECTION 3: DESIGNING AND IMPLEMENTING A QUALITATIVE RESEARCH STUDY

By the end of this section, learners will be able to:

- Describe qualitative data collection methods
- Analyze and interpret qualitative data
- Develop an outline for a qualitative research report
- Discuss relevant ethical and cultural considerations in each phase of the qualitative research process

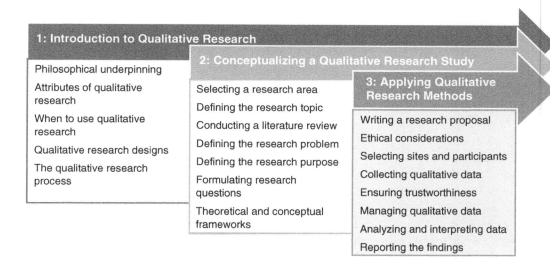

INTRODUCTION

This final section pulls it all together as it discusses the application of qualitative research methods, taking into account the technical, methodological, ethical, cultural, and logistical considerations. This section specifically discusses the process of designing and implementing the qualitative research methods and procedures to answer the research questions. This section concludes with a discussion of the principles for reporting and disseminating qualitative research findings.

WRITING A QUALITATIVE RESEARCH PROPOSAL

As with any type of research, qualitative research requires a clearly formulated research plan that provides details on the proposed research methods and procedures to guide the implementation of the study. The research proposal or protocol represents the research plan. It presents background information on the problem and the philosophical, theoretical, and conceptual frameworks guiding the study and provides a detailed account of the planned research procedures from the beginning to the end of the study. While a qualitative research proposal communicates the planned course of action in sufficient detail, it is built with flexibility to accommodate the emergent, inductive, and dynamic nature of qualitative research as discussed throughout this section. The structure and contents of a research proposal are both variable across disciplines and institutions; however, the basic elements of a qualitative research proposal are depicted in Table 3.2.

TABLE 3.2. The Structure and Contents of a Qualitative Research Proposal

Title
- The title of the study (include the specific topic and qualitative design)
- Authors, credentials, and affiliations
- Institution the proposal is submitted to
- Date produced or submitted

Table of Contents

Introduction
- Statement of the broad and specific problem
- Background information on the problem (i.e., summary of the literature review)
- Statement of the purpose, aims, or objectives of the study
- Research questions
- The structure/organization of the report (for longer reports such as dissertations)

TABLE 3.2. (Continued)

Literature review (can be included in the introduction section if not a required section)
- Related literature
- Conceptual framework

Methodology
- Description of the study setting and context
- Philosophical paradigm
- Theoretical/interpretive framework
- Qualitative design and rationale for the design selection
- Researcher's role and relevant background (i.e., reflexivity/positionality statement)
- Participants and other data sources
    - Sample, sampling methods, and sample size
    - Accessing the study site and participants
    - Recruitment methods (e.g., email, phone) and procedures
    - Incentives or compensation (if applicable)
- Data collection
    - Data collection methods and procedures (include duration)
    - Description of data collection tools and equipment
    - Informed consent process
- Data management procedures
    - Storage, digitization, transcription, verification, translation
    - Ethical considerations in data handling and storage
- Data analysis procedures
    - Unit of analysis
    - Analysis methods, procedures (e.g., coding, derivation of themes), and personnel
    - Software
- Ethical considerations and protection of human participants
- Strategies for ensuring the trustworthiness of the findings

Dissemination
- The target audiences of the research findings (including rationale)
- The proposed dissemination methods for each audience and the aspects/sections of the research to share
    - Can include potential academic journals and scientific conferences to disseminate the report

References

Appendices
- Data collection tools
- Templates of authorization letters for accessing sites
- Recruitment scripts or materials
- Consent documents
- Research timeline
- Proposed budget

Once finalized, the research proposal undergoes two major types of review and approval prior to the implementation of the study. The first consists of a scientific review and approval by a research committee (e.g., dissertation committee) and/or funding agency, while the second consists of an ethical review and approval by an authorized ethics or institutional review board, as discussed in Module 1.

ETHICAL CONSIDERATIONS

After a scientific review and approval of the research proposal, any research study involving human participants must undergo an ethics review and approval to ensure that it meets the highest ethical standards for research. Ethics and institutional review boards are responsible for reviewing research proposals to evaluate compliance with ethical codes for conducting research with human participants. They particularly ensure that participants are protected from any potential risks or harm and that they acquire the benefits associated with the study. As discussed more extensively in Module 1, the landmark ethical codes for conducting research such as the Nuremberg Code and the Belmont Report were triggered by historical unethical research practices such as the Nazi medical experiments and the Tuskegee Study of Untreated Syphilis in the Negro Male from 1932 to 1972. The Belmont report is particularly an important reference for biomedical and social-behavioral research studies globally as it outlines the following internationally accepted ethical principles for conducting research with human participants (United States National Commission for the Protection of Human Subjects of Biomedical and Behavioral Research, 1978): (a) respect for persons; (b) beneficence (and nonmaleficence); and (c) justice. These ethical principles must be upheld throughout the qualitative research process and, more importantly, when designing the study, collecting data, analyzing, and disseminating the findings.

The principle of *respect for persons* refers to the protection of an individual's autonomy to make informed decisions. This principle is primarily embodied in the informed consent document, which must be formally administered to participants prior to collecting any data from them and renegotiated throughout the qualitative research process. In keeping with the principle of respect for persons, the informed consent document provides sufficient information about the study, including an overview of the study, voluntary participation with no penalty for nonparticipation, participants' rights to withdraw from the study at any time without any penalty, as well as the researcher's obligation to maintain confidentiality or anonymity throughout the study to the extent permitted by the law.

The principle of *beneficence* obliges researchers to maximize the potential benefits of the study to the participants and the society. The benefits of the study can be maximized by ensuring the methodological integrity of the study and by reporting and disseminating the findings to those with the capacity to act on them. Ethics committees require that the researcher conduct a risk–benefit assessment of their proposed study, where they must demonstrate that the potential benefits outweigh the potential risks associated with the study. In compliance with this principle, the informed consent form must provide participants with accurate information about the potential risks and benefits associated with the study. This includes information that the study may not benefit the participants directly but may be beneficial to the community, the profession, or the society. The following is an example of a statement of benefits taken from an informed consent form:

> *The information collected from this study may not benefit you directly. The information learned from this study will inform activities to improve maternal health services.*

The principle of *nonmaleficence* is closely related to beneficence; it requires researchers to assess, prevent, and mitigate the potential risks or harms associated with the study. This includes a careful assessment and transparent communication of any anticipated physical, psychological, social, professional, financial/economic, or legal harm that individuals may incur for participating in the study. Qualitative research often makes use of open-ended questions that allow participants to elaborate on their experiences and perspectives, some of which may be sensitive or personal. As such, any breach of confidentiality and anonymity may have adverse psychological, social, financial, or professional consequences for participants. Overall, the potential risks associated with the study should not outweigh the potential benefits of the study. A study is determined to pose minimal risk to participants when the probability and magnitude of the potential risks are not greater than those normally encountered on a regular day. Many qualitative research studies that do not include an intervention are minimal risk research and may be eligible for an expedited ethics review. A study is said to present greater than minimal risk when the probability and magnitude of the potential risks are significantly higher than encountered on a normal day but still acceptable when taking into account the benefits of the study. Greater than minimal risk studies often require a strong scientific justification, a full ethics committee review, and additional measures to protect participants. The following is an example of a statement of the potential risks taken from a qualitative research protocol:

> *There are no known risks associated with this study. However, discussions about health and social issues may be frustrating for participants with negative experiences. Participants will be informed that they can end their participation at any time without losing any benefits. The potential risk to the research participants is minimal and not more than they would encounter in everyday life.*

The ethical principle of *justice* ensures that the study does not exploit, manipulate, or discriminate against certain individuals or populations. This is important in qualitative research since participants are often selected purposively based on their knowledge or experience with the phenomenon being investigated. Even for such sampling methods, the selection of participants must be fair and justified, and the benefits and burdens associated with the study must be fairly distributed across the participants and the society. This principle places an emphasis on protecting vulnerable populations that have historically been at higher risk for exploitation, coercion, manipulation, and deprivation of benefits in research activities, such as socioeconomically disadvantaged individuals, pregnant women, children, incarcerated individuals, and individuals with disabilities. The inclusion of vulnerable populations in research, especially in greater than minimal risk research, often receives more scrutiny from the ethics review committee and warrants further justification and protective measures for participants.

The Informed Consent Form and Process

Before the interview, focus group, or observation, the researcher begins by administering and obtaining informed consent from participants as indicated by the Ethics/Institutional Review Board. The informed consent form complies with the ethical principle of autonomy or respect for persons because it provides potential participants with general information about the study to enable informed decisions about whether or not to participate. The informed consent document (Box 3.6) is written in nontechnical language, at the reading level of participants, and in a language they can understand. It typically contains the following key information that must be highlighted during the consent process:

- An invitation to participate in the research study
- An overview of the study
- What participation entails
- Potential risks and benefits
- How results will be utilized
- Audio or video recording
- Duration of participation
- Incentives or compensation
- Measures to ensure confidentiality or anonymity
- Secure data handling and storage
- Voluntary participation with no penalty for nonparticipation
- Participants' rights to discontinue participation anytime, for any reason, with no questions asked and no penalties
- Contact persons for questions, concerns, or complaints about the study
- Names and signatures of the participants (if signed consent) and of the researcher

There are different types of informed consent documents depending on the level of potential risks associated with the study and on the characteristics of participants:

- *Signed informed consent:* requires a written signature from the participant. While some institutions require signed consent for all research with human participants regardless of the overall potential risk, signed consent is commonly used for invasive research studies or those classified as greater than minimal risk.
- *Waiver of signed consent or waiver of documentation of informed consent:* a waiver of signed consent is used in minimal risk research that does not collect sensitive personally identifiable information, does not involve any research procedures for which signed consent is normally required, and/or involves a group for which signing forms is not the norm. In this case, the participant is still given a consent form, but they issue a verbal, implied, or electronic consent to take part in the study rather than a written consent (University of California San Francisco, n.d.). For verbal consent, the participant verbally indicates whether or not they agree to participate in the study after reading the consent form. Online or electronic consent often involves clicking Agree or Continue after reading the information about the study in an email or on a website. The implied consent is one in which participants are given information about the

study and implicitly grant their permission by completing an anonymized sociodemographic survey prior to the interview or focus group. While still containing all the information required of a consent form, these unsigned consent forms (e.g., Box 3.6) tend to be shorter than signed informed consent forms.

- *Waiver of consent:* involves research that does not require obtaining any type of consent from participants, such as research studies involving secondary data that have already been collected and deidentified.
- *Assent and parental permission consent document:* the term consent is used when referring to adult participants who are capable of making an informed decision while assent is obtained from children within a particular age range to indicate their agreement to take part in a study. Research studies involving children are often required to obtain a signed parental permission consent document in addition to the assent obtained from the child.

BOX 3.6 An Unsigned Consent Template

[Title of the Study]

Date:
Dear_____,

You are being invited to participate in a research study that **[explain the purpose of the study]**. This study is conducted by **[insert name and position of the researcher]** of/at the **[insert name of the institution]**. Your participation will include **[insert data collection methods (e.g., an interview)]**. For this, you will be asked to **[explain what participants will be asked to do (e.g., provide information)]**. There are no known risks for your participation in this research study. The information collected may not benefit you directly. The information collected in this study may be helpful to others. The information you provide will **[explain what the information will be used for]**. Your completed **[insert data collection method or output]** will be stored in a secure location at **[site of file storage]**. Your participation will take approximately **[insert duration]**.

Individuals from the **[insert name of sponsoring department, school, or institution]**, the **[insert the name of the Institutional Review Board (IRB)/ethics committee]** and other regulatory agencies may inspect these records. In all other respects, however, the data will be held in confidence to the extent permitted by law. Should the data be published, your identity will not be disclosed.

Taking part in this study is voluntary. By answering survey questions [if applicable] you agree to take part in this research study. You do not have to answer any questions that make you uncomfortable or prosecutable by law. You may choose not to take part at all. If you decide to be in this study you may stop taking part at any time, for any reason, with no questions asked. If you decide not to be in this study or if you stop taking part at any time, you will not lose any benefits for which you may qualify.

If you have any questions, concerns, or complaints about the research study, please contact: **[insert name and phone number of the researcher]**

If you have any questions about your rights as a research subject, you may call **[insert contact information of the IRB/ethics committee]**. You can discuss any questions about your rights as a research subject, in private, with a member of the **[insert the name of the IRB or research ethics committee]**. You may also call this number if you have other questions about the research, and you cannot reach the research staff, or want to talk to someone else. The **[insert name of IRB/ethics committee]** is an independent committee made up of **[describe the general composition of the IRB/ethics committee—for example university staff, people from the community]**. The **[insert name of IRB/ethics committee and its host institution]** has reviewed this research study.

If you have concerns or complaints about the research or research staff and you do not wish to give your name, you may call **[insert phone number]**.

Sincerely,

Signature of the investigator   Signature of co-investigator/collaborators

Source: *Adapted from* University of Louisville Human Subjects Protection Office (n.d.).

Informed consent must be administered and acquired face-to-face to the extent possible unless using an online data collection method, where it can be secured electronically. For face-to-face data collection, the researcher begins by handing out a copy of the consent document in a language they can understand and gives them time to read the document. Alternatively, the researcher can read aloud this document in its entirety as participants read along from their copies. After reading the consent form and prior to participants confirming their participation, the researcher must ensure that participants understand the informed consent document by asking questions regarding its content using an interactive but noninterrogative technique such as the teach-back technique. For example, the researcher can ask: "Can you remind me who you can contact if you have any questions or complaints about this study?" Those who agree to participate after reading the consent form are asked to indicate their consent (signed or verbal) as required by the Ethics/Institutional Review Board.

The process of obtaining consent in qualitative research follows a relational rather than transactional ethical framework. Unlike most quantitative studies where informed consent is only obtained prior to the initiation of the study, informed consent in qualitative research is a dynamic and continuous process given its emergent, evolving, and interactive nature (Byrne, 2001; Klykken, 2021). This is based on the premise that participants continue to evaluate and enhance their understanding of the research project as they experience its processes, thus can provide a more informed consent compared to the predata collection phase (Byrne, 2001; Klykken, 2021). This is especially applicable to qualitative approaches requiring prolonged or multiple interactions with participants, such as ethnography, narrative research, or Photovoice.

The continuous informed consent process involves obtaining formal informed consent at the beginning of the study and renegotiating consent using both explicit and implicit techniques throughout the study as it evolves around emergent ideas (Klykken, 2021). Examples of explicit renegotiation techniques include reminding participants about the purpose of the study, reiterating its voluntary nature, and reassessing participants' willingness to continue participation at different phases of the study. Implicit techniques require close attention to participants' actions, behaviors, questions, and interactions that could indicate continuous consent or desire to withdraw from the study. Klykken (2021) provides a detailed reflection on the implementation of continuous consent throughout an ethnographic study, where she obtained formal prefield work informed consent but renegotiated consent during and after fieldwork using more informal explicit and implicit methods.

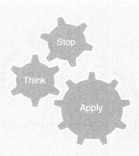

Evaluating an Informed Consent Form

1. Conduct an online search of a signed informed consent template. Review the content of the form and place a check mark next to the elements it contains.

- An invitation to participate in the research study
- An overview of the study
- What participation entails (any procedures)
- Potential risks
- Benefits
- How results will be utilized
- Audio or video recording
- Duration of participation
- Payments or compensation for participation
- Measures to ensure confidentiality or anonymity

(Continued)

(Continued)

- Secure handling and storage of data
- Voluntary participation with no penalty for nonparticipation
- Participant's rights to discontinue participation
- Contact persons for questions, concerns, or complaints about the study
- Names and signatures of the participants and the researchers/investigators

2. Discuss any missing elements in the form you evaluated and describe what information you would provide to improve the consent template.

SELECTING THE STUDY SITES AND PARTICIPANTS

Sampling Methods and Sample Size

In qualitative research, recruitment and selection, data collection, analysis, and interpretation occur concurrently. There are various sampling methods used in selecting the units to be included in the study, such as the study sites, participants (for interviews and observations), processes/events/activities (for observations), and documents (for document reviews). Overall, sampling methods fall within two main categories: probability sampling (Module 2) and nonprobability sampling. Probability sampling, which is used in quantitative research, involves the random selection of a representative sample to generate generalizable findings. Conversely, qualitative research employs nonprobability sampling methods, in which the units are sampled based on their ability to generate an in-depth understanding of the phenomenon given their specific characteristics or connections to the phenomenon. The following are common nonprobability sampling methods used in qualitative research: purposive sampling, convenience sampling, snowball sampling, quota sampling, maximum variation (heterogenous) sampling, homogenous sampling, and theoretical sampling. A study can use a single or combination of these sampling methods. The combination can involve a concurrent application of more than one sampling method or a sequential combination, where one sampling method is used to select the first-level unit (e.g., study sites) and another sampling method is used to select the second-level unit (e.g., participants within the selected study sites), and so on.

Purposive sampling is also known as purposeful, selective, or criterion sampling. This sampling technique entails strategically and purposefully selecting participants with specific backgrounds, experience, knowledge, or involvement in the phenomenon of interest, to provide a holistic and rich understanding of the phenomenon. The researcher specifies the essential criteria for inclusion into the study (inclusion criteria) on the basis that the units (i.e., participants, sites, events, or documents) meeting these criteria will generate a broad range of perspectives or experiences needed to answer the research questions and to achieve the purpose of the study. For instance, as part of a community-based participatory research class, a group of doctoral public health students were interested in exploring the health and social issues affecting refugees from a Sub-Saharan African country, who had newly resettled in an urban city in a southern state within the United States. They defined the following inclusion criteria for their study: (a) English-speaking adults (18 years or older) residing in [name of city]; (b) originally from [country of origin]; (c) arrived in the United States as a refugee within the past five years; and (d) able and willing to share their experiences living in the United States.

Convenience sampling (also known as haphazard sampling) entails sampling units that meet the inclusion criteria and are readily accessible and available to the researcher considering the location, time/availability, and other resources required to access them (Merriam, 2009). While this sampling technique reduces potential barriers in accessing the sample, it may miss the most information-rich units that cannot be accessed conveniently and produce a limited understanding of the phenomenon. This method is useful for studies such as rapid assessments, where the researcher needs quick and easy access to participants, sites, and documents, or when the information-rich units are difficult to locate. For instance, a group of health promotion and epidemiology students enrolled in a qualitative research class teamed up to conduct a study exploring the conceptualization of "social justice" by members of the School of Public Health within their university. They were particularly interested in comparing the meanings within and across departments as well as among students, staff, and faculty members of the School of Public Health. Considering the limited time frame and resources to complete this project, the student researchers decided to sample individuals from the main School of Public Health building (one of two buildings) since they were more readily and conveniently accessible.

Snowball sampling, also known as chain referral sampling, initially samples a small group of participants, documents, or observations and relies on this initial sample to assist in identifying additional individuals, documents, or sites that can provide further insights into the phenomenon. This is simply done by asking participants if they know anybody else who meets the criteria and would be interested in participating in the study. The sample size grows as additional units meeting the criteria are identified or referred to the researcher by the initial sample. This method is useful for studying rare, stigmatized, relatively unknown, or hidden phenomena involving units that are difficult to access such as homeless individuals, commercial sex workers, people who inject drugs, survivors of human trafficking, and undocumented immigrants.

Quota sampling is a sampling technique in which the researcher determines different subgroups from the population of interest based on specific characteristics and samples units from each subgroup to ensure that they are adequately represented in the final sample. This is similar to stratified sampling in quantitative research. For instance, to capture multiple perspectives regarding a community-based public health program, the potential participants may be purposively sampled from the following sub-groups or categories of program stakeholders: (a) program managers or coordinators; (b) program staff/implementers; and (c) program beneficiaries.

Maximum variation sampling (also known as heterogenous sampling) aims to achieve a heterogenous sample by purposefully selecting units that differ or vary from each other as much as possible on selected dimensions. For example, a study may sample community members with various sociodemographic characteristics (e.g., age, gender, socioeconomic status) to assess diverse perceptions of the health impacts of gold mining activities.

Homogenous sampling is the opposite of maximum variation sampling. It seeks to sample participants sharing similar characteristics. This is particularly useful when the study seeks to explore a topic in more depth.

Theoretical sampling is an iterative, emergent, and evolving sampling procedure used in grounded theory. Unlike the aforementioned sampling procedures, the units are not selected at once but rather individually, one after the other. The previous interview/document/observation informs decisions related to the selection of the next participant/document/event, until theoretical saturation is achieved.

Qualitative research primarily seeks to achieve an in-depth understanding of a phenomenon rather than a generalization of the findings. Essentially, it seeks depth rather than breadth. As such, qualitative research is less focused on the sample size and more concerned about the richness and depth of the information collected. Unlike quantitative research, there is no formula for calculating the sample size in qualitative research. Participants, sites, documents, and activities are purposively sampled until data or thematic saturation. Saturation is achieved when subsequent data collection sessions no longer produce new insights, the relationships between categories have been established, and the research questions have been answered (Charmaz, 2014; Green and Thorogood, 2018). In grounded theory, this concept is known as theoretical saturation, where the main constructs and interrelationships have been identified, and a grounded theory related to the phenomenon being investigated has been constructed. The sample size to reach data saturation depends on a combination of factors, including the research questions, study design, data collection methods, and the information richness of participants. For instance, a narrative study can be conducted with one participant, while a grounded theory design may require a larger sample size of 20 or more participants to reach theoretical saturation. Given the emergent nature of qualitative research, the sample size may change (i.e., reduce or increase) as the data collection and analysis uncover new information. As such, the exact sample size cannot be determined until the completion of the data collection and analysis. In addition, the researcher should consider their resources when making decisions related to the sample size.

As mentioned earlier in this module, institutional requirements for research often conflict with the principles of qualitative research because these requirements are largely influenced by the positivist tradition. For instance, Ethics/Institutional Review Boards often require the specification of the sample size in the research proposal and the ethics review application. To comply with such requirements while staying true to the nature of qualitative research, our past qualitative research proposals have provided an estimation of the maximum number of potential participants/documents/activities/events/sites to be sampled (e.g., up to 50 participants will be sampled) or an overestimation of the expected sample size. For instance, if the expected sample size to reach theoretical saturation is 30 participants, the researcher may initially propose a sample size of 60 participants with a statement that the sample size may be adjusted during data collection and analysis given the emergent nature of qualitative research. We propose providing a maximum sample size or an overestimation of the expected sample size in the research proposal because having a final sample size that is higher than initially proposed may require the submission of an amendment (i.e., update/modification) to the ethics review application yet an amendment is often not required when the final sample size is lower than originally proposed. While the amendment does not take as long as an initial review, it may delay or interrupt the research process. It is important to consult with the local ethics or institutional review board to verify which practice aligns with their local code of ethics.

Negotiating Entry into the Study Sites

In many settings, special permission or authorization is required from gatekeepers at multiple levels to access the study sites for recruitment and data collection purposes. As part of the recruitment plan, the researcher must define their strategy for negotiating access to the study sites and potential participants. This plan should include an identification of the potential gatekeepers such as government officials, public health authorities, site supervisors, and community or religious leaders. For instance, based on the authors' international public health research experience, local health authorities within the Ministry of Health and community leaders (e.g., village chiefs) are first consulted to negotiate the terms of entry into their community. Informal contact with potential gatekeepers may be initiated in the planning phase to convey the researcher's intention to conduct the study within the setting and inquire about the local procedures for accessing the sites and potential participants. However, the official request for permission begins after receiving the ethical approval or clearance for the study.

The researcher can secure written or verbal authorization from the gatekeepers to access the study sites and potential participants within their respective jurisdictions. However, obtaining formal written authorization is preferable and required by many institutions since it minimizes roadblocks during field work. There are several procedures involved in requesting and obtaining written authorization from gatekeepers. First, the researcher sends a letter/email providing an overview of the study and requesting access to the study site(s). This not only provides information on the study but also legitimizes the researcher and the study, thus creating trust (Vuban and Eta, 2019). This letter typically contains the following elements:

- An official letterhead (e.g., university letterhead) or stamp
- The researcher's name, position, affiliation
- The title of the research study
- An overview of the purpose of the study and the data collection methods
- A statement that the research was reviewed and approved by an ethics committee (attach the approval letter from the local ethics committee)
- The request to access the study sites for research purposes
- The request to schedule an in-person meeting (if needed)
- The researcher's dated signature with appropriate credentials and affiliation
- Signature slots for the appropriate gatekeepers to indicate their permission

The initial letter is often followed by an in-person meeting with the gatekeepers, during which the researcher provides further information on the study, answers their questions, and secures their approval to access the study sites and potential participants. In some cases, this process starts with an in-person meeting during which the researcher presents the letter. Governments and other organizations often have standard permission forms that they issue to researchers who meet their requirements once they have reviewed and approved the request. Alternatively, the gatekeepers may directly place their signature of approval in the designated signature slots within the initial letter sent by the researcher. In some cultural contexts or settings, verbal permission obtained from local authorities or community leaders is as valuable as written permission, thus sufficient to provide access to the study sites and participants for recruitment and data collection purposes (Vuban and Eta, 2019). After receiving approval from authorities at higher levels of the hierarchy, the researcher should be ready to schedule additional meetings with gatekeepers at the lower level to formally introduce themself and present the approval letters from the higher officials. The gatekeepers may have additional requirements for the researcher as a condition for their approval, such as debriefing or submitting a copy of the final research report. Researchers should comply with these additional guidelines or requirements provided that they do not conflict with any procedures covered by the ethical approval, in which case Ethics/Institutional Review Boards must be consulted and amendments filed as needed.

Negotiating access to study sites and potential participants often requires navigating complex administrative, bureaucratic, and cultural procedures and uncertain time frames. Given the uncertainty surrounding this process, the researcher must allocate sufficient time to this process and develop contingency plans if original plans do not work. The researcher should leverage their local connections or stakeholders to identify and reach gatekeepers within each site. Local stakeholders are often familiar with the local processes, policies, costs, and cultural contexts for securing such permission, thus may be helpful in following up or speeding up the process. Bernard (1994) cautions against using stakeholders and gatekeepers with a controversial history or questionable reputation or agenda in their communities since associations with untrusted gatekeepers may raise the community's suspicions of the researcher and create mistrust in the research activities. As much as possible, the researcher should associate themselves with gatekeepers and stakeholders who are neutral, trusted, and respected in their communities to establish a trusting relationship with the communities upon entry.

The permission granted by these local authorities or gatekeepers only gives a greenlight to begin the research activities within their respective sites and should not be mistaken for participant consent. The researcher is still expected to recruit and obtain consent from each participant as indicated in their research protocol.

Recruitment and Selection Process

Once the ethical approval and the permission to access the study sites are secured, recruitment and data collection activities can begin. Recruitment involves identifying and locating potential participants, inviting them to participate in the study, and screening those expressing interest and willingness to participate in the study. The recruitment strategy should specify how potential participants will be identified, invited to participate, and screened. Participants can be identified by the researcher, their personal or professional connections, gatekeepers, or other participants. Since qualitative research seeks information-rich individuals using nonprobability sampling techniques, gatekeepers, local stakeholders, and other participants are instrumental in identifying potential participants who may be eligible for the study. Once identified, participants can be recruited into the study using direct or indirect methods. Direct recruitment methods are those in which the researcher directly interacts with the potential participants, such as face-to-face, mail/letter, email, or phone. Conversely, indirect methods are more passive because the potential participants are not directly approached by the researcher but rather contact the researcher if interested after viewing the recruitment materials such as flyers, posters, public announcements, social media, or mass emails. The recruitment advertisements used in print or electronic materials should address the following questions:

- What is happening (i.e., data collection method and topic?)
- Who can join (i.e., inclusion criteria)?
- When is the event happening (i.e., date and time)?
- Where is it happening (i.e., the venue)?
- How can I join (i.e., the contact information)?
- Are there any incentives?

The recruitment strategy and any materials used must be reviewed and approved by the Ethics/Institutional Review Board. To enable informed decision-making, the potential participants should be informed about the research study, its voluntary nature, confidentiality, rights to terminate participation at any time without consequences, and audio recording of interviews (see recruitment script in Box 3.7).

BOX 3.7 Sample Participant Recruitment Script

Dear _____,

My name is Jane Doe. I am a public health student at State University. I am conducting a research study to understand the work and experiences of CHWs in Eagle County. You are invited to participate in this study. You may participate if (a) you have been or are currently a CHW, or if you are involved in any activity related to training and managing CHWs in Eagle County, (b) you are over 18 years old, and (c) are comfortable communicating in English or Spanish.

Participation in this study is voluntary. You may choose not to take part at all. If you agree, you will be asked to take part in an audio recorded interview. Your involvement is anticipated to take approximately 60 minutes. Your identity will remain confidential, meaning your identity and the name of your workplace will not be revealed during or after the study.

(Continued)

> (Continued)
>
> If you participate, you will not have to answer any questions that make you uncomfortable. You may stop taking part at any time. If you decide not to be in this study or if you stop taking part at any time, you will not lose any benefits for which you may qualify. People who participate in this research study will receive a 25$ gift card to thank them for their time.
>
> Do you have any questions? If you would like to participate in this research study or if you have questions later, please contact me at: +100,000,000,000 or jane.doe@stateuniversity.edu.
>
> Thank you!
>
> Sincerely,
>
> Jane Doe
> Doctoral Candidate
> Department of Public Health
> State University

Those expressing an interest to participate in the study should be screened to ensure that they meet the study's inclusion criteria. Potential participants' names and contact information may be collected for recruitment and data collection purposes provided that this is addressed in the ethical approval and confidentiality is maintained throughout the study. Each participant can be assigned a unique nonidentifying identification number, code, or pseudonym. To protect confidentiality, a master list linking participants to their nonidentifying code should be securely stored in a locked cabinet or password-protected electronic document that is separate from other research documents, as discussed in more detail later in this section. The researcher and participants who agree to take part can identify a mutually acceptable date, time, and location that ensures convenience, privacy, and safety for data collection purposes.

Incentives and Compensation

Recruiting an adequate number of information-rich participants into the study is a challenging endeavor. Participants may be difficult to locate, may have other priorities, or may lack interest or motivation to participate in the study. Evidence has shown that providing incentives encourages and increases participation into the study (Kelly et al., 2017). However, there have been controversies and debates surrounding the use of incentives in medical and public health research. When incorrectly used, incentives can potentially cloud participants' judgments regarding the risks associated with the study, leading them to choose differently despite their original aversion (Grant and Sugarman, 2004). There have been reports of the unethical use of incentives to exploit vulnerable individuals by recruiting them into research studies with greater than minimal risk yet with little to no benefits to the participants (Grant and Sugarman, 2004). On the other hand, in some cultural contexts, it may be considered culturally insensitive or even unethical for a study not to provide any form of incentive or not to reciprocate the information, efforts, and time given by participants who practically share their lives and stories with the researcher. In such cultural contexts, an incentive is considered a form of reciprocity among other forms (e.g., disseminating the report) and not as a compensation or wage. Since qualitative research often involves prolonged and/or multiple interactions with participants, the researcher should consider giving a culturally appropriate form of monetary or nonmonetary incentive, depending on the local ethical guidelines, sociocultural norms, and the nature of the study.

In their thorough analysis of the debates surrounding incentives, Grant and Sugarman (2004) argue that the mere act of providing incentives is not the ethical issue but rather the manner and conditions in which they are used. They argue that incentives are ethically questionable when used within the following contexts: (a) dependency of the participant on the researcher; (b) the study presents greater than minimal risk; (c) the research is degrading; and (d) participants are strongly averse to the study but can consent only if given high incentives. The use of incentives should adhere to the legal and ethical codes for research, avoiding any form of manipulation, coercion, bribery, blackmail, or other violations of the principles of justice and respect for persons. Voluntary participation into the study is a critical concern when using incentives. The principle of respect for persons requires that these incentives be given without coercion or undue influence (United States National Commission for the Protection of Human Subjects of Biomedical and Behavioral Research, 1978). Excessive, inappropriate, and unwarranted incentives are particularly questionable and not ethically permissible. The goal of providing incentives should be to motivate not coerce individuals to participate in the study. The appropriate amount for the incentive is determined based on multiple pieces of information, including the daily wage in the country and previous research studies or organizational practices in the area. Incentives should be distinguished from compensation. While incentives are given as bonuses to motivate individuals, compensation is paid to individuals for products or services rendered to the project (Grant and Sugarman, 2004).

COLLECTING QUALITATIVE DATA

Data collection in qualitative research is a systematic and iterative process of gathering data to answer the research questions and achieve the purpose of the study. Qualitative research data are primarily obtained by asking, listening, observing, and reviewing to gain insights into a phenomenon of interest (Merriam, 2009). Merriam (2009, pp. 85–86) asserts that data are not waiting to be collected, they are rather "noticed by the researcher, and treated as data" to achieve the purpose of the research. Rather than numerical form, qualitative data take the form of: (a) direct quotations of people's experiences, opinions, feelings, and knowledge, as elicited in interviews, focus groups, and audiovisual materials; (b) detailed descriptions of people's activities, behaviors, and actions from observations or visual materials; and (c) excerpts, texts, or images from documents and visual materials (Patton, 2002, p. 4). There are a variety of data collection methods in qualitative research, the most common of which are interviews, focus groups, observations, and document review/document analysis.

Interviews

Interviews are the most common method of data collection in qualitative research. They serve a primary role in most qualitative research designs such as grounded theory, phenomenology, narrative, and case study research, where they can be used with other data collection methods. Qualitative interviewing is an interactive and research-oriented conversation between a researcher and a participant, in which the researcher poses questions to understand participant's perspectives, experiences, and meanings related to the phenomenon being investigated (Kvale, 1996; Kvale and Brinkmann, 2015). During the interview, the researcher and the participant co-create knowledge by reconstructing behaviors, experiences, feelings, knowledge, sensory responses, and opinions that cannot be observed (Patton, 2002).

When developing and planning an interview, researchers need to (Patton, 2002) select the structure of interview, determine the type of information to collect or type of questions to ask, determine the length of the interview, develop the interview guide, and determine the location or setting of the interview.

Structure of the Interview

In terms of structure, interviews can take three major forms: structured, semistructured, and unstructured.

A *structured interview* strictly adheres to a predetermined set of detailed questions, with little to no deviations from the interview guide. All participants are asked the same set of questions in the same sequence, with little to no variation across the interviews. This type of interview does not enable the use of probes or follow-up questions to explore new concepts or ideas that are identified during the interview. This standardized interview format can contain both close-ended and open-ended questions.

Types of Interviews
- Structured interview
- Semistructured interview
- Unstructured interview

A *semistructured interview* is the most common type of interview in qualitative research. It utilizes an interview guide with predefined interview topics or general open-ended and close-ended questions that focus but not restrict the interview. This format enables participants to elaborate extensively on their experiences and perceptions, while offering the flexibility for the researcher to ask new relevant questions that explore emerging concepts during the interview. A semistructured interview is particularly suitable for exploratory studies or when there is a dearth of information on the topic being investigated (Merriam, 2009; Salazar et al., 2015).

Unlike structured and semistructured interviews, an *unstructured interview* has no specific predetermined questions and is usually initiated with one broad open-ended question that sparks a conversation between the researcher and participant. An unstructured interview is also known as informational conversational interview because questions emerge spontaneously from the natural course of the interaction or conversation between the researcher and the participant. It is commonly used in ethnographic studies, where it occurs as an extension of the participant observations (Patton, 2002). While the interview itself may be unstructured or conversational, it is purposeful and intentional in that the researcher conducts the interview with the research purpose and central research question(s) in mind. The questions asked during the interview should align with the central research questions posed at the beginning of the study to achieve the purpose of the study.

Selecting an appropriate interview structure depends on the researcher's philosophical paradigm, the purpose of the study, and the research questions. Semistructured and unstructured interviews are more suitable for exploring topics for which little is known and when seeking a rich understanding of the phenomenon. Unstructured interviews are particularly suitable for ethnographic and grounded theory studies, where researchers aim to enter the process without any preconceived notions. On the other hand, structured interviews may be more suitable for deductive approaches when responses are to be classified into predetermined frameworks, when the topic area is well developed, when the goal is to compare responses, or when used in conjunction with other data collection methods.

Types of Interview Questions

There are different types of interview questions varying in breadth or scope, information elicited, directness, and purpose. In terms of breadth or scope, interview questions can be close-ended or open-ended. *Close-ended questions* have a limited set of possible responses that usually consist of a single word (e.g., yes, no) or phrase (Table 3.3). Close-ended questions are directive and restrictive because the questions posed predetermine the scope of the responses, generating very specific rather than elaborate responses. While close-ended questions are more common in quantitative research, they are sometimes used in qualitative research when specific or precise responses are required (e.g., sociodemographic information), when the research aims to classify responses into predetermined frameworks or categories, or when the study aims to compare responses across participants. Conversely, *open-ended questions* (Table 3.3) allow participants to provide more elaborate responses, capturing complex ideas or concepts that cannot be explored through close-ended questions. By asking *what, how,* and *why* questions, they produce rich and thick narratives that enable an in-depth exploration of a topic. It is advisable that qualitative research primarily utilize open-ended questions and reserve close-ended questions for the specific purposes listed earlier (e.g., clarification, classification). As such, close-ended questions can be used in combination with open-ended questions, as an opening to open-ended questions, a follow-up to open-ended questions (e.g., to verify or clarify), or as standalone questions within the mix.

In terms of the information elicited, Patton (2002) identified the following types of interview questions (Table 3.4):

- *Experience and behavior questions:* elicit information regarding a person's actions, behaviors, activities, and experience with the phenomenon

- *Opinions and values questions:* examine opinions, judgments, and values—essentially, what people *think* and *believe* about an issue

- *Feelings questions*: elicit participants' emotional responses to the phenomenon—how they *feel* rather than what they think about an issue

TABLE 3.3. **Examples of Close-Ended and Open-Ended Questions**

Close-ended question	Open-ended questions
Did you receive quality care during your most recent delivery?	- What are your thoughts about the care you received during your recent delivery? - How would you describe the care you received during your most recent delivery?
Is an action plan developed as part of the perinatal death review process?	- How are the findings from a perinatal death review used? - What happens after a perinatal death review?
Do you think the mining sector has a role in addressing women's health in your community?	- What do you think is the role, if any, of the mining sector in addressing women's health in your community?

TABLE 3.4. Examples of Types of Interview Questions in Terms of the Information Elicited

Types of interview questions	Examples
Experience and behavior questions	- What typically happens during a perinatal death review session? - What do you do to cope with grief?
Opinions and values questions	- What are your thoughts about the process of signing up for health insurance? - What are the beliefs about female genital mutilation in your culture?
Feelings questions	- How did you feel when you heard that you were being resettled to a new country? - How do you feel about living in this neighborhood?
Knowledge questions	- What do you know about HIV pre-exposure prophylaxis (PrEP)? - How do you prepare the oral rehydration solution for your child with diarrhea?
Sensory questions	- What do you smell when entering this building? - What were your observations when visiting the health center?
Background and sociodemographic questions	- What is your race/ethnicity? Age? Gender? Level of education? Income?

- *Knowledge questions*: elicit factual information to examine what people *know*, rather than feel or think, about the topic being investigated

- *Sensory questions*: ask what participants have seen, heard, smelled, tasted, or felt through touch

- *Background and demographic questions*: identify participants' sociodemographic characteristics (e.g., age, education, occupation) to determine how they compare with others in the sample. Sociodemographic questions can be close-ended (i.e., predetermined categories) or open-ended. While close ended questions are easy to analyze and summarize, open-ended sociodemographic questions are recommended because they respect participants' autonomy to describe or categorize themselves rather than forcing their identities into researcher-imposed and often poorly conceptualized categories (Hughes et al., 2016; Patton, 2002). This practice embraces diversity and inclusion and enhances the integrity of the research findings by producing a more accurate description of participants' complex identities (Hughes et al., 2016).

Interviews often comprise a combination of the aforementioned types of questions to enable a rich understanding of the phenomenon. The interview questions can be framed in past, present, and/or future tense, depending on the time period of focus (Patton, 2002).

In terms of directness, interview questions can be direct or indirect. *Direct questions* are straight to the point. Meaning, they introduce the topic in a direct manner or directly ask the participant to elaborate on their personal experience or perceptions related to the topic. The following are examples of direct open-ended and close-ended questions:

- How has gold mining in your community impacted you?
- Are you satisfied with the prenatal care services offered by your community health center?

Kvale and Brinkmann (2015) suggest delaying direct questions to when the topic is naturally brought up by the respondent during the interview or when rapport has already been established between the researcher and participant, which usually happens toward the middle or end of the interview. Doing so enables more open responses and lowers any guards that respondents may have when asked a direct question before they are ready.

Conversely, *indirect questions* introduce the topic in an indirect and general manner. Some indirect questions are projective in that they ask for the participant's general views on a topic without directly asking for their personal views. For instance, rather than directly asking the participant how gold mining activities have impacted them personally or whether they are satisfied with the prenatal care services, indirect questions may ask:

- How do you think gold mining activities have impacted people in your community?

- Do you think women in your community are satisfied with the prenatal care services offered by your community health center?

When asking such projective indirect questions, the researcher hopes that as respondents report on general perceptions, they can also reflect, report, or make inferences about their personal experiences or perceptions. However, such questions can be a dead end, as exemplified by the following response: "I am not sure what others think about this issue." As such, indirect questions can be followed up with more direct questions such as: What about you? What has been your experience? How has gold mining affected you personally?

The decision to use direct or indirect questions should take into account the sensitivity of the topic and participants' cultural context. Direct questions are not appropriate for sensitive topics because they may be perceived as invasive, causing participants to be more guarded or to provide socially desirable responses. In addition, direct questions may not be well received in cultures with indirect communication styles, where people generally imply or suggest what they mean rather than telling it like it is. In such contexts, direct questions are more likely to be perceived as disrespectful or to raise suspicion of the researcher's intention. Even within such cultures, there are often personal differences and subcultures that the researcher/interviewer should familiarize themselves with when planning the study. For instance, while cultures with indirect communication styles are more open to indirect questions, younger participants may be more receptive to direct questions than older participants. It is important that the interview questions are reviewed and pretested in a small sample of potential participants, as discussed later in this section.

Finally, Kvale (1996) identifies the following types of interview questions based on their role throughout the interview: introductory, follow-up, probing/specifying, interpreting/clarification, structuring, and silence.

- *Introductory questions:* opening questions designed to kickstart the interview and create a natural and rich discussion on the topic. Example: Can you tell me about your community? What do you like about it?

- *Follow-up questions:* questions asked to follow-up on the participant's response to the main question. Example: You mentioned that you dislike living in this community, what is it that you do not like about living in this community? This also includes verbal and nonverbal cues (e.g., a nod) that encourage a participant to elaborate further on the question asked.

- *Probing and specifying questions:* elicit more in-depth information, explanation, or an example to illustrate the participant's response. Example: Can you give me an example of a time you felt unsafe in this community? How did you react? What did you do about it?

- *Interpretation questions:* allow the researcher/interviewer to clarify their understanding and interpretation of the participant's answer to ensure that it is interpreted as originally intended. Example: Do you mean that the neighborhood crime rates prevent you from participating in outdoor activities in the evening?

- *Structuring questions:* transition questions or statements that indicate the end of one section of the interview or introduce the beginning of a new section of the interview. Example: Now, I would like to ask you questions about children's health programs and services here in your community.

- *Silence:* Allows both the researcher and the participant to process or reflect on the question or response. Silent gaps also provide an opportunity for the participant to provide new information.

Developing an Interview Guide

In qualitative research, the researcher is the primary research instrument as mentioned earlier in this module. As part of this role, the researcher can develop tools such as interview, observation, and document review guides or protocols, to guide and focus their investigation. Both structured and semistructured interviews use an interview guide, also known as an interview schedule, interview protocol, or topic guide, that is prepared in advance with variable level of detail. A structured interview uses a structured guide with a detailed and extensive list of questions from which the interviewer does not deviate. Conversely, a semistructured interview guide includes a more general set of questions and probes to guide the interviewer, while allowing the flexibility to spontaneously generate further questions or probes during the interview. The interview guide generally comprises questions that elicit information on participants' experience and behaviors, opinions and values, feelings, knowledge, sensory impressions, and sociodemographic characteristics (Patton, 2002). Sociodemographic questions can be embedded within an interview guide or administered separately to the participant at the beginning or end of the interview. We recommend asking sociodemographic questions at the end of the interview and creating a separate tool to ensure confidentiality and encourage open and frank responses.

Unlike quantitative surveys, most qualitative interview guides are uniquely developed by each researcher for their participants and specific research context. However, in some cases, one may adapt parts of an existing interview guide from a similar study to their context and participants. In such cases, these data collection tools should be adapted or adopted with permission from the authors, unless permitted for public use (Module 5). Any tool that is adopted or adapted from another source must be properly cited. The development and validation of an interview guide is an iterative process consisting of several rounds of feedback and revision. The interview guide undergoes face and content validation, during which subject matter experts, methodology experts, participants, and other stakeholders systematically review and provide feedback on the interview questions. This validation process ensures that at face value, the interview examines what it was intended to examine (face validity), includes topics that adequately represent the phenomenon being investigated (content validity), and that the questions are clearly formulated, understandable, ethical, and culturally appropriate. Figure 3.11 depicts an interview guide development and validation process adapted from Carrico et al. (2013) and Prescott (2011).

The first step in developing an interview guide is to conduct a *literature review* to identify the key concepts, topics, or questions that can be further explored in the interview. Next, the researcher develops an *initial set of interview questions* reflecting the purpose of the research study and the research questions. This initial interview guide is then submitted for *expert review and feedback* focusing on its content, language, and clarity. The expert panel can comprise subject matter and qualitative research experts such as members of a dissertation/thesis committee, peers, or practitioners. This step may require several rounds of review and revision, until both the researcher and experts are satisfied with the initial interview guide. For researchers collecting data in another language, the interview guide undergoes a *translation and verification* process discussed later in this section, after which the translated version or both original and translated versions are submitted for *review by local experts or stakeholders* to ensure the accuracy of the translation and the local relevance of the questions. This is followed by another round of revisions based on local experts' feedback. The original and translated (if applicable) versions of the interview guide can be submitted for ethics review and approval along with other research documents, as discussed earlier in this section.

Once approved by the ethics committee, the interview guide can be pretested and refined prior to initiating the actual data collection. *Pretesting* is a process of validating a data collection tool by administering it to a small sample of individuals that are as similar as possible to the target population to examine its performance prior to the actual data collection. Two important components of pretesting are the analysis of responses and participant debriefing sessions to determine whether they understand and interpret the questions correctly, how they respond to the questions, whether the current formulation of the questions elicits comprehensive responses, the time it takes to complete the interview, and the questions to be discarded or modified because of their ambiguity or sensitivity.

FIGURE 3.11. *Interview guide development and validation process.*

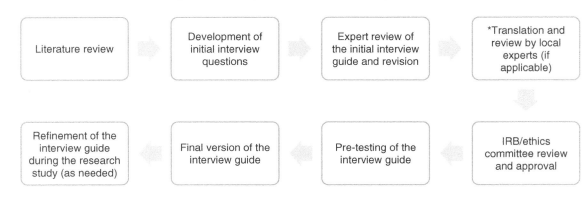

Pretesting is different from pilot testing which tests the entire study rather than a data collection tool in a small sample of the target population. Pilot testing is essentially a mini trial version of the full study. There is no prescribed sample size for pretesting and pilot testing because decisions should be made based on the complexity of the tool as well as the resources available (Chaudhary and Israel, 2014). For instance, pretesting the interview guide in less than 10 individuals may generate sufficient insights into the interview guide's performance. The interview guide should be revised accordingly, after which it is ready for use in actual data collection. In qualitative research, the interview guide can be *refined as needed during the study*, particularly following the completion of the first few interviews.

Conducting an Interview

Once the interview guide has been finalized, the researcher recruits the participants, schedules and prepares for the interviews, and conducts the interviews on the scheduled dates and times. The interviews should take place in mutually agreed upon and convenient venues for both the researcher and participants, taking into account safety, privacy, accessibility, comfort, and silence/levels of distraction. The duration of the interview depends on the nature and complexity of the topic, the number of questions, and the participants' and researcher's availability. The duration of the interview can be determined during pretesting and should be communicated in advance when scheduling the interview. Interviews typically last 45–60 minutes.

On the day of the interview, the researcher starts by introducing themselves and their role in the study (Figure 3.12). Next, they administer the informed consent document to the participant, emphasizing information about the purpose of the study, its confidential nature, the voluntary nature of participation, the respondent's right to withdraw at any time, whether the interview is audio recorded, and the potential risks and benefits associated with the study. The interviewer assesses the participant's understanding of the informed consent document using a series of questions related to its content. The participant can formally indicate their consent once they demonstrate an understanding of the informed consent document, suggest that they have no further questions, and express the willingness to continue with the study. The interviewer then provides an overview of the interview process, including its expected duration and the general rules.

The interviewer should notify the participant about the start of the interview and audio recording so as not to capture any information that they do not wish to be recorded, as exemplified by the following statement: "As discussed earlier, now I'm going to start the audio recording, so I do not miss important information from our interview, is that okay?" Audio recording is useful for data analysis as it preserves an accurate account of participants' experiences and generates portable data for easier storage and multiple hearings (Merriam, 2009; Nikander, 2008). During each interview, the interviewer takes notes capturing pertinent points, new questions, ideas, and nonverbal cues to supplement the data. The interview should end with closing statements that summarize the key points, ask the participant if there is anything else they would like to add or discuss on the topic, and thank them for their participation. It is also important to notify the participant when the audio recording is stopped as this indicates the official end of the interview itself. After the interview, the participant can complete the sociodemographic questions, although some researchers may opt to begin with these questions. This segment is usually not audio recorded, but responses are written on the designated form either by the interviewer or the participant. After each interview, the interviewer should reflect on the interview and identify emergent themes or categories from the interview, comparing them with the previous interviews that have already been completed. This practice is part of the preliminary analysis since qualitative data analysis occurs concurrently with data collection. Box 3.8 provides some basic tips for conducting interviews.

FIGURE 3.12. *The qualitative research interview process.*

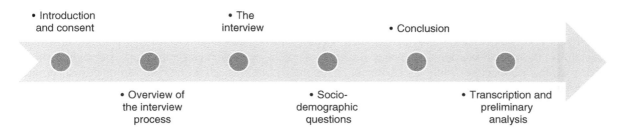

> **BOX 3.8** **Tips for Conducting a Qualitative Interview**
> - Establish trust and rapport. Example: small talk prior to the interview.
> - Avoid loaded, biased, or leading questions that may influence responses.
> - Come prepared: familiarize yourself with the topic, the interview guide, and the audio recording equipment to ensure a smooth flow.
> - Create a friendly, welcoming, and comfortable environment.
> - Ask one question at a time, with each question expressing a single idea
> - Acknowledge the participant's response using culturally appropriate verbal or nonverbal feedback (e.g., a nod, mmmm noise).
> - Respect the participant's time. Time the interview and politely ask for an extension if possible and necessary
> - Be mindful of your body language (e.g., do not cross your legs; maintain eye contact where culturally appropriate).
> - Be respectful. Do not coerce the participant into answering any questions because an interview is voluntary.
> - Consider the cultural context of the interview. For example, some cultures may prefer an interviewer of the same gender and others may require a third "silent" person in the room to ensure safety.
> - Consider the power differentials between the interviewer and the participant.
> - Do not challenge or question the participant's response during the interview; rather, probe and seek clarification.
> - Practice active listening—a conscious, purposeful, and involved type of listening that captures the depth of the message being communicated.
> - Do not share your own experiences and perspectives during the interview.
> - Start transcription and analysis as early as possible rather than waiting for all interviews to be completed.
> - Do not answer any participant questions or requests for factual information related to the topic during the interview.

While interviews typically generate in-depth data, they can be resource and labor-intensive since multiple interviews are often required to generate diverse data and to reach theoretical saturation. Focus group discussions are more efficient in exploring diverse perspectives within a shorter time frame than individual interviews.

Focus Groups

Focus groups are facilitated, semistructured group discussions that elicit collective perceptions, experiences, and meanings related to a specific phenomenon. Unlike interviews that involve one-on-one interactions between the researcher and the participant, focus groups center on interactions between participants to generate rich data and capture areas of divergence and convergence (Nyumba et al., 2018). These group interactions stimulate new ideas and offer an opportunity to triangulate participants' accounts. The researcher therefore assumes the role of a facilitator rather than the primary role of an investigator who drives the interactions. A focus group facilitator's role is to stimulate focused and meaningful interactions between participants, manage the group dynamics, and ensure a positive and open environment for dialogue. The facilitator specifically asks questions, probes, listens actively, and redirects or refocuses the conversation. Another member of the research team can assume the role of a notetaker who captures nonverbal cues and pertinent information from the focus group. Splitting the roles enables the facilitator to maintain active listening throughout the focus group, though this is not always possible.

Focus groups generally convene 6–12 purposively selected participants, with discussions generally lasting 90–120 minutes. However, large focus groups often produce independent or side conversations and an inequitable participation in the main discussion (Nyumba et al., 2018). As such, we recommend convening six to eight participants to capture diverse perspectives while also maintaining an orderly and focused discussion. Multiple focus group sessions can be conducted to reach data saturation (Nyumba et al., 2018). The final number of participants is often unknown until the actual focus group session since not all who confirm their participation are able to attend. The final sample size may therefore be larger or smaller than desired for a focus group. To avoid a sample size that is smaller than desired, Rabiee (2004) suggests overrecruiting by 10–25% of the desired sample size. From our experience, sending additional reminders closer to the scheduled focus group day (e.g., the eve) also works in securing a near-possible estimate of the final number of participants. Given this uncertainty, researchers should be prepared to break-up larger groups into separate concurrent focus group sessions, if possible. This may require an additional facilitator, extra copies of the focus group guide, a spare meeting space, and additional audio recording equipment as part of the contingency plan.

The composition of the focus group depends on the purpose of the research study. Focus groups can be homogenous or heterogenous. Homogenous focus groups comprise participants with similarities in certain sociodemographic characteristics. For instance, a health insurance literacy study by Ali et al. (2018) organized multiple focus group sessions in the study sites, two of which were homogenous in terms of age group (under 30 years old and over 65 years old) to capture unique experiences related to different types of health insurance coverage. A heterogenous focus group comprises participants with diverse sociodemographic characteristics and backgrounds. Homogenous focus groups tend to have more positive group dynamics and interactions since participants are more likely to have similar experiences and perceptions and less likely to argue or disagree. Such group dynamics reduce power imbalances and enhance the level of openness and comfort. Despite these advantages, homogenous groups limit the opportunity to explore diverse perspectives and experiences related to the phenomenon and may result in a one-sided or narrow understanding of the phenomenon. To gather diverse data, multiple homogenous focus group sessions may be required, where individuals with similar characteristics are grouped into one session. Having multiple, separate focus groups may be more culturally appropriate in some cultural contexts and may reduce the influence of power imbalances among participants. Conversely, heterogenous focus groups are more likely to create debates and, in some cases, tensions among participants. While debates can generate rich, divergent data, tensions can be time-consuming and counterproductive since some participants may be discouraged to voice their opinions or may feel silenced by those higher on the power hierarchy. Facilitators of heterogenous focus groups should therefore be mindful of these group dynamics and create an environment where participants respectfully express diverse ideas. The concepts of homogeneity and heterogeneity fall on a continuum rather than a dichotomy. In addition, these concepts are complex because individuals are multidimensional beings and the intersectionality of their identities influence how they perceive, experience, and ascribe meanings to phenomena. The degree of homogeneity or heterogeneity should depend on the purpose of the study and the focus group itself.

Homogenous  **Heterogenous**

While focus groups are more efficient than interviews in capturing diverse perspectives, there are several inherent limitations. First, focus groups are not suitable for exploring sensitive topics since participants may be reluctant to disclose personal or sensitive information in group settings. Individual interviews and other less invasive data collection methods may be appropriate to explore such topics. In addition, focus groups are not appropriate for all cultural and political contexts. While they may be more readily embraced in some cultures, they may violate sociocultural norms or be mistaken for political opposition in other contexts. For instance, in some cultures, it is disrespectful or culturally inappropriate for younger participants to oppose the views of older participants or for women to express their opinions in the presence of men (Halcomb et al., 2007). In addition, participants from cultures that value saving face may not readily express views that they perceive will harm their reputation or that of their loved ones in a group setting (Halcomb et al., 2007). It is critical that the researcher examine the cultural context prior to selecting an appropriate data collection method. Last, confidentiality is a common concern for focus groups. Though researchers are aware of the ethical obligation of maintaining the confidentiality, there is potential for breach of confidentiality by focus group participants themselves who may not perceive this ethical obligation. It is important to remind participants that the information disclosed within the focus group should be kept confidential and that participants have the right to withhold any information that they do not wish to disclose in the focus group.

The focus group process is similar to the interview process described earlier in this section. The groups are also guided by a semistructured topic guide or discussion guide similar to the interview guide. Box 3.9 outlines the focus group process.

> **BOX 3.9** Overview of a Focus Group Session
>
> **Preparation**
>
> - Check the functionality of the audio or visual recording equipment.
> - Arrange the seats into a semicircle (U and V shape) such that participants can face each other.
> - Welcome participants and complete the sign-in sheets (if applicable).
>
> **Introduction and Consent**
>
> A. Welcome participants and thank them for their attendance.
> B. Introduce the research team and explain their roles, for example, facilitator, notetaker.
> C. Explain the purpose of the focus group.
> D. Secure participant consent:
>   - Provide copies of the consent form to participants.
>   - Read or ask participants to read the consent form.
>   - Take questions.
>   - Assess participants' understanding and correct misinformation.
> E. Ask participants to indicate consent.
> F. Administer or ask participants to complete the sociodemographic form.
>
> **Overview of the focus group process and ground rules**
>
> A. Explain the focus group steps and process.
> B. Explain the ground rules:
>   - Avoiding interruptions or cross-talks when one person is speaking
>   - Stepping up, stepping back: Step up listening and step back speaking when you normally speak a lot, step up speaking and step back listening when you are normally quiet (Cornell University Cooperative Extension, n.d.)
>   - Understanding that there are no right or wrong answers but that participants speak from personal experience
>   - Avoiding distractions such as electronic devices and side conversations
>   - Maintaining confidentiality among group members
> C. Giving directions to the restrooms
>
> **Focus Group Discussion** [90–120 minutes; audio recorded if possible]
>
> **Conclusion**
>
> - Ask participants if there is anything else they would like to add.
> - Stop the audio recording.
> - Announce the end of the focus group.
> - Thank participants for their participation.
>
> **Debriefing (facilitator and notetaker), transcription, and preliminary analysis**
>
> *Source:* Adapted from Center for Community College and Student Engagement. (2017). *Focus group guide*. Center for Community College Student Engagement -The University of Texas at Austin. Retrieved from https://www.ccsse.org/focusgrouptoolkit/Focus_Group_Guide.pdf

While focus groups and interviews were traditionally conducted in-person or face-to-face, there has been an increase in virtual platforms, such as video conferencing, online chatrooms, and online discussion boards, that attempt to replicate the in-person interview and focus group experience while connecting individuals from diverse geographical locations. While virtual interviews and focus groups reduce expenses related to travel and space rentals, virtual platforms come with inherent challenges that may affect the group dynamics and quality of interactions including connectivity, Internet accessibility, and potential confidentiality issues. As such, the advantages and disadvantages of using virtual platforms for interviews and focus groups must be carefully evaluated.

Observations

Observation in qualitative research is an interactive process in which the researcher uses their senses to explore a phenomenon of interest within its natural setting (Creswell, 2013; Merriam, 2009). Observations are recommended under the following circumstances (Merriam, 2009):

- When the phenomenon under study is observable
- When participants are unable or unwilling to discuss the issue
- When awareness on the issue cannot be developed through other data collection methods
- When self-reported behaviors may differ from actual behaviors
- When complementary data are needed to achieve a holistic and in-depth understanding of the phenomenon

Observations enable a firsthand experience of the processes, activities, behaviors, and interactions related to the phenomenon. They can be used as a stand-alone data collection method or in conjunction with other data collection methods to enhance the understanding of the phenomenon being investigated. Observations are central but not limited to ethnographic studies, where they can be conducted in the physical setting or the online/virtual setting.

When planning for observations, there are four major technical decisions or considerations with regards to the nature of the observation: (a) what to observe; (b) whether the observation will be overt or covert; (c) whether the observer will be a passive observer or an active participant in the activity or event; and (d) whether the observation is structured, semistructured, or unstructured. In terms of what to observe, observations generally elicit information on elements within the following categories proposed by Merriam (2009):

1. *Physical setting*: The physical environment in which the activity or event is taking place, including the materials used during the activity

2. *Participants:* Roles and characteristics of participants involved in the event or process being observed, including who was present and who was not

3. *Activities and interactions:* The sequence and characteristics of the observed process including interactions between different actors

4. *Conversations:* A summary of the nature of conversations between participants throughout the implementation of the activity

5. *Subtle factors:* Less obvious factors such as unplanned/informal activities, nonverbal cues, or what did not happen during the observations

6. *Researcher's behavior*: The researcher's role, thoughts, and reactions and how the researcher affected the observed activity

The researcher can assume one of the following major roles as an observer, from covert to overt and from participation to nonparticipation in the event being observed: complete participant, complete observer, participant as observer, nonparticipant/observer as participant. A *complete participant* is fully integrated and engaged in the activity and conceals their identity as an observer/researcher so as not to alter participants' behaviors. On the other hand, a *complete observer* does not participate in the activity or event but observes covertly without being seen or noticed. These covert observation methods aim to reduce the Hawthorne or observer effect, which refers to an individual's tendency to alter their behavior as a result of being observed. However, covert methods involve some level of deception, yet research studies involving deceptive methodologies or incomplete disclosure have lower chances of receiving ethical clearance or approval. In unique circumstances where such studies are required, the researcher must provide a scientific justification for the use of deception by demonstrating that there is no equally effective nondeceptive alternative, and they must comply with additional demands to protect the participants. In contrast, the *participant as observer* and *nonparticipant/observer* are both overt observation methods. The *participant as observer* is actively involved in the activity and discloses his/her identity as an observer. The *nonparticipant/observer as participant* observes overtly as a researcher without being directly involved in the activity. Such overt methods minimize potential ethical issues but are more subject to the observer effect. A qualitative researcher may shift roles during observations, as dictated by the study. Where appropriate for the study and permissible by the ethics committee and participants, the researcher can audio or video record the activity being observed in lieu of or in addition to conducting a face-to-face observation. While audio or video recordings can facilitate data analysis, they may be subject to ethical and legal issues, especially if used in covert observations.

Like qualitative interviews, observations can be unstructured, semistructured, or structured. Unstructured observations are purposeful but not guided by an observation protocol. The observer is open to discovering emergent issues related to the phenomenon being studied. Contrastingly, both semistructured and structured observations utilize an observation protocol with predetermined criteria to guide and focus the observations, with variations in the level of detail. The structured observation protocol provides highly detailed predetermined observation criteria or prompts, making it useful for observing specific and well-defined procedures and for ensuring consistency across observation sessions and/or observers. One such example is a checklist that can be used for observing the delivery of public health interventions or services such as immunizations or community health education sessions. However, a semistructured observation guide contains more general criteria or prompts that guide the observations while offering the flexibility to observe new criteria or new elements within the criteria. The observation guide should capture both reflective and descriptive notes pertaining to the physical setting, participants, activities and interactions, conversations, subtle factors (e.g., unplanned/informal activities, nonverbal cues), and the researcher's behavior, as set forth by Merriam (2009).

In addition to technical decisions related to the type and structure of the observation, there are several logistical considerations when planning observations, including the population to observe, the specific activities or events to observe, as well as the observation sites and their accessibility. The observation sites have to be purposefully selected based on the location of the target population and the activity or event being observed. Depending on the site, the researcher may need to secure informal or formal, written permission (formal preferred) to access and gain entry into the observation sites. As discussed earlier in this section, it is important to identify local gatekeepers or local connections who can facilitate access and entry into the observation sites given their connections to these sites. Achieving an in-depth understanding of the phenomenon may require extended observations and multiple visits to multiple sites. Observers assuming more active roles or participation in the activity being observed need to establish trust and rapport with the participants being observed prior to engaging in the activities and observations.

During the observation, the observer takes notes of pertinent findings. These observation notes can be used to craft more detailed reflective and descriptive observations notes, also known as field notes, immediately following the event to provide a rich and vivid account of the observed activities. These notes can also be supplemented by images, videos, or audio recordings where ethically and legally permitted. Reflective observation notes capture the researcher's personal experience, reactions, and perceptions regarding the observed activities, while descriptive notes summarize the key aspects of the process, setting, activities, interactions between personnel, and characteristics of participants being observed (Creswell, 2013; Merriam, 2009).

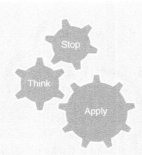

Conducting a Mini Observation

Find a familiar or public setting where you can safely and legally observe an activity without participating in it. This could be your library, church, public transportation, or work or school building. Observe the setting for 10 minutes and take descriptive notes of your observations summarizing key aspects of the *physical setting, participants, activities, and interactions.*

Then, write reflective notes capturing your personal experience, feelings, reactions, and perceptions regarding the activities you observed.

Document Review

Document review or document analysis denotes a systematic and iterative process of reviewing, evaluating, analyzing, and interpreting various types of documents to understand a phenomenon of interest (Bowen, 2009). Documents are a good source of data in qualitative research because they are often easily accessible, less costly to retrieve (i.e., cost-efficient), less obtrusive or unaltered by the research process, and take less time to collect (i.e., time-efficient). They provide rich insights when the phenomenon under study cannot be observed or when participants cannot fully recall the details (Bowen, 2009). Documents can be used as a stand-alone or primary data collection method or they can be used to augment and corroborate evidence from interviews, focus groups, and observations. Documents often provide background and contextual information, shedding light on the socioeconomic, cultural, structural, historical, or political context of a phenomenon. In addition, reviewing existing documents can highlight areas or questions warranting further exploration in subsequent interviews or observations. There are several types of documents that can be used in qualitative research. Merriam (2009) outlines the following types of documents:

- *Public documents*: Official or publicly accessible documents produced by organizations, governments, and institutions to report on their processes, structures, and results/outcomes. Examples of public documents include census reports, records from civil and vital registration systems, government and organizational annual reports, operating manuals, and newspapers. Public documents are often accessible without special permission or authorization and are often reliable sources of information on each organization.

- *Personal/private documents*: Personal/subjective narratives or accounts that reflect an individual's perceptions, feelings, experiences, actions, and behaviors related to a phenomenon. Examples of personal documents include journals, diaries, social media posts, medical records, autobiographies, activity logs, and personal albums and videos. While such documents provide a firsthand account of an individual's own perceptions, experiences, and meanings, they may not be an accurate representation of what actually happened and may not be readily accessible to the researcher for personal and ethical reasons (Merriam, 2009).

- *Physical materials*: Physical objects, materials, or artifacts relevant to the study and found in the study setting, such as tools, pieces of art, posters, utensils, and billboards.

- *Audiovisual and digital documents*: Include a variety of audio or visual materials in physical or digital forms such as photographs, images, videos, films, chats, and emails. Audiovisual materials can be public or private. They often have the capacity to capture activities and behaviors more vividly. However, using these documents for research purposes presents potential ethical and legal issues related to confidentiality, privacy, and copyright that researchers have to prevent. Accessing such documents may also require special permission or authorization from the owners.

Prior to undertaking the document analysis, the researcher has to fulfill steps within the following phases adapted from the steps outlined by O'Leary (2014):

1. *Define the objectives of the document review*. The researcher should clearly determine the role of the document review/analysis in answering the research questions defined earlier in the research process. Essentially, the researcher should determine the information or data needed from the document review.

2. *Identify and list relevant documents to explore*. Having decided on the objectives of the document review, the researcher systematically identifies and creates a list of relevant documents, remaining open to discovering all documents that could potentially provide insights into the research questions. Only relevant and reasonably accessible documents should be considered for review (Merriam, 2009). Additional documents can be identified as the researcher interacts with the participants during data collection.

    When selecting the documents to review, the researcher should consider several ethical, cultural, and linguistic factors that can potentially limit or challenge access to the desired documents. For instance, documents containing personally identifiable information such as medical records are difficult to access and often require additional measures from the researcher, such as data use agreements and justifications of the need for accessing such documents in the ethics review application. Sensitive and culturally significant documents (e.g., cultural artifacts) may not be readily accessible to researchers since they are often intentionally withheld or hidden from outsiders to preserve their cultural significance. Establishing trust and rapport with participants and gatekeepers through prolonged immersion in the study setting has been shown to facilitate access to such documents for research purposes as seen in ethnographic studies. However, the researcher must weigh the risks and benefits of accessing such significant documents. For instance, the researcher can reflect on whether accessing and publishing findings on sensitive documents or artifacts will benefit or harm the community and whether the benefits outweigh the risks. Finally, when conducting international or cross-cultural research, researchers should also be mindful of the linguistic barriers and make necessary plans to translate the documents.

3. *Develop a plan for accessing the documents.* For each of the documents listed, the researcher must identify the potential sources (e.g., organization, individual), locations (physical or online), and contact persons or gatekeepers that will provide access to the documents. Keep in mind that accessing documents that are not publicly accessible requires permission or authorization from the organization's designated gatekeeper or from the author.

4. *Develop strategies for evaluating the authenticity, credibility, and completeness of the documents.* Authenticity and credibility can be assessed by asking questions related to a document's source or origin, the reasons it was produced, the author, any official markers, the date produced, and the context in which it was produced (Merriam, 2009). More specifically, the researcher can ask the following questions to assess the document's authenticity (Guba and Lincoln, 1981; Merriam, 2009; O'Leary, 2014):

    a. Who is the author or creator of the document?

    b. Is this document a primary (firsthand account) or secondary (secondhand account) source?

    c. When was the document produced (if applicable)? Has it been modified or updated?

    d. Why was the document created? (Take note of any potential biases.)

    e. Who is the intended audience?

    f. Is the document complete or is there missing information?

    The individuals or organizations responsible for producing or storing these documents can be interviewed to provide additional background information on the documents.

5. *Define the process for reviewing, coding, and analyzing the content of the documents. I*nvolves reading and rereading each document and annotating or taking notes of excerpts or sections that are relevant and meaningful to the research questions. When reviewing and analyzing each document, researchers can take both descriptive and reflective/analytical notes. Descriptive notes summarize the document's content and analytical/reflective notes capture the researcher's analysis, reflections, and interpretations. The document and the document review notes can be analyzed using both content and thematic analysis, which involve coding and organizing codes into broader categories or themes reflecting patterns in the data as discussed in more detail in the data analysis portion of this section. Additional data collection forms can be used, especially if the document analysis component includes collecting quantitative information to supplement the qualitative data acquired from the documents, as commonly practiced in case study research and qualitative evaluation studies.

Once the document review strategy is defined, the document review process begins. The researcher begins by systematically locating all relevant and accessible documents that could potentially provide insights into the research questions. Permission or authorization to access each document should be secured from gatekeepers as needed. Once granted, the researcher retrieves and gathers the documents and evaluates their relevance, authenticity, and credibility using the predetermined questions. While the documents may contain sufficient information to permit this evaluation, the gatekeepers or key informants can provide additional information regarding the background of the documents. This initial screening process enables the researcher to exclude documents that are deemed irrelevant or unreliable such that only those meeting the initial criteria undergo the full review and analysis process. If possible, the researcher can secure permission to make copies or take photographs of nonsensitive documents as this facilitates the data analysis process. However, this may not be possible for sensitive documents or those containing personally identifiable information, which may have to be reviewed in their respective locations. Systematic document review and analysis requires extended periods of time, multiple site visits, and in some cases, key informant interviews.

As with any data collection method, document review/analysis has inherent limitations. Since the documents were developed prior to the research study and not specifically for research purposes, these documents may not yield sufficient information to answer the research questions (Merriam, 2009). The documents may be incomplete, missing, illegible, inaccurate, or inaccessible. This is especially true in settings with limited use of technology in recordkeeping. In such settings, the researcher may have to sort through piles of papers and notebooks to secure the documents needed for their research, and when secured, some pieces may be missing or misplaced.

Field Notes

Field notes are written by the researcher during data collection, regardless of the data collection method used. They serve as a supplementary source of data because they document the researcher's vivid thoughts in real time and provide contextually rich information that is useful during data analysis and interpretation. The field notes are often handwritten notes when the researcher is actively collecting data, after which they can be transcribed electronically soon after each data collection session. Field notes can be descriptive, reflexive, and methodological. Descriptive notes provide a concrete and detailed description of what the researcher sees, hears, smells, tastes, and experiences during data collection. Essentially, they describe the context, physical setting, participants, behaviors, activities, interactions, verbal and nonverbal cues/communication, and other relevant factors, with no interpretation by the researcher. On the other hand, reflexive notes document the researcher's thought process and interpretation of the elements described in the descriptive notes. This includes their actions and reactions in the field, their feelings, thoughts/ideas, impressions, and analysis of what is happening. Since data collection and analysis occur concurrently in qualitative research, reflexive field notes also document the researcher's developing analytical ideas including the potential codes and themes/patterns as the data are being collected. Descriptive and reflexive notes should be clearly distinguished from each other using schemes that the research deems appropriate. For instance, one can create a two-column table, with descriptive notes in one column and reflexive notes in another column. Alternatively, one can add subheadings or color codes distinguishing descriptive from reflexive notes. Finally, field notes also capture any methodological decisions or modifications made by the researcher over the course of the data collection, along with the rationale for such decisions. This enables the researcher to maintain an audit trail that ensures transparency throughout the study and can be included in the report.

ENSURING THE TRUSTWORTHINESS OF THE FINDINGS

Just as in quantitative research, qualitative researchers are responsible for ensuring that their studies meet standards of rigor. Qualitative research has often been incorrectly evaluated against positivist criteria designed for quantitative research. The concepts of reliability and validity in qualitative research have been highly debated, and distinct concepts like trustworthiness, accuracy, or authenticity have been proposed for qualitative research. Depending on the specific qualitative approach used and the researcher's epistemological standing, there are numerous validation strategies to ensure the accuracy and credibility of the study findings. Lincoln and Guba's (1985) trustworthiness criteria are the most widely adopted. These criteria involve establishing the credibility, dependability, transferability, and confirmability of the research findings.

Credibility

Credibility refers to the plausibility or truthfulness of the research findings—that is, whether the findings presented by the researcher accurately represent participants' experiences and context. There are several practical measures for ensuring credibility such as data triangulation, respondent validation, adequate engagement in data collection, and reflexivity. *Data triangulation* involves the use of multiple data sources to corroborate the findings (Creswell, 2013; Merriam, 2009). *Member checking* or *respondent validation* is considered the most important technique for ensuring credibility (Lincoln and Guba, 1985). It entails sharing the preliminary findings and analysis with the study participants for their evaluation and feedback. A sample of participants are usually recontacted to provide feedback on preliminary findings, clarify misinterpretations, provide additional input, or ensure that their voices are accurately represented. *Reflexivity* involves maintaining a reflexive stance regarding one's position in relation to the study and documenting one's personal assumptions, biases, expectations, and potential influence on the study. *Peer examination, review,* or *debriefing* involves inviting external peers to critically examine or scrutinize the research process, methods, data analysis, interpretation of findings, and conclusions (Anney, 2014; Creswell, 2013; Merriam, 2009). For students, this is already integrated into the thesis or dissertation process, where advisors and dissertation/thesis committee members provide scholarly guidance and feedback (Anney, 2014; Merriam, 2009). The *adequate engagement in data collection* refers to the researcher's active involvement in field research activities, where they directly engage with the participants to better understand their experiences and the study context (Creswell, 2013; Merriam, 2009).

Dependability

Dependability refers to the stability or consistency of the study findings in relation to the data collected (Korstjens and Moser, 2018; Merriam, 2009). Merriam (2009, p. 221) asserts that "the question then is not whether findings will be found again but whether the results are consistent with the data collected." Dependability can be established using triangulation, peer examination, reflexivity, and audit trails. An audit trail is a detailed account of the research procedures and methodological decisions made throughout the study. A study's audit trail is primarily housed in the methodology section, where the researcher provides a transparent account of the research procedures to ensure that they are verifiable (Bowen, 2009). This is facilitated by a reflective journal capturing descriptions of events, reflections, questions, and decisions made throughout the research process (Lincoln and Guba, 1985; Merriam, 2009). *Interrater reliability* or *interrater agreement* is a form of peer examination in which two or more researchers code the same excerpts of selected transcripts to determine their level of agreement on the code application. Alternatively, individual researchers may use the code–recode strategy in which they code the transcripts and recode them after leaving them for some time to compare the level of agreement between both coding sessions. New types of qualitative data analysis software such as Dedoose enable researchers to set-up the inter-rater reliability test and automatically generate a numerical report indicating the level of agreement between multiple coders.

Transferability

Transferability refers to the possibility that the findings can be extrapolated or applied to similar settings based on the reader's judgment. In qualitative research, transferability is problem-oriented and naturalistic as opposed to the statistical generalizability in quantitative research. Transferability is focused on applying lessons learned from one setting to a similar setting while taking into careful consideration the contextual and heterogenous nature of knowledge (Kvale, 1996; Merriam, 2009; Patton, 2002). The reader, not the researcher, assesses whether the findings are applicable to their contexts (Merriam, 2009) based on the researcher's description of the study setting, participants, context, boundaries, findings, and limitations.

Confirmability

Confirmability is the extent to which findings can be confirmed by others. It is concerned with establishing that the research findings do not reflect the researcher's preferences or imagination (Anney, 2014; Korstjens and Moser, 2018). It occurs when credibility, transferability, and dependability have been established (Thomas and Magilvy, 2011). Confirmability can be achieved through previously described techniques, particularly triangulation, audit trail, peer review, and reflexivity.

MANAGING QUALITATIVE DATA

Once collected, the raw data are processed in preparation for data analysis. Data management involves a combination of manual and computer-assisted techniques to process, organize, store, and protect the research data in compliance with the ethical codes for conducting research. Data management comprises various activities including digitization, transcription, verification, deidentification, translation, labeling, classification, and safe storage to facilitate retrieval during data analysis.

Digitization

All physical research documents should be verified for quality, labeled, and classified by content (e.g., interview transcripts, field notes) and kept in sealable envelopes within locked cabinets to which only the research team has access. As much as possible, the research documents should be digitized or converted into electronic files as they are collected, to facilitate storage, sorting, retrieval, and analysis (Merriam, 2009). More specifically, observation notes, field notes, and interview or focus group transcripts can be entered in Microsoft Word or similar applications, while paper documents can be scanned or photographed and uploaded on a computer. Additionally, audio or video recordings should be transferred from the recording devices to a password-protected computer following each interview, focus group, or observation, after which they can be erased from the recording device. All electronic files should be stored in properly labeled folders on a password-protected computer or encrypted device that is accessible only to the researcher or research team. All electronic documents to be analyzed can then be uploaded into a qualitative data management and analysis software, if using any. Ethics committees often require keeping the research outputs or raw data in secure locations for a specified time frame (e.g., three years, five years), after which the physical documents can be shredded and the electronic data erased using special software. Researchers are expected to comply with their ethics committee's specific requirements.

FIGURE 3.13. Qualitative data processing tasks.

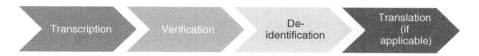

Data management is not merely a technical task; it also involves interpretive and analytical tasks such as transcription, verification, deidentification, and translation (Figure 3.13). These tasks require critical judgments and decisions and, in some cases, the construction of meaning among those involved.

Transcription, Verification, Deidentification

The transcription of audio recorded interviews or focus groups is an interpretive process that translates verbal interactions between researchers and participants into textual form for analytical purposes (Bailey, 2008; Kvale and Brinkmann, 2015). Transcription is considered a preliminary step in data analysis because it involves judgments regarding data interpretation and representation while enabling the researcher to gain an intimate familiarity of the data through repeated listening. Ideally, all audio recordings should be transcribed verbatim (word-for-word), capturing as much detail as possible including any punctuations, pauses, and contextual information such as laughter and other verbal cues. It is recommended that researchers transcribe their own interviews or focus groups as soon as possible because this enhances familiarity with the data, enables them to identify analytical structures and patterns, and minimizes transcription errors. However, transcription is a time-consuming process because it involves listening and relistening to the audio recording. For instance, it can take 4–8 hours to transcribe a 45–60-minute audio recording, which can easily produce a 30 page document (McGrath et al., 2019; Sutton and Austin, 2015). Alternatively, the researcher can transcribe the first few interviews or focus groups and send the remainder to professional transcribers. Researchers with time constraints and sufficient funds can send all audio recordings for professional transcription. While hiring professional transcribers allows the researcher to devote more time to other data analysis tasks, it comes at a higher cost and a higher potential for transcription errors. Once completed, the transcripts must undergo a verification process, where the researcher verifies all or a sample of the transcripts against their original audio recordings to identify and correct any discrepancies, misinterpretations, and inaudible passages. Ensuring the validity of the transcripts enhances the quality of the data analysis and research findings (MacLean et al., 2004).

Maintaining confidentiality or anonymity is a prime ethical concern during data management. All transcripts must be deidentified by removing personal identifiers such as names, specific locations, or job titles and replacing them with pseudonyms or general descriptions (e.g., a community health center, a health care provider). Each participant can be assigned a unique nonidentifying number or name, which can be used on the transcripts and other research documents. A master list linking participants to their assigned name or number should be securely stored in a separate location from the deidentified data and made only accessible to the research team. Any breaches in data security must be immediately reported to the ethics or institutional review board.

Translation

Translation from one language to another adds another layer of interpretation and representation to the transcription process (Bailey, 2008; Nikander 2008) since it involves operating between languages and sociocultural contexts (Halai, 2007; Torop, 2002). Crystal (1991, p. 346) defines translation as a process in which "the meaning and expression in one language [source] is tuned with the meaning of another [target] whether the medium is spoken, written or signed." Given the centrality of interpretation and understanding of meaning in qualitative research, translation should be carefully considered to minimize the loss of meaning and enhance the validity of the research findings. Effective translation ideally requires an understanding of the study's terminology (Piazzoli, 2015), familiarity with the sociocultural context, fluency in both source and target languages, and experience or training in translation. To ensure accuracy in translation, Brislin (1970) recommends assigning at least two bilingual translators who are sufficiently briefed on the study and its terminology. Translations should aim to maintain conceptual equivalence, also known as cultural equivalence, across both languages and sociocultural contexts rather than a literal word-for-word translation

(Squires 2008, 2009). Brislin's (1970) classic model of translation has been widely applied in cross-cultural and international research. This model generally consists of the following key steps: (a) forward translation of the research documents from the source language to the target language by one bilingual translator; (b) back-translation of the documents from the target language back to the source language by a separate bilingual translator; and (c) verification of original documents against translated versions and corrections of discrepancies by both bilingual translators until agreement is reached and no errors are noted in the translated documents. While this process generates high quality translations, it may not be feasible with limited time and funding. Thus, researchers often use modified versions or adaptations of this model to suit their resources. At the minimum, we recommend the following: (a) forward translation of all documents by a professional translator or the bilingual researcher; (b) back-translation of a small sample of documents from the target language back to the source language by a separate bilingual translator unless major errors are discovered in the sample transcripts, in which case all documents should be back-translated (Strauss and Corbin, 1998); and (c) verification of the original documents against the translated versions and corrections of discrepancies by the main translator. Others omit the back translation (step 2) and involve an independent individual in the verification step (step 3).

ANALYZING AND INTERPRETING QUALITATIVE DATA

Qualitative data analysis is a complex and systematic process of organizing, consolidating, reducing, and interpreting data from interviews, observations, documents, and other sources to understand the phenomenon being investigated (Merriam, 2009). Wolcott (2009) breaks down the data analysis or "transformative process" into the following interrelated activities:

- Description: What is happening here?
- Analysis: What are the interrelationships among the concepts, themes, and patterns?
- Interpretation: What does it mean (i.e., relationship to the research questions)?

In qualitative research, data collection, analysis, and interpretation are interactive, simultaneous, and iterative processes. Data analysis begins with the first interview, observation, or document review to enable the refinement of the data collection and further exploration of emerging ideas (Merriam, 2009). While data analysis occurs concurrently with data collection, the analysis becomes more intensified toward the end of data collection, when data saturation is reached (Merriam, 2009).

There are a variety of qualitative data analysis approaches and methods that can be used to analyze data acquired from interviews, focus groups, documents, and other sources. Qualitative data analysis can be broadly grouped into deductive and inductive analytic approaches. The inductive analytic approach identifies the codes and themes from the data and does not apply any predetermined codes or preexisting frameworks on the data. Conversely, the deductive analytic approach fits the data within preexisting coding frameworks derived from existing theories. Braun and Clarke (2006) classify the analytic methods in qualitative research into two main categories. The first category comprises qualitative data analysis methods that are bounded to specific theoretical or epistemological frameworks and have limited flexibility such as discourse analysis, conversation analysis, phenomenological analysis, narrative analysis, and grounded theory analysis. The second category comprises those that are not bounded within theoretical or epistemological positions, and are therefore applicable to various qualitative research designs, theoretical, and epistemological positions (Braun and Clarke, 2006). Thematic analysis belongs to this second category of independent and flexible qualitative analytic methods, making it widely applicable across qualitative designs, data collection methods, as well as theoretical and epistemological positions. Overall, the decision regarding the analysis approach and method to use in a study should take into account the research questions, qualitative design, data collection methods, as well as the researcher's technical skills and resources, among other factors.

While there are some nuances across the qualitative analysis techniques, this section describes in more detail the inductive thematic analysis method given its flexibility and extensive use in the fields of health and social sciences. Thematic analysis was first introduced by Glaser and Strauss (1967) for constructing grounded theory, but it has been widely applied to other qualitative approaches given its rigorous, iterative, comparative, and interactive nature (Charmaz, 2014; Merriam, 2009). It enhances the analytic understanding of perceptions, experiences, actions, and processes in relation to the phenomenon while keeping the researcher grounded in the data. The final output of this analysis is not necessarily a theoretical model, unless used in a grounded theory study. This analysis technique can be used to derive the meaning of participants' experiences in phenomenology, to generate practical lessons and recommendations in case study research, or to acquire a deeper understanding of the meanings ascribed to cultural norms and practices in ethnography.

A hallmark feature of inductive thematic analysis is the *constant comparative method*, an inductive process that involves systematically comparing the data against each other to identify convergent and divergent patterns of meaning across the data. It culminates in a development of categories or themes that are grounded in participants' construction of the phenomenon. In other words, the constant comparative method entails comparing the data with the data, the codes with other codes, the codes with the categories, and the categories with each other until saturation (Kenny and Fourie, 2015). Data analysis using this approach begins with breaking down raw data into the smallest units (word, line, segment) of information that are relevant and meaningful on their own (known as *codes*) and labeling them during a process known as *coding*. Charmaz (2014) describes codes as the skeletal framework of the analysis. Coding with gerunds or verbs (words ending in -ing) rather than nouns or topics is also known as process coding (Saldaña, 2009). Process coding permits the researcher to remain grounded in participants' perspectives and to focus on the processes or actions within the data (what is happening, how, why?). For instance, the codes "experiencing stigma," "feeling stigmatized," "combatting stigma" provide more specific and deeper insights into the participants' experience or perceptions than the codes "stigma" or "stigmatization." The inductive thematic analysis process ends with classifying codes into broad categories or themes that reflect recurring patterns of meaning across the data.

The inductive thematic analysis can be conducted in the following major phases (Figure 3.14) (Charmaz, 2014):

1. An initial phase that involves open line-by-line coding

2. A focused phase that involves recoding the interview transcripts, documents, and observation notes using the most salient and frequent initial codes

3. A thematic phase that involves the identification of themes within the data

This analysis process is not linear; rather, it is an iterative process that requires moving back and forth through the data and making analytic adjustments accordingly (Charmaz, 2014).

The *initial coding phase* begins with an immersion in the data, closely reading and scrutinizing each interview transcript, document, observation note, and field note to reexperience the interactions with participants and gain a deeper understanding of the data. Merriam (2009) considers this familiarization with the data as a rudimentary analysis that informs subsequent levels of analysis. Next, depending on the sample size, a subset or all the interview transcripts, documents, and observation notes are coded line by line. When working in teams, assigning at least two team members to the same set of transcripts generates a rich set of initial codes and enables rich discussions between coders when consolidating the codes in the next phase. Line-by-line coding is particularly useful in the early analysis phase as it enables the researchers to capture all possible data segments that are potentially relevant to the research questions and to discern relationships between the data by making repeated comparisons (Charmaz, 2014; Merriam, 2009). This process generates a comprehensive list of initial codes from the interview transcripts, document reviews, and observations, which are then processed and consolidated in the subsequent phase. The number of initial codes depends on the scope and nature of the study, the volume of the data, and the researchers' analytical skills.

After generating the initial codes, the researcher engages in the *focused/selective coding phase*. First, the initial codes are compared with the data and with other initial codes to identify their interrelationships. Similar initial codes are combined into larger conceptual categories and assigned new labels. The process of consolidating the initial codes and developing focused codes can be time-consuming and laborious as it requires sifting through large volumes of data. For instance, the Community Research Louisville team (n.d.) employed an interactive and collaborative technique for developing focused codes that consisted of printing each coder's initial codes on colored papers with a unique color assigned to each coder, cutting the codes into small pieces of paper, and manually sorting, comparing, and grouping the initial codes into categories. This can also be done electronically using Microsoft Word or qualitative

FIGURE 3.14. *The inductive thematic analysis process.*

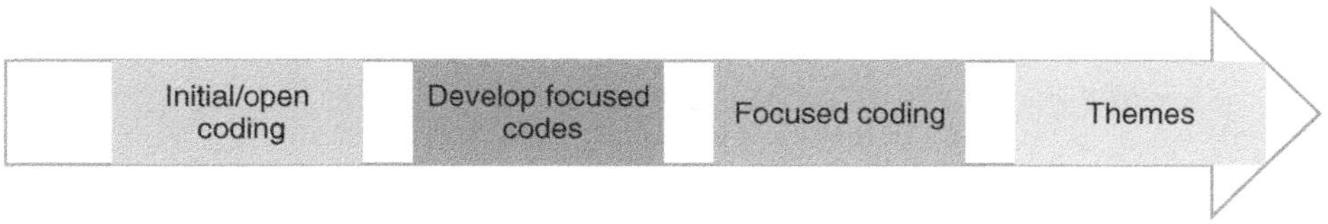

data management software with interactive platforms for teamwork. Not all initial codes become focused codes. Only initial codes or categories that are frequent across the data, significant or relevant to the research questions, and possess high analytic power are elevated as *focused codes* (Charmaz, 2014). Once all focused codes are determined, the next step is to develop a qualitative codebook containing these focused codes and their respective descriptions. If using a qualitative analysis software, this qualitative codebook can be uploaded into the software to facilitate electronic code application. This is still an inductive process since the focused codes in the codebook are derived from the data itself rather than from the literature or existing theoretical frameworks. In addition, this codebook can evolve as the analysis progresses. Qualitative codebooks are useful guides especially when data analysis involves multiple researchers and multiple documents. Next, the focused codes from the codebook are applied to all the interview transcripts, documents, and observation notes, including the clean versions of the documents that were initially coded. In keeping with the constant comparative method, the focused codes are iteratively compared with the data and refined accordingly by merging them into other codes, creating new codes, or creating sub codes. Any changes, revisions, or updates to the codes should also be made to the qualitative codebook after discussions or meetings among the coders.

The final phase consists of *identifying the major themes* within the data. This marks the official beginning of the interpretative analysis of the data (Braun and Clarke, 2006). The researchers begin by carefully examining the applied focused codes and their corresponding excerpts to identify broad patterns of meanings in relation to the research questions. To facilitate this task when using a software, one option is to export the coded transcripts, documents, and observation notes from the qualitative data management software (e.g., Dedoose™) into Microsoft Word. The focused codes, their corresponding coded excerpts, and the analytical narrative of the excerpts can then be arranged into a table (e.g., Table 3.5).

The focused codes and their corresponding excerpts are then sorted and combined into broader categories or themes and subthemes that reflect divergent and convergent patterns of meaning. The identification of the themes depends on the researcher's judgment. This should not be based on prevalence or frequency across the data but rather on whether the theme/pattern conveys something meaningful or significant in relation to the phenomenon and to the research questions (Braun and Clarke, 2006). Each theme should capture variations and nuances related to the patterns they represent. These themes are iteratively reviewed against the data and refined to ensure that they accurately represent the relationships and meanings within the data and answer the research questions. The themes should be distinct from each other yet linked in such a way that when put together, they tell a coherent story about the data and the research questions in relation to the phenomenon of interest. The researcher then develops an analytical narrative for each theme and subtheme to convey the meaning and story of the theme in relation to the research questions. This

TABLE 3.5. Example of Focused Codes, Corresponding Excerpts, and Analytic Narrative

Focused codes	Corresponding quotes/excerpts	Analytical narrative
Feeling isolated Seeking social connectedness	▪ "You know, there's a great sense of feeling isolated and being isolated and not being connected." ▪ "I think another thing is helping people get connected in whatever way that works--so that's providing people an opportunity to kinda engage in the activity, to get them to think to actually be involved, as opposed to focusing on their…you know past and you know…just being isolated. That's been important." ▪ "So the relationship is really important but a relationship that helps people to see the best of themselves and work toward the future."	Survivors of abuse often feel a sense of isolation and disconnect from their society. Positive relationships and social support from family members, community members, and service providers are vital elements in their healing and recovery as they enable them to "think differently" and "work toward the future" rather than focusing on their past.

constitutes the researcher's interpretation of the theme that is grounded in the data. Braun and Clarke (2006) propose the following questions to guide the development of analytical narratives that are beyond a mere description of the content:

- What does this theme mean?
- What are the underlying assumptions?
- What are the implications of this theme?
- What are the possible explanations or conditions that may have given rise to it (within the data)?
- Why do participants talk about or view this theme in this particular way?
- What is the overall story of this theme in relation to the research question and the topic?

Finally, the researcher names each theme and subtheme with a label that concisely reflects its meaning or narrative. Since qualitative research studies often collect quantitative information on the sample's characteristics, simple descriptive statistics (e.g., frequencies and proportions) can be generated using qualitative, mixed methods, or quantitative data analysis software to provide an overview of the sociodemographic characteristics of the sample.

The researcher should maintain analytic memos throughout data analysis. Analytic memos articulate the researcher's analytic ideas, reflections, questions, interpretations, and decisions throughout data collection and more importantly, during data analysis. Analytic memos primarily focus on data analysis while field notes primarily focus on data collection when the researcher is in the field. In other words, analytic memo writing starts during data collection because of the concurrent nature of data collection and analysis in qualitative research but extends beyond data collection, when data analysis is intensified. Analytic memos specifically capture the researcher's reflections on the code selection, recurring patterns or themes, and interpretations of the key findings as they collect, transcribe, read/review, and code the data. Both field notes and memos are also considered data and can be coded during data analysis.

Qualitative Data Analysis Software

While qualitative coding and analysis can be done manually with physical copies of the documents, computer-assisted qualitative data analysis enables faster and more efficient data management and analysis. Qualitative data analysis software are designed to facilitate storing, organizing, sorting, retrieving/locating, annotating, and analyzing qualitative data and, in many cases, mixed methods data. Table 3.6 provides a list of common qualitative data management and analysis software, which typically offer similar features with a few nuances. Researchers should seek training or review tutorials issued by these platforms to ensure their optimal utilization and maximize their benefits to the research study.

TABLE 3.6. **Common Qualitative Data Management and Analysis Software**

Software	Description
ATLAS.ti	- Computer-based (Mac and Windows) - Supports qualitative and mixed methods data analysis
Dedoose	- Web-based and computer-based: can be used online on any device or downloaded as a desktop app - Supports qualitative and mixed-methods data analysis
Nvivo	- Computer-based (Mac and Windows) - Supports qualitative and mixed-methods data analysis
MAXQDA	- Computer based- (identical on Mac and Windows) - Supports qualitative and mixed-methods data analysis

TABLE 3.6. (Continued)

Software	Description
QDA Miner	▪ Computer-based (Mac and Windows) ▪ Supports qualitative and mixed-methods data analysis
Taguette	▪ Web-based and computer-based (Mac, Windows, Linux) ▪ Supports qualitative data analysis ▪ Free and open source
Coding Analysis Toolkit (CAT)	▪ Web-based: Mac, Windows, Linux ▪ Supports qualitative data analysis ▪ Free and open source
HyperRESEARCH	▪ Computer-based: Windows, with reduced functionality on Mac ▪ Supports qualitative data analysis
Quirkos	▪ Computer-based: Windows, Mac, Android or Linux; also has cloud storage so that data can be accessed on any device ▪ Supports qualitative data analysis

REPORTING AND DISSEMINATING THE RESEARCH FINDINGS

The research study culminates in reporting and disseminating the findings to diverse audiences in various formats to inform further research, public health practice, and policies. The findings should be widely and strategically disseminated to academic audiences (e.g., peer-reviewed publications) and more importantly, nonacademic audiences including practitioners, community members, policymakers, and media personnel (Figure 3.15). While researchers have

FIGURE 3.15. *Disseminating qualitative research findings.*

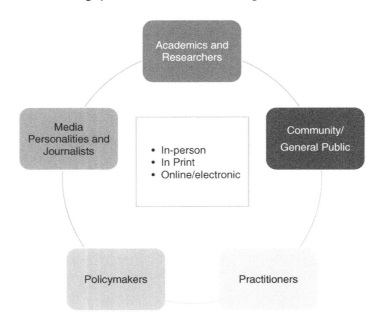

traditionally limited their dissemination to academic audiences to contribute to the scholarly debate on the topic, disseminating the research findings to nonacademic audiences with the capacity to act on them promotes the translation of research findings into practice or policy through policy advocacy and participatory action within communities and organizations. Module 5 discusses various methods and tools for disseminating findings to both academic and nonacademic audiences.

Develop a Dissemination Plan

Propose a research topic of your choice and answer the following questions related to your dissemination plan:

1. What is your proposed research topic [propose a tentative title]?
2. In one sentence, what is the purpose of your study?
3. Who are the primary and secondary audiences for your research findings?
4. What are the best dissemination methods to communicate your findings with each audience?

Writing a Qualitative Research Report

A formal research report is often the preliminary or primary method for reporting the research findings to the organization that commissioned the study and the stakeholders within these organizations. While quantitative research has widely accepted reporting standards or guidelines for a research report, there is no consensus on criteria for reporting qualitative findings but rather a variety of approaches given the diversity of qualitative research designs operating within multiple philosophical frameworks. Hays and Singh (2012) assert that the technique used in writing the qualitative research report is largely shaped by the qualitative researcher's writing philosophy, which itself is rooted in their broader philosophical orientation. They particularly identify four qualitative writing philosophies, with the first two (i.e., holy trinity and translation approaches) having positivist/postpositivist undertones and the last two (i.e., emergence of qualitative criteria and criteria as relative and emerging) expressing interpretivist/constructivist orientations (Hays and Singh, 2012):

1. *The holy trinity approach*: Models qualitative reports after quantitative reports and guidelines and incorporates positivist/postpositivist language that conveys the objectivity of the researcher and the research process

2. *Translation approach:* Reflects gold standard writing guidelines or criteria that have been translated from quantitative into qualitative standards (e.g., measures of rigor such as credibility, transferability) while conveying the subjectivity of the researcher and the research process

3. *Emergence of qualitative criteria*: Acknowledges that there are multiple approaches and criteria for reporting qualitative findings that are unique to qualitative research and selects the most effective writing approach that suits the context of one's research

4. *Criteria as relative and emerging*: Does not utilize specific established criteria in writing the report; the report reflects the recursive and iterative nature of the qualitative research process and provides a detailed description of the research processes and the researcher's role using a suitable approach

Rather than prescribing a specific approach, we acknowledge that the approach used is driven by each researcher's beliefs about the truth or reality (i.e., epistemology, axiology, ontology), by the specific qualitative research design, and the research questions. Qualitative researchers often espouse a combination of the writing philosophies identified by Hays and Singh (2012). As such, each researcher should reflect on their philosophical paradigms, their writing philosophies, as well as the strengths and limitations of these philosophies in relation to their research study. Researchers should be ready to justify the writing philosophy or technique used in representing the research process, findings, and their role in the study. Regardless of the approach used, a qualitative researcher should adhere to the following fundamental principles when writing a qualitative research report: (a) maintain transparency about the processes and their complexities; (b) maintain transparency about the researcher's positionality; (c) remain grounded in the data, staying true to the collective accounts of participants, observations, and documents; and (d) clearly distinguish the participants voice from the researcher's voice or interpretation and from the literature.

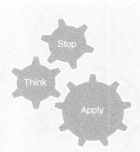

Define your Writing Approach

Review and reflect on the qualitative writing philosophies proposed by Hays and Singh (2012), as presented in this section. After your reflection, answer the following questions:

- Which writing philosophies best describe yours?
- Discuss the relationship between your writing philosophy and your general philosophical paradigm or orientation.
- Develop a basic outline for a qualitative research report based on your writing philosophy.

Reporting guidelines provide a set of standards or criteria related to the content and structure of a research report for different research designs. These guidelines are developed by panels of methodological experts, drawing on the evidence and on their collective experiences (Simera et al., 2010). They are often used by peer reviewers and publishers for evaluating the quality of research reports submitted to them and by writers to develop quality and comprehensive research reports. While there are several reporting guidelines for quantitative designs, only a few have been developed for qualitative designs. The Consolidated Criteria for Reporting Qualitative Research (COREQ) and Standards for Reporting Qualitative Research (SRQR) are common qualitative reporting guidelines. The COREQ is a reporting guideline for qualitative studies involving interviews and focus groups (Tong et al., 2007). It contains a checklist of 32 items within the following three domains: research team and reflexivity, study design, and analysis of findings. COREQ specifically requires that researchers report on their personal characteristics (e.g., credentials, experience), their relationships with the participants, the theoretical framework and qualitative approach, participant selection (e.g., sampling and recruitment), study setting, data collection procedures, data analysis procedures, as well as the findings (themes and participant quotations) (Tong et al., 2007). The SQRQ contains similar items but structures the main report around the common AIM (RaD) acronym (abstract, introduction, methods, results, discussion), with additional guidelines related to the title and abstract (O'Brien et al., 2014). The SQRQ lists the following items to include in a qualitative research report: statement of the problem and research questions, qualitative approach, theoretical framework, philosophical paradigm, researcher characteristics and reflexivity, study context, sampling strategy, ethical issues related to human subjects, data collection methods, instruments and technologies, units of study, data processing, data analysis, strategies to enhance the trustworthiness of the study and findings, the findings and interpretation, a discussion of the findings within the context of the literature, and the limitations of the study (O'Brien et al., 2014).

Table 3.7 presents the general components of a qualitative research report based on the established qualitative reporting guidelines, the literature, and on our collective qualitative research experiences. The final report builds on

TABLE 3.7. **The Structure and Contents of Qualitative Research Report**

Title
- The title of the study (include the specific topic and qualitative approach used)
- Authors, credentials, and affiliations
- Institution the report is submitted to
- Date produced or submitted

Acknowledgments (technical, material, or financial support received)

Table of Contents

Abstract
- A structured summary (150–500 words) of the research study, with the following headings: introduction/background, methods, results, conclusions
- Relevant keywords at the end of the abstract (optional)

Introduction
- Statement of the problem in context
- Background information on the problem (i.e., summary of the literature review)
- Statement of the purpose, aims, or objectives of the study
- Research questions
- The structure/organization of the report (typically for longer reports)

Literature review (can be included in the introduction section if not a required section)
- Related literature
- Conceptual Framework

Methodology
- Description of the study setting and context
- Philosophical paradigm
- Theoretical/interpretive framework
- Qualitative design/approach and rationale for the design selection
- Researcher's role and relevant background (i.e., reflexivity/positionality statement)
- Participants and other data sources
    - Sample, sampling methods, and sample size
    - Accessing the study site and participants
    - Recruitment methods (e.g., email, phone) and procedures
    - Incentives or compensation if applicable
- Data collection
    - Data collection methods and procedures (include duration)
    - Description of data collection tools and equipment
    - Informed consent process
- Data management procedures
    - Storage, digitization, transcription, verification, translation
    - Ethical considerations in data handling and storage
- Data analysis procedures
    - Unit of analysis
    - Analytical method, procedures (e.g., coding, derivation of themes), and personnel
    - Software

(Continued)

TABLE 3.7. (Continued)

- Ethical considerations and human subjects protection
- Strategies for ensuring the trustworthiness of the findings

Findings
- Sociodemographic characteristics of participants or units
- Rich, thick description and interpretation of the findings (i.e., themes, analytic narratives, quotes, excerpts)

Discussion
- Restate the main contributions/findings of the study
- Compare, contrast, and explain with prior research or theories from the literature
- Strengths and limitations of the study
- Implications and recommendations for practice, policy, and future research

Conclusion
- Concisely restate the purpose of the study and response to the research questions.
- Emphasize the significance or unique contribution of the study
- Reiterate the main recommendations for policy, practice, and/or future research

References

Appendices
- Supplementary materials such as data collection tools, informed consent forms, or letters

the research proposal, adding the following three major sections: findings, discussion, and conclusions. However, since qualitative research is a dynamic and evolving process, the sections of the research proposal, particularly the methods section, should be revised prior to being incorporated into the final research report to ensure that the final report accurately reflects the actual procedures that were conducted. In addition, the tense should be changed from the future tense used in sections of the research proposal to past tense, indicating that the study has been completed. The components of a research report and the various dissemination methods are discussed extensively in Module 5.

The findings section of a qualitative research report goes beyond a mere description of the themes. It is rather an analytical and interpretive narrative that tells a compelling story of the themes within the data in relation to the research questions (Braun and Clarke, 2006). The analytical points in the narrative must be grounded in the data and substantiated by carefully selected and unedited excerpts from the data such as participants' vivid quotes, document excerpts, or photographs. This demonstrates that in qualitative research, the researcher's interpretation is not restricted to the discussion section as it is already integrated into the findings section in a balanced account comprising the researcher's interpretation of the data and the data excerpts supporting their interpretation (Wu et al., 2016). In addition, the findings section can incorporate visuals or graphics (e.g., models, diagrams) that illustrate the connections between the themes or concepts of the study. As such the findings section of a qualitative research report is typically longer than the results section of a quantitative research report.

Whether to combine the findings and discussion sections in a qualitative research report or to present them as two distinct sections remains debated in qualitative research circles. The choice to combine or separate these two sections depends on a combination of factors including the qualitative design used, the researcher's judgment and writing philosophy, the purpose of the study, and the organization or publisher's requirements. We recommend separating the findings and discussion sections, where the findings section provides a rich description and interpretation of the data while the discussion section expands the interpretation of the findings within the context of the existing literature. Combining these sections can make it challenging to distinguish between the findings from the data and the findings from the literature. It also prevents the researcher and the readers from clearly visualizing and appreciating the richness and uniqueness of the data. For those who decide to combine both sections, we recommend that the narrative make a clear distinction between the data excerpts and analytical narratives grounded in the data, and the existing literature.

In addition to comparing the findings with the existing literature, the discussion section typically highlights the study's significant contribution to the literature and to the field, presents the strengths and limitations of the study, and discusses its implications on practice, policy, and future research. Limitations are methodological or design-related weaknesses that can influence the quality of the study and its findings. The discussion of the limitations includes a statement of the important limitations, their potential influence on the quality or trustworthiness of the study, and practical strategies for mitigating these limitations in future studies. Providing a transparent account of the limitations and their potential influence on the research study is an ethical obligation because it guides the reader's evaluation of the research findings and conclusions, as well as their relevance, applicability/transferability, and utility. When discussing the limitations of qualitative research studies, it is important to avoid measuring the quality of qualitative research designs against the standards of rigor for quantitative research. For instance, generalizability is not considered a limitation in qualitative studies because by design, qualitative research intends to seek depth rather than breadth or generalizability. Examples of limitations that can affect the trustworthiness of the study findings include the composition of the focus group (e.g., homogenous), social desirability bias, lack of access to the original documents with a firsthand account, resource constraints (time and finances), or data collection and analytical flaws.

Box 3.10 presents some general writing tips that are specific to qualitative research.

BOX 3.10 General Tips When Writing a Qualitative Research Report

- A qualitative research report can be written in first person. The first person is accepted in qualitative research because it recognizes the researcher's subjectivity and reflective stance.
- Qualitative research prefers the term *findings* rather than *results* because the former emphasizes the exploratory nature of qualitative research whereas the latter denotes finality (Hays and Singh, 2012).
- In the findings section, the researcher's analytical and interpretive narrative must be grounded in and supported by the participants' narratives or excerpts from other data sources used in the study.
- The main themes and subthemes are typically used as headings and subheadings within the findings section. Note that the themes are the patterns within the data and not the research questions nor the interview questions.
- When referring to the themes, use the terms *developed* or *identified* rather than *emerging* or *discovered* because the last two terms do not recognize the researcher's active role in the analysis process and in identifying the themes within the data (Braun and Clarke, 2006).
- Ensure that the selected quotes accurately and adequately support the theme or narrative to which they are linked (Wu et al., 2016).
- Use each quote only once in the report.
- Use quotes and other excerpts from the data to support but not replace the analytic narrative.
- Use quotes of moderate length to preserve their context.

 ## SUMMARY

This section discussed the technical, methodological, ethical, cultural, and logistical considerations of designing, implementing, and disseminating a qualitative research study.

In qualitative research, recruitment, data collection, analysis, and interpretation occur concurrently. Since qualitative research is more concerned about the richness and depth of the information than the sample size, it employs nonprobability sampling, in which the units are purposively selected based on their ability to generate rich insights into the phenomenon.

Interviews, focus groups, observations, and document reviews are the primary data collection methods in qualitative research. An interview is a structured, semistructured, or unstructured research-oriented conversation between a researcher and a participant. A focus groups is a facilitated group discussion that elicits participants' collective experiences and meanings related to a phenomenon. When conducting observations, the researcher

(continued)

(continued)

can assume one of the following roles, ranging from covert to overt and from participation to nonparticipation in the event being observed: complete participant, complete observer, participant as observer, and nonparticipant/observer as participant. Document review is a systematic evaluation, analysis, and interpretation of various types of documents related to a phenomenon. Researchers must administer and obtain informed consent from participants prior to data collection.

Qualitative data analysis can be broadly grouped into deductive and inductive analytic approaches. The inductive analytic approach identifies the codes and themes from the data rather than applying preexisting codes or frameworks. Conversely, the deductive analytic approach fits the data within preexisting coding frameworks derived from existing theories. Qualitative data analysis generally begins with coding the data and ends with classifying codes into broad categories or themes that reflect recurring patterns of meaning across the data.

Lincoln and Guba's (1985) trustworthiness criteria are the most widely adopted standards of rigor in qualitative research. These criteria involve establishing the credibility, dependability, transferability, and confirmability of the research process and findings.

The research study culminates in reporting and disseminating the findings to academic and nonacademic audiences. While a qualitative research report generally follows the standard scientific reporting format, the findings section of a qualitative research report goes beyond a mere description of the findings and presents the researcher's analytical and interpretive narrative that is grounded in and supported by the data.

Now that I have reached the end of this section, I am able to:

Course objective	Strongly agree	Somewhat agree	Neutral	Somewhat disagree	Strongly agree
Describe qualitative data collection methods					
Analyze and interpret qualitative data					
Develop an outline for a qualitative research report					
Discuss relevant ethical and cultural considerations in each phase of the qualitative research process					

REFERENCES

Agee, J. (2009). Developing qualitative research questions: A reflective process. *International Journal of Qualitative Studies in Education*, 22(4), 431–447. http://doi.org/10.1080/09518390902736512

Ali, N. M., Combs, R. M., Muvuka, B., & Ayangeakaa, S. D. (2018). Addressing health insurance literacy gaps in an urban African American population: A qualitative study. *Journal of Community Health*, 43(6), 1208–1216. http://doi.org/10.1007/s10900-018-0541-x

Anney, V. N. (2014). Ensuring the quality of the findings of qualitative research: Looking at trustworthiness criteria. *Journal of Emerging Trends in Educational Research and Policy Studies*, 5(2), 272–281.

Ataro, G. (2020). Methods, methodological challenges and lesson learned from phenomenological study about OSCE experience: Overview of paradigm-driven qualitative approach in medical education. *Annals of Medicine and Surgery (London)*, 49, 19–23. http://doi.org/10.1016/j.amsu.2019.11.013

Bailey, J. (2008). First steps in qualitative data analysis: Transcribing. *Family Practice*, 25(2), 127–131. http://doi.org/10.1093/fampra/cmn003

Baxter, P., & Jack, S. (2008). Qualitative case study methodology: Study design and implementation for novice researchers. *Qualitative Report*, 13(4), 544–559.

Bernard, H. R. (1994). *Research methods in anthropology: qualitative and quantitative approaches* (2nd ed.). Sage Publications.

Bowen, G. A. (2009). Document analysis as a qualitative research method. *Qualitative Research Journal*, 9(2), 27–40. http://doi.org/10.3316/QRJ0902027

Braun, V., & Clarke, V. (2006). Using thematic analysis in psychology. *Qualitative Research in Psychology*, 3(2), 77–101. http://doi.org/10.1191/1478088706qp063oa

Brislin, R. W. (1970). Back-translation for cross-cultural research. *Journal of Cross-Cultural Psychology*, 1(3), 185–216. http://doi.org/10.1177/135910457000100301

Bryant, A. (2017). *Grounded theory and grounded theorizing: pragmatism in research practice*. Oxford University Press.

Byrne, M. (2001). The concept of informed consent in qualitative research. *AORN Journal*, 74(3), 401–403. http://doi.org/10.1016/s0001-2092(06)61798-5

Calba, C., Goutard, F. L., Hoinville, L., Hendrikx, P., Lindberg, A., Saegerman, C., & Peyre, M. (2015). Surveillance systems evaluation: A systematic review of the existing approaches. *BMC Public Health*, 15, 448. http://doi.org/10.1186/s12889-015-1791-5

Cardwell, F. S., & Elliott, S. J. (2013). Making the links: Do we connect climate change with health? A qualitative case study from Canada. *BMC Public Health*, 13(1), 208. http://doi.org/10.1186/1471-2458-13-208

Carrico, C., Boynton, M., Matusovich, H. M., and Paretti, M. C. (2013). *Development of an interview protocol to understand engineering as a career choice for Appalachian youth*. Paper presented at the American Society of Engineering Education, Atlanta, GA. https://www.asee.org/public/conferences/20/papers/6810/view

Centers for Disease Control and Prevention. (2020). *National Diabetes Statistics Report, 2020*. Atlanta: GA: Centers for Disease Control and Prevention, U.S. Dept of Health and Human Services; https://www.cdc.gov/diabetes/pdfs/data/statistics/national-diabetes-statistics-report.pdf.

Charmaz, K. (2006). *Constructing grounded theory*. Sage Publications.

Charmaz, K. (2014). *Constructing grounded theory* (2nd ed.). Sage.

Chaudhary, A. K., and Israel, G. D. (2014). *The Savvy Survey #8: Pilot Testing and Pretesting Questionnaires*. Department of Agricultural Education and Communication; UF/IFAS Extension. Gainesville, FL https://edis.ifas.ufl.edu/pd072

Collins, C. S., & Stockton, C. M. (2018). The central role of theory in qualitative research. *International Journal of Qualitative Methods*, 17(1), 1609406918797475. http://doi.org/10.1177/1609406918797475

Community Research Louisville. (n.d.). Community Research Louisville. https://communityresearchlouisville.com

Connelly, F. M., & Clandinin, D. J. (1990). Stories of experience and narrative inquiry. *Educational Researcher*, 19(5), 2–14. http://doi.org/10.3102/0013189x019005002

Connelly, F. M., & Clandinin, D. J. (2006). Narrative inquiry. In F. Erickson, J. Green, G. Camilli, & P. Elmore (Eds.), *Handbook of complementary methods in education research* (pp. 477–487). Routledge.

Conway, L., Wolverson, E., & Clarke, C. (2020). Shared experiences of resilience amongst couples where one partner is living with dementia-a grounded theory study. *Frontiers in Medicine*, 7, 219–219. http://doi.org/10.3389/fmed.2020.00219

Corbin, J. M., & Strauss, A. L. (2008). *Basics of qualitative research: techniques and procedures for developing grounded theory* (3rd ed.). Sage Publications, Inc.

Corbin, J. M., & Strauss, A. L. (2015). *Basics of qualitative research: techniques and procedures for developing grounded theory* (4th ed.). SAGE.

Cornell University Cooperative Extension. (n.d.). *Group Ground Rules*. https://cpb-us-e1.wpmucdn.com/blogs.cornell.edu/dist/f/575/files/2016/07/newlogo-YG-Group-Ground-Rules-zvfel4.pdf

Creighton, G., Oliffe, J. L., Ferlatte, O., Bottorff, J., Broom, A., & Jenkins, E. K. (2018). Photovoice ethics: Critical reflections from men's mental health research. *Qualitative Health Research*, 28(3), 446–455. http://doi.org/10.1177/1049732317729137

Creswell, J. W. (2013). *Qualitative inquiry and research design: choosing among five approaches* (3rd ed.). SAGE Publications.

Creswell, J. W., & Creswell, J. D. (2018). *Research design: qualitative, quantitative, and mixed methods approaches* (5th ed.). SAGE.

Crowe, S., Cresswell, K., Robertson, A., Huby, G., Avery, A., & Sheikh, A. (2011). The case study approach. *BMC Medical Research Methodology*, 11, 100. http://doi.org/10.1186/1471-2288-11-100

Crystal, D. (1991). *The Cambridge encyclopedia* (2nd ed.). Cambridge University Press.

Donabedian, A. (1966). Evaluating the quality of medical care. *Milbank Memorial Fund Quarterly*, 44(3), Suppl:166-206.

Flyvbjerg, B. (2006). Five misunderstandings about case study research. *Qualitative Inquiry*, 12(2), 219–245. http://doi.org/10.1177/1077800405284363

Glaser, B. G., & Strauss, A. L. (1967). *The discovery of grounded theory; strategies for qualitative research*. Aldine Pub. Co.

Grant, R. W., & Sugarman, J. (2004). Ethics in human subjects research: Do incentives matter? *Journal of Medicine and Philosophy*, 29(6), 717–738. http://doi.org/10.1080/03605310490883046

Green, J., & Thorogood, N. (2018). *Qualitative methods for health research* (4th ed.). SAGE Publications.

Guba, E. G., & Lincoln, Y. S. (1981). *Effective evaluation*. Jossey-Bass Publishers.

Guba, E. G., & Lincoln, Y. S. (1994). Competing paradigms in qualitative research. In *Handbook of qualitative research* (pp. 105–117). Sage Publications, Inc.

Guest, G., Namey, E. E., & Mitchell, M. L. (2013). *Collecting qualitative data: a field manual for applied research*. SAGE Publications.

Halai, N. (2007). Making use of bilingual interview data: Some experiences from the field. *Qualitative Report*, 12(3), 344–355.

Halcomb, E. J., Gholizadeh, L., DiGiacomo, M., Phillips, J., & Davidson, P. M. (2007). Literature review: Considerations in undertaking focus group research with culturally and linguistically diverse groups. *Journal of Clinical Nursing*, 16(6), 1000–1011. http://doi.org/10.1111/j.1365-2702.2006.01760.x

Hall, J. M. (2011). Narrative methods in a study of trauma recovery. *Qualitative Health Research*, 21(1), 3–13. http://doi.org/10.1177/1049732310377181

Hannes, K., & Parylo, O. (2014). Let's play it safe: Ethical considerations from participants in a photovoice research project. *International Journal of Qualitative Methods*, 13(1), 255–274. http://doi.org/10.1177/160940691401300112

Harper, D. (2002). Talking about pictures: A case for photo elicitation. *Visual Studies*, 17(1), 13–26. http://doi.org/10.1080/14725860220137345

Hays. D. G., & Singh, A. A. (2012). *Qualitative inquiry in clinical and educational settings*. Guilford Press.

Herrmann, A., Hall, A., & Proietto, A. (2018). Using the health belief model to explore why women decide for or against the removal of their ovaries to reduce their risk of developing cancer. *BMC Women's Health*, 18(1), 184. http://doi.org/10.1186/s12905-018-0673-2

Holmes, A. G. (2014). *Researcher positionality: A consideration of its influence and place in research*. Hull.

Hughes, J. L., Camden, A. A., & Yangchen, T. (2016). Rethinking and updating demographic questions: Guidance to improve descriptions of research samples. *Psi Chi Journal of Psychological Research*, *21*, 138–151.

Hulton, L. A., Matthews, Z., & Stones, R. W. (2000). *A framework for the evaluation of quality of care in maternity services*. University of Southampton.

Kelly, B., Margolis, M., McCormack, L., LeBaron, P. A., & Chowdhury, D. (2017). What affects people's willingness to participate in qualitative research? An experimental comparison of five incentives. *Field Methods*, *29*(4), 333–350. http://doi.org/10.1177/1525822x17698958

Kenny, M., & Fourie, R. J. (2015). Contrasting classic, straussian, and constructivist grounded theory: Methodological and philosophical conflicts. *Qualitative Report*, *20*, 1270–1289.

Khisa, A. M., Omoni, G. M., Nyamongo, I. K., & Spitzer, R. F. (2017). 'I stayed with my illness': A grounded theory study of health seeking behaviour and treatment pathways of patients with obstetric fistula in Kenya. *BMC Women's Health*, *17*(1), 92–92. http://doi.org/10.1186/s12905-017-0451-6

Klykken, F. H. (2021). Implementing continuous consent in qualitative research. *Qualitative Research*. http://doi.org/10.1177/14687941211014366

Knight, R., Fast, D., DeBeck, K., Shoveller, J., & Small, W. (2017). "Getting out of downtown": A longitudinal study of how street-entrenched youth attempt to exit an inner city drug scene. *BMC Public Health*, *17*(1), 376. http://doi.org/10.1186/s12889-017-4313-9

Korstjens, I., & Moser, A. (2018). Series: Practical guidance to qualitative research. Part 4: Trustworthiness and publishing. *European Journal of General Practice*, *24*(1), 120–124. http://doi.org/10.1080/13814788.2017.1375092

Kvale, S. (1996). *InterViews: An introduction to qualitative research interviewing*. Sage Publications.

Kvale, S., & Brinkmann, S. (2015). *InterViews: Learning the craft of qualitative research interviewing* (3rd ed.). Sage Publications.

Lännerström, L., Wallman, T., & Holmström, I. K. (2013). Losing independence—the lived experience of being long-term sick-listed. *BMC Public Health*, *13*, 745–745. http://doi.org/10.1186/1471-2458-13-745

Liebenberg, L. (2018). Thinking critically about photovoice: Achieving empowerment and social change. *International Journal of Qualitative Methods*, *17*(1), 1609406918757631. http://doi.org/10.1177/1609406918757631

Lincoln, Y. S., & Guba, E. G. (1985). *Natrualistic inquiry*. SAGE Publications.

MacLean, L. M., Meyer, M., & Estable, A. (2004). Improving accuracy of transcripts in qualitative research. *Qualitative Health Research*, *14*(1), 113–123. http://doi.org/10.1177/1049732303259804

Maxwell, J. A. (2009). Designing a qualitative study. In L. Bickman & D. J. Rog (Eds.), *The SAGE handbook of applied social research methods* (2nd ed., pp. 214–253). SAGE Publisher. http://doi.org/10.4135/9781483348858.n7

McGrath, C., Palmgren, P. J., & Liljedahl, M. (2019). Twelve tips for conducting qualitative research interviews. *Medical Teacher*, *41*(9), 1002–1006. http://doi.org/10.1080/0142159X.2018.1497149

Merriam, S. B. (2009). *Qualitative research: a guide to design and implementation*. Jossey-Bass.

Miles, M. B., & Huberman, A. M. (1994). *Qualitative data analysis: an expanded sourcebook* (2nd ed.). Sage Publications.

Morse, J. M. (2016). Underlying ethnography. *Qualitative Health Research*, *26*(7), 875–876. http://doi.org/10.1177/1049732316645320

Moustakas, C. E. (1994). *Phenomenological research methods*. Sage.

Muvuka, B. (2019). *Uncovering the stories behind the numbers: A case study of maternal death surveillance and response in Goma, Democratic Republic of Congo*. Electronic Theses and Dissertations (Paper 3194).

Muvuka, B., & Harris, M. J. (2019). A rapid assessment of the impacts of gold mining on women's health and quality of life in Ashanti region, Ghana. *Journal of Public Health Issues and Practices*, *2*, 138. http://doi.org/10.33790/jphip1100138

Neubauer, B. E., Witkop, C. T., & Varpio, L. (2019). How phenomenology can help us learn from the experiences of others. *Perspectives on Medical Education*, *8*(2), 90–97. http://doi.org/10.1007/s40037-019-0509-2

Nikander, P. (2008). Working with transcripts and translated data. *Qualitative Research in Psychology*, *5*(3), 225–231. http://doi.org/10.1080/14780880802314346

Nyumba, T. O., Wilson, K., Derrick, C. J., & Mukherjee, N. (2018). The use of focus group discussion methodology: Insights from two decades of application in conservation. *Methods in Ecology and Evolution*, *9*(1), 20–32. http://doi.org/10.1111/2041-210x.12860

O'Brien, B. C., Harris, I. B., Beckman, T. J., Reed, D. A., & Cook, D. A. (2014). Standards for reporting qualitative research: A synthesis of recommendations. *Academic Medicine*, *89*(9), 1245–1251. http://doi.org/10.1097/ACM.0000000000000388

O'Leary, Z. (2014). *The essential guide to doing your research project* (2nd ed.). SAGE.

Patton, M. Q. (2002). *Qualitative research and evaluation methods: integrating theory and practice* (3rd ed.). Sage Publications.

Piazzoli, E. C. (2015). Translation in cross-language qualitative research: Pitfalls and opportunities. *Translation and Translanguaging in Multilingual Contexts*, *1*(1), 80–102. http://doi.org/10.1075/ttmc.1.1.04pia

Polkinghorne, D. E. (2007). Validity issues in narrative research. *Qualitative Inquiry*, *13*, 471–486.

Prescott, F. J. (2011). *Validating a Long Qualitative Interview Schedule*. WoPaLP, (5). Budapest, Hungar.

Rabiee, F. (2004). Focus-group interview and data analysis. *Proceedings of the Nutrition Society*, *63*(4), 655–660. http://doi.org/10.1079/pns2004399

Rafiq, M. Y., Wheatley, H., Mushi, H. P., & Baynes, C. (2019). Who are CHWs? An ethnographic study of the multiple identities of community health workers in three rural districts in Tanzania. *BMC Health Services Research*, *19*(1). 712. http://doi.org/10.1186/s12913-019-4563-6

Reed, N. P., Josephsson, S., & Alsaker, S. (2020). A narrative study of mental health recovery: Exploring unique, open-ended and collective processes. *International Journal of Qualitative Studies on Health and Well-Being*, *15*(1), 1747252–1747252. http://doi.org/10.1080/17482631.2020.1747252

Reichel, M., & Ramey, M. A. (1987). *Conceptual frameworks for bibliographic education: Theory into practice*. Libraries Unlimited.

Rieger, K. L. (2019). Discriminating among grounded theory approaches. *Nursing Inquiry*, *26*(1), e12261. http://doi.org/10.1111/nin.12261

Roglic, G., & World Health Organization. (2016). *Global report on diabetes*. World Health Organization.

Salazar, L. F., Crosby, R. A., & DiClemente, R. J. (2015). *Research methods in health promotion* (2nd ed.). Jossey-Bass, a Wiley brand.

Saldaña, J. (2009). *The coding manual for qualitative researchers*. Sage Publications.

Sbaraini, A., Carter, S. M., Evans, R. W., & Blinkhorn, A. (2011). How to do a grounded theory study: A worked example of a study of dental practices. *BMC Medical Research Methodology*, *11*(1), 128. http://doi.org/10.1186/1471-2288-11-128

Shaffer, R. (1983). *Beyond the dispensary*. African Medical and Research Foundation.
Simera, I., Moher, D., Hoey, J., Schulz, K. F., & Altman, D. G. (2010). A catalogue of reporting guidelines for health research. *European Journal of Clinical Investigation*, *40*(1), 35–53. http://doi.org/10.1111/j.1365-2362.2009.02234.x
Smith, S., Eatough, V., Smith, J., Mihai, R., Weaver, A., & Sadler, G. P. (2018). 'I know I'm not invincible': An interpretative phenomenological analysis of thyroid cancer in young people. *British Journal of Health Psychology*, *23*(2), 352–370. http://doi.org/10.1111/bjhp.12292
Snipes, S. A., Thompson, B., O'Connor, K., Shell-Duncan, B., King, D., Herrera, A. P., & Navarro, B. (2009). "Pesticides protect the fruit, but not the people": Using community-based ethnography to understand farmworker pesticide-exposure risks. *American Journal of Public Health*, *99*(S3), S616–S621. http://doi.org/10.2105/ajph.2008.148973
Squires, A. (2008). Language barriers and qualitative nursing research: Methodological considerations. *International Nursing Review*, *55*(3), 265–273. http://doi.org/10.1111/j.1466-7657.2008.00652.x
Squires, A. (2009). Methodological challenges in cross-language qualitative research: A research review. *International Journal of Nursing Studies*, *46*(2), 277–287. http://doi.org/10.1016/j.ijnurstu.2008.08.006
Stake, R. E. (1995). *The art of case study research*. Sage Publications.
Strauss, A., & Corbin, J. (1998). *Basics of qualitative research: Techniques and procedures for developing grounded theory*. Sage Publications.
Strauss, A. L., & Corbin, J. M. (1990). *Basics of qualitative research: grounded theory procedures and techniques*. Sage Publications.
Sultana, F. (2007). Positionalities and knowledge: Negotiating ethics in practice. *ACME: An International Journal for Critical Geographies*, *6*(3), 374–385.
Sun, N., Wei, L., Shi, S., Jiao, D., Song, R., Ma, L., . . . Wang, H. (2020). A qualitative study on the psychological experience of caregivers of COVID-19 patients. *American Journal of Infection Control*, *48*(6), 592–598. http://doi.org/10.1016/j.ajic.2020.03.018
Sutton, J., & Austin, Z. (2015). Qualitative research: Data collection, analysis, and management. *Canadian Journal of Hospital Pharmacy*, *68*(3), 226–231. http://doi.org/10.4212/cjhp.v68i3.1456
Teherani, A., Martimianakis, T., Stenfors-Hayes, T., Wadhwa, A., & Varpio, L. (2015). Choosing a qualitative research approach. *Journal of Graduate Medical Education*, *7*(4), 669–670. http://doi.org/10.4300/jgme-d-15-00414.1
Thomas, E., & Magilvy, J. K. (2011). Qualitative rigor or research validity in qualitative research. *Journal for Specialists in Pediatric Nursing*, *16*(2), 151–155. http://doi.org/10.1111/j.1744-6155.2011.00283.x
Timonen, V., Foley, G., & Conlon, C. (2018). Challenges when using grounded theory: A pragmatic introduction to doing GT research. *International Journal of Qualitative Methods*, *17*(1), 1609406918758086. http://doi.org/10.1177/1609406918758086
Tindana, P. O., Rozmovits, L., Boulanger, R. F., Bandewar, S. V. S., Aborigo, R. A., Hodgson, A. V. O., . . . Lavery, J. V. (2011). Aligning community engagement with traditional authority structures in global health research: A case study from northern Ghana. *American Journal of Public Health*, *101*(10), 1857–1867. http://doi.org/10.2105/AJPH.2011.300203
Tong, A., Sainsbury, P., & Craig, J. (2007). Consolidated criteria for reporting qualitative research (COREQ): A 32-item checklist for interviews and focus groups. *International Journal for Quality in Health Care*, *19*(6), 349–357. http://doi.org/10.1093/intqhc/mzm042
Torop, P. (2002). Translation as translating as culture. *Sign System Studies*, *30*(2), 593–605.
Tummers, L., & Karsten, N. (2012). Reflecting on the role of literature in qualitative public administration research: Learning from grounded theory. *Administration & Society*, *44*(1), 64–86. http://doi.org/10.1177/0095399711414121
United States National Commission for the Protection of Human Subjects of Biomedical and Behavioral Research. (1978). *The Belmont report: ethical principles and guidelines for the protection of human subjects of research*. US Department of Health and Human Services.
University of California San Francisco. (n.d.). Consent guidelines. https://irb.ucsf.edu/verbal-electronic-or-implied-consent-waiver-signed-consent
Vuban, J. A., & Eta, E. A. (2019). Negotiating access to research sites and participants within an African context: The case of Cameroon. *Research Ethics*, *15*(1), 1–23. http://doi.org/10.1177/1747016118798874
Walliman, N. (2005). *Your research project: a step-by-step guide for the first-time researcher* (2nd ed.). Sage Publications.
Wang, C., & Burris, M. A. (1994). Empowerment through photo novella: Portraits of participation. *Health Education Quarterly*, *21*(2), 171–186. http://doi.org/10.1177/109019819402100204
Wang, C., & Burris, M. A. (1997). *Photovoice: Concept, methodology, and use for participatory needs assessment*. Health Education & Behavior, *24*(3), 369–387. http://doi.org/10.1177/109019819702400309
Wang, C. C., & Redwood-Jones, Y. A. (2001). Photovoice ethics: perspectives from Flint Photovoice. *Health Education & Behavior*, *28*(5), 560–572. http://doi.org/10.1177/109019810102800504
Wolcott, H. F. (2009). *Writing up qualitative research* (3rd ed.). SAGE.
Wu, Y. P., Thompson, D., Aroian, K. J., McQuaid, E. L., & Deatrick, J. A. (2016). Commentary: Writing and evaluating qualitative research reports. *Journal of Pediatric Psychology*, *41*(5), 493–505. http://doi.org/10.1093/jpepsy/jsw032
Yin, R. K. (2003). *Case study research: Design and methods* (3rd ed.). Sage Publications.

CHAPTER 4

MODULE 4: RESEARCH METHODOLOGY—MIXED METHODS APPROACHES

INTRODUCTION

Modules 2 and 3 provided an overview of different types of research, but most important they identified quantitative (Module 2) and qualitative (Module 3) approaches to research. They described a plan that consists of the steps leading to data collection, data analysis, and interpretation to answer the research question. Qualitative and quantitative methods are often compared as different philosophical worldviews in which quantitative approaches provide more valid research outcomes and qualitative research generalizable and are therefore of little value. However, this approach does not acknowledge or take advantage of the strengths and weaknesses of each approach. The mixed methods approach described in this module leverages a developing research approach and the embodiment of the philosophical perspectives of both quantitative and qualitative research and combines them in a mixed methods design that ranges from a convergent method to a more complex combination of approaches as well as embedding them in existing evaluation studies of experimental or quasi-experimental designs. Excerpts from Case Study 4.1 are used to illustrate many of the concepts in this module.

By the end of this module, learners will be able to:

- Compare mixed methods research designs
- Apply mixed methods approaches to a research project
- Discuss a mixed methods approach to evaluation

Integrated Research Methods In Public Health, First Edition. Muriel Jean Harris and Baraka Muvuka.
© 2023 John Wiley & Sons, Inc. Published 2023 by John Wiley & Sons, Inc.
Companion website: www.wiley.com/go/harris/integratedresearchmethods

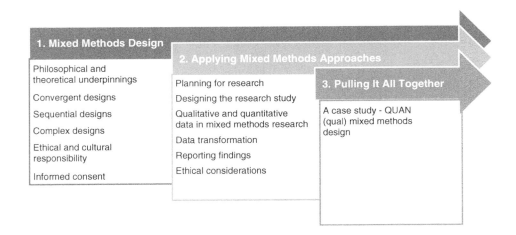

SECTION 1: MIXED METHODS DESIGN

By the end of this section, learners will be able to:

- Distinguish between the philosophies that undergird mixed methods research
- Describe the different approaches to mixed methods research
- Discuss key features that influence mixed methods research

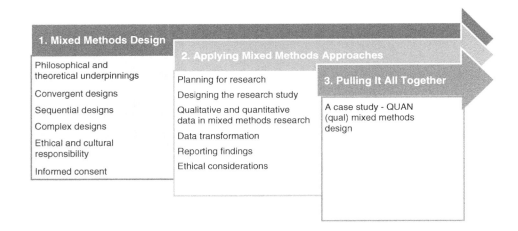

INTRODUCTION

Although mixed methods research generally refers to a single study, it can also be adopted across several studies that are addressing the same research question yet use multiple methods. Mixed methods research has been adopted across a variety of academic fields, and many find potential in using mixed methods approaches due to the ability of mixed methods designs to deal with complexity, flexibility, and transdisciplinary research (Bergman, 2018). Similar to the research approaches described in this book, the research question drives the selection of the method used in mixed methods designs. In general, quantitative methods are used to answer questions that relate to distribution, causality, generalizability, and the size of the phenomenon. Qualitative methods are used to explore or describe the phenomenon in deeper ways and to develop a theory that articulates the relationship between concepts. Mixed methods research allows us to combine these approaches and provide insights into the answer to the research question in ways that are often impossible with just using one or the other.

The worldview that supports a development of the mixing of qualitative and quantitative methods to collect data and ultimately to answer a more complex research question is still developing. However, Creswell and Plano Clark (2018) describe it as "composed of beliefs and assumptions about knowledge that informs the study" (p. 35).

PHILOSOPHICAL UNDERPINNING

Quantitative methods are rooted in positivism/postpositivism, whereas qualitative methods align with an interpretivist or constructivist model (Creswell and Creswell, 2018). Mixing the methods provides the benefit of offsetting each other's weaknesses and playing off their strengths. Kumar (2014) defined mixed methods as the use of two or more methods—either quantitative or qualitative or both—for the whole or part of a research process that contributes the mixed/multiple methods approach (p. 23) without necessarily presenting a paradigm perspective. Researchers in mixed methods have operated within four theoretical and research-based approaches such as pragmatism, transformative-emancipative, dialectics, and critical realism (Shannon-Baker, 2016). However, Creswell and Plano Clark (2018, p. 36), propose four worldviews for use in mixed methods research that are associated with the four paradigm perspectives: (1) postpositivist; (2) constructivist; (3) pragmatist; and (4) transformative.

The positivist approach is somewhat rigid in its design and interpreting the data is based on a preconceived notion that drove the development of the study in the first place. On the other hand, a mixed methods design can incorporate a more organic and holistic approach to answering the research question. Using different methods gives the researcher a comparative framework from which to see the results (Denzin, 1989). This perspective allows them to take a more pragmatic approach (Onwuegbuzie and Johnson, 2006) that moves between the inductive and the deductive paradigms with a focus on communication and shared meaning to create practical solutions (Morgan, 2007). It provides an opportunity for the researcher to ask new kinds of questions (Arnon and Reichel, 2009).

The critical realism perspective supports the view that qualitative and quantitative data support each other rather than being divergent like a dialectic perspective. It reflects a constructivist epistemology rooted in understanding each individual's perceptions (Creswell and Plano Clark, 2011; Model, 2009) and provides a complete understanding of the perspective while bringing both types of data together in a context-based framework for assessing causality (Maxwell and Mittapalli, 2010; Shannon-Baker, 2016) and providing opportunities for theory development.

The more pragmatic approach recognizes the usefulness of postpositivist and constructivist approaches for understanding the world around us, even if sometimes the results are contradictory (Onwuegbuzie and Johnson, 2006). The pragmatist draws on what works best to answer the research question, valuing both postpositivist and constructivist ways of knowing (Creswell and Plano Clark, 2018). This research approach considers how quantitative and qualitative data can be used to their best advantage. Researchers such as Teddlie and Tashakkori (2009) believe that pragmatism is the best philosophical basis for mixed methods designs, notwithstanding other perspectives in this debate. The alternative transformative approach provides the researcher with an additional decision regarding the purpose of the research.

The last the approaches discussed here is the transformative approach. It requires the inclusion of marginalized voices throughout the research process while addressing issues of power, privilege, and voice and paying attention to subgroups to promote social change (Mertens, 2010; Shannon-Baker, 2016). Participatory research falls within the transformative philosophy and incorporates social justice components that may be integrated using both qualitative or quantitative data (Bartholomew and Lockard, 2018).

In addition to considering mixed methods research within a single paradigm, an alternative approach is to bring together two or more paradigms and to recognize for its unique perspective while identifying divergent data, supporting cross-perspective research, and promoting equal weight between groups and a balanced and qualitative–quantitative approach (Johnson and Stefurak, 2013). For example, the dialectic perspective recognizes the value of incorporating geographic information system (GIS) applications and data into mixed methods research to bring together different epistemologies (Frels et al., 2011).

In the literature, the term *mixed method research* is used in a variety of ways to refer to qualitative and quantitative approaches for the purposes of combining methods, philosophies, and theoretical frameworks (Onwuegbuzie and Johnson, 2006). Creswell and Plano Clark (2018) identify seven reasons for using mixed methods that are associated with the choice of the approach focusing on the problem to be solved. To facilitate the later analysis and interpretation of data from a mixed methods designs study, it is important to clearly define the intent for using the approach in the methods section of the paper. In early discussions of the use of mixed methods approaches, Green (2007) included the need to:

- Triangulate to converge, corroborate, and provide correspondence on the methods
- Complement one method with the other to provide elaboration, enhancement, illumination, and clarification of the results
- Use one method to inform the other
- Extend the range of inquiry by using different methods

Mixed methods can be used to examine different aspects of a single research question or use separate but related research questions that reflect qualitative and quantitative approaches Schoonenboom and Johnson (2017).

THEORETICAL FRAMEWORKS IN MIXED METHODS RESEARCH

In quantitative research, theory is used to identify the variables in a postpositivist approach. However, in a transformative–emancipatory position, it is critical to include stakeholder and community member engagement. In qualitative research, the theory is generated in the grounded theory approach (Charmaz, 2014), which values stakeholder engagement as part of its philosophical approach. Although qualitative research in public health often starts with identifying variables that form the basis of the inquiry, using semistructured interviews and focus groups approaches will reveal additional variables, which may form the basis of a new or expanded theoretical framing. Similar to Creswell and Plano Clark's (2018, p. 45) steps for social science research, public health behavioral science incorporates the following research-based, conceptual theoretical framework to guide the study (noting the adaptations for mixed methods research):

- Conduct a literature review to identify the variables for the study.
- Confirm the research questions.
- Confirm the philosophical views guiding the researcher and the study to answer the research question.
- Develop the conceptual/theoretical framework showing the hypothesized relationships of the independent and dependent variables that may incorporate racial or feminist positions.
- Identify the approach that best provides the data to answer the research questions.
- Specify the mixed methods framework (convergent, sequential, or complex), and confirm the data collection methods for the study.
- Collect the data.
- Analyze the data as appropriate for the approach adopted.
- Report on the findings in line with the mixed methods approach that was adopted.

Mixed methods approaches may be used to increase the validity of a study through three phases of triangulation (Silverman, 2001): (1) methodological and a strategy for increasing validity; (2) a deeper or a more comprehensive understanding of an issue or a situation under study; or (3) a source of additional knowledge and just not for the purposes of confirming existing results (Flick, 2017). Another advantage of mixed methods is to provide the opportunity for new conceptual perspectives, expanding the team of researchers and providing the basis for triangulation either within one method or between methods. This approach has the potential to lead to a systematic triangulation perspective that results in combining the theoretical and epistemological backgrounds of both qualitative and quantitative research (Flick, 2017). In addition to methodological triangulation, there is the issue of data triangulation with its several forms of data. Factors important in choosing a mixed methods design include the expected outcomes of the study and the approach to mixing qualitative and quantitative data, yet Hesse-Biber and Guest's concern is the application of mixed methods research without questioning the appropriateness for the study (Flick, 2017). Creswell and Plano Clark propose a rationale for considering when to use the mixed methods approach to explain initial results, explore a phenomenon for the development of a survey instrument, and use the methods to corroborate findings, but they expand Green's (2007) rationale to include involving participants in developing, implementing, and evaluating programs (Table 4.1).

Using a mixed methods approach has both strengths and weaknesses. Strengths include that the research approach may provide a more comprehensive understanding of the phenomenon but at the same time be more challenging to describe the methods and report on the findings. Another advantage is being able to combine the approaches, but researchers question the validity of utilizing a randomly selected sample for the quantitative portion of the study and a purposive sample to explain or clarify the results. Additional limitations may include the need to assemble teams with both skill sets and expertise, an extension of the timeline, and increase in cost. Consider the length of time needed to first conduct a set of focus groups or individual interviews in a sequential mixed methods approach before then designing a survey. However, a convergent design where the methods are used concurrently may not have a similar time limitation, although there may be other factors to consider in its implementation (Table 4.2).

TABLE 4.1. Rationale for Selecting Mixed Methods Research Approaches

Rationale for Conducting a Mixed Methods Research Study When there is a need to:

Obtain more complete and corroborated results

Explain initial results

Explore the phenomenon before developing an instrument to ensure appropriate and adequate understanding of the context

Enhance a quantitative study with a qualitative method

Describe different kinds of cases followed by a comparison of the cases in terms of criteria

Involve participants in the research in the design of the study and in adopting the findings for change

Develop, implement, and evaluate a program

Adapted from Creswell and Plano Clark (2018).

TABLE 4.2. Strengths and Weaknesses of Mixed Methods Research

Strengths	Weaknesses
Research is more comprehensive in understanding the phenomenon.	It can be more challenging to describe the methods and report the findings from qualitative and quantitative data separately.
The results of one set of data can be validated using the results from another set of data.	Validity of the study could be compromised by the alternative approach in the synthesis of the results.
Both inductive and deductive philosophies can be applied to answering the research question providing opportunities for triangulation thus enhancing the accuracy and validity of the research findings.	Opportunities for publishing mixed methods research are more limited than publishing qualitative or quantitative research alone.
Results can be communicated in multiple formats that include both qualitative and quantitative data and ways of visualizing the data.	It can be more expensive and time-consuming to collect both types of data.

In an earlier typology for the combination of quantitative and qualitative data in triangulation, Morse (1991) proposed dominant and complementary notations where the more dominant method is represented by all capitals (QUAN/QUAL) and the complementary method is represented by small letters (qual/quan). The objective of triangulation is to use a combination of methodological or theoretical approaches to answer a research question and thus increase confidence in the conclusions. It is a means of bringing qualitative and quantitative data together intentionally in a research process (Creswell and Plano Clark, 2017). Morse proposed various combinations of data in equivalent and sequential combinations as a means of triangulation where the underlying theory dictates which to use first, qualitative or quantitative approaches.

Limitations of bringing both qualitative and quantitative approaches together can be minimized by incorporating reliability and validity controls—for example, taking randomly selected samples from the same populations in both the qualitative and quantitative portions of the study. However, triangulating findings may also occur at the method level, when philosophical underpinnings of the different methods may be ignored.

The mix of methods and approach is guided by key questions about the appropriateness of a mixed methods design (Palinkas et al., 2011), much the same as would be the case in postpositivist and constructivist research (Modules 2 and 3 of this book), including:

- What is the rationale for conducting a mixed methods study?
- Why would a convergent or sequential use of the data be appropriate?

Creswell and Creswell (2018) offer several approaches for conducting mixed methods research, including convergent, explanatory, and exploratory sequential designs and the less common complex design. The complex design proposes embedding the standard mixed methods within an existing experimental intervention or evaluation study. These designs may contain convergent or sequential components. In the conceptualization of the study from the research questions, the researcher determines the:

1. Nature of the study
2. Qualitative and quantitative data collection required to answer the research questions
3. Approach that would be most appropriate for combining the different data within the study (convergent or sequential)
4. Steps in the procedure that would be appropriate for collecting quantitative and qualitative data

A one-dimensional conceptualization of the combinations of data to achieve a mixed methods design could be a combination of qualitative data (Qual), quantitative data (Quan), or quantitative plus qualitative data (Figure 4.1).

Multiple researchers have adopted the use of mixed methods designs, yet there is little clarity in how to integrate the different types of data (Bartholomew and Lockard, 2018). However, Creswell and Plano Clark (2018) propose three core designs, the second and third of which are sequential: convergent, exploratory, and explanatory. In addition, the data may be integrated at multiple levels in each of the designs and through multistage, intervention, case study, and participatory frameworks in complex designs.

Integration at the methods level can occur through (a) linking databases, (b) building a database that informs the data collection of the other, (c) merging the two databases for analysis, (d) embedding, in which the data collection and analysis are linked together at multiple points (Fetters et al., 2013). It may also occur through narrative, data transformation, and joint display of results or during the discussion of findings from the study (Bartholomew and Lockard, 2017; Fetters et al., 2013).

FIGURE 4.1. *Mixed methods study design options for combining qualitative and qualitative data.*

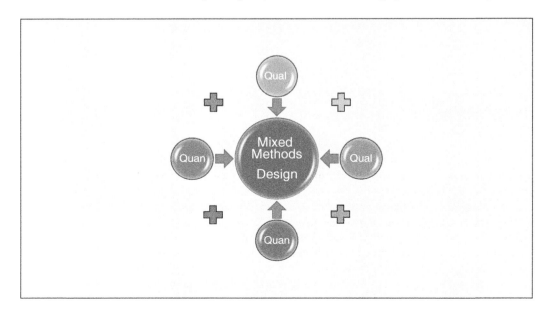

CONVERGENT/CONCURRENT DESIGNS

In equivalent designs, there is the simultaneous collection of quantitative and qualitative data followed by the analysis of the data. The result of the analysis is compared to determine the convergence or divergence of the findings. The data may be combined to make either qualitative aspects of the research more dominant (QUAL + quan) or quantitative aspects of the research more dominant (QUAN + qual) or where there is no distinction of dominance (QUAL + QUAN); therefore, both are notated in capital letters. This is the most familiar of the mixed methods designs and is used when the researcher believes that collecting additional data from an alternative source will enhance the validity of their study or explain the findings from the study. In another recently conducted study to understand issues of trust between a funding agency and a minority-owned early childhood intervention program, the author conducted interviews and concurrently collected data on a Likert-like scale that assessed specific aspects of trust, yet the qualitative data was the more dominant (QUAL + quan).

> **Case Study 4.1**
>
> A recent study conducted by the authors utilized a mixed methods approach with a convergent mixed methods design. The purpose of the study was to assess the factors that influenced women's early entry into prenatal care (PNC). This evaluation considered women in general but specifically Hispanic women's facilitators and barriers to their utilization the federally qualified health center's (FQHC) services. In addition, it reviewed pregnancy-related educational materials provided to women. The evaluation research questions were:
>
> - What were the experiences of patients, providers, and staff at the FQHC?
> - What were the barriers to the implementation and utilization of the services?
> - What is the information/education needs of patients?
>
> This study adopted a mixed methods case study design for its evaluation, allowing researchers to study a complex phenomenon within the natural contexts in which it exists while drawing from multiple data sources (Baxter and Jack, 2008). It incorporated the use of the FQHC's database, surveys, observations, document review, and GIS mapping to answer the research questions. The research team collected data at four participating prenatal clinic sites.

The convergent design brings together the results of the quantitative and qualitative data analysis, with the basic idea of getting a complete understanding of the problem and in some cases to validate one set of results against the other. In the use of surveys, a mixed method design is adopted when a closed-ended question is followed immediately by an open-ended question that asks the respondent to describe or explain their previous response.

For example, do you believe that gun violence is a structural or systemic issue that must be addressed using a multifaceted approach? Answer prompt—Yes/No

- If yes, why do you believe that gun violence is a structural or systemic issue?
- If no, what do you believe influences gun violence?

Another example of a mixed methods design would be a study where a quantitative survey is conducted in the same sitting with an individual or group following the collection of qualitative data. Notations like the one shown in Figure 4.2 help to explain relationships between the methods.

FIGURE 4.2. *Convergent design.*

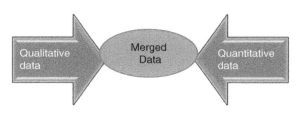

Strategies suggested for merging the two sets of results include:

- Identify shared content in the two data sets and compare, contrast, or synthesize the findings in a discussion or in a table.
- Identify differences and similarities within one set of data based on the other.
- Create a joint display of the data.
- Transform qualitative data to quantitative data and compare the results with the existing quantitative data (Creswell and Plano Clark, 2018).

In a study based in Turkey, Demir and Pismek (2018) conducted a convergent parallel mixed methods research study combining quantitative and qualitative data with the methods bearing equal weight (QUAL+QUAN) and analyzed independently with results interpreted together (Figure 4.3). In this study, eight teachers (four males and four females) were interviewed using a semistructured interview form, and data were collected using a structured observation form to triangulate the data from the interviews (qualitative data). Data from 5,104 survey responses were used in the analysis (quantitative). Traditional approaches were used in the analysis of the data. Descriptive analysis of the samples, one-way and factorial analysis of variance (ANOVAs), and Pearson's correlations were used for the quantitative data, and NVivo was used to code and analyze the qualitative data from semistructured interviews. Traditional approaches for validating the data methods were used throughout the research study.

Demir and Pismek (2018) showed a comparison of qualitative and quantitative results from their study of controversial issues in social studies classes. Their results shows that 71.62% of teachers who completed the survey believed they should or should not be influenced by their ideologies, which compared well to seven out of eight teachers in the qualitative study. Only one person (K6) and 28.38% did not believe that ideologies influence how lessons are taught (Demir and Pismek, 2018) (Table 4.3).

FIGURE 4.3. *Example: mixed methods study design.*

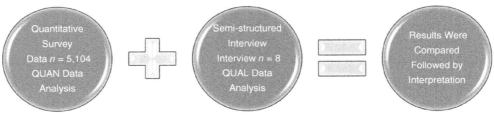

Adapted from Demir and Pismek (2018).

TABLE 4.3. **Comparisons of Qualitative and Quantitative Results**

Survey item	Qualitative data	Quantitative data			
		n_1	%	n_2	%
Those who think that ideologies should influence how lessons are taught	K1, K2, K3, K4, K8	5	62.5	2,534	49.64
Those who think that ideologies should not influence how lessons are taught	K5, K7	2	25.0	1,121	21.97
Those who think that ideologies do not influence how lessons are taught	K6	1	12.5	1,449	28.38
Total	8	8	100	5,104	100

Demir and Pismek (2018, p. 131).

SEQUENTIAL DESIGNS

In sequential designs one method follows the other with qualitative data or quantitative data being collected and analyzed first in either an exploratory or explanatory research project. The sequential analysis of data may occur in multiple phases in a variety of combinations with the data being reported separately.

In the more complex designs one data set is embedded in another larger data collection framework either concurrently or in phases (Creswell and Creswell, 2018). This is characteristic of evaluation studies, where the individual mini-research studies may be embedded in a larger evaluation pretest–posttest research designed study as described later in this module. See Case Study 4.2 in this module.

Exploratory Sequential Design

In Phase 1 of the exploratory sequential design model, qualitative data are collected initially, and their analysis informs the development of a quantitative study in Phase 2. This approach may be used to strengthen the development of the quantitative research study. In describing the proposed study protocol for investigating communication behaviors, Hagiwara et al. (2018) initiated the process with video elicitation interviews of a subset of Black patients about their physician's communication behavior. This was followed by the specification of the measurement units associated with the behaviors. These were then integrated into surveys in an exploratory sequential mixed model design. The publication suggests that the study adopted a QUAL-QUAN-QUAN approach, although the specific notation shown here was not used (Figure 4.4).

The sequential design has two options that dictate the order of the data collection: exploratory and explanatory. The *sequential exploratory design* generally starts with qualitative data to help identify variables that may be used as the basis for the development of a quantitative survey or other quantitative data collection tool in a traditional two-phase study (Figure 4.5).

FIGURE 4.4. *Three-phased sequential mixed methods exploratory design.*

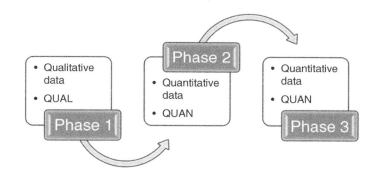

FIGURE 4.5. *Qualitative data to inform survey development followed by validation of the findings in a two-phase exploratory sequential mixed methods model.*

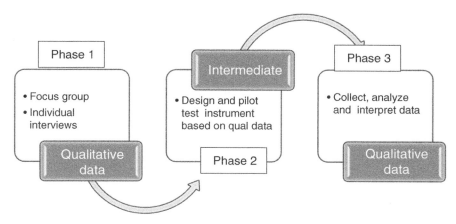

FIGURE 4.6. *Explanatory flowchart.*

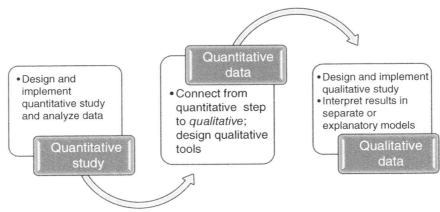

Adapted from Creswell and Plano Clark (2018 p. 79).

Explanatory Sequential Design

The *explanatory sequential design* starts with the collection of quantitative data in the first phase of the study and is followed by a qualitative study. The purpose may be to validate the findings from the first study or to explain unexpected or contradictory results (Creswell and Plano Clark, 2018). In the explanatory design the research must consider design characteristics of each phase of the study separately. In a model described by Creswell and Plano Clark (2018), there are potentially four steps: (1) design and implement the quantitative strand; (2) use specific strategies to connect from the quantitative results; (3) design and implement a qualitative component using individuals from the step 1 sample; and (4) interpret the results summarizing them separately or discussing how the qualitative results supported or helped explain the quantitative results (Figure 4.6).

Phase 1 of this model is the collection and analysis of quantitative data followed by the collection and analysis of qualitative data in phase 2. It builds on the results of the quantitative data and provides a deeper explanation and contextual information related to the results of the phase 1 study. This approach could be useful in understanding and incorporating marginalized voices in culturally sensitive ways in the implementation of a pragmatic approach to mixed methods research as suggested by Creswell and Plano (2011) and drawing on the work of Bagele Chilisa (2012).

A study to understand diabetes-related distress characteristics of urban African American adults with type 2 diabetes adopted a two-phase approach: phase 1 is a purposive sample of adults who completed a survey; and phase 2 is a subset of the participants in phase 1 who participated in follow-up focus groups for the primary purpose of providing context to the survey results derived from phase 1 (Hood et al., 2018) (Figure 4.7).

There are limitations with using sequential approaches that have to do with how the institutional review board (IRB) process is set up and their expectations of what needs to be included in a research proposal as well as the very nature of the mixed methods sequential approach. The exploratory design requires that a qualitative approach is used, yet the qualitative approach is not prescribed in the same terms as a quantitative constructivist approach and does not have the required level of definition that is expected by the IRB. Also, the postpositivist approach anticipates the development of the research question, the conceptual framework, and the methodology from the literature review, which in the exploratory model must wait until the qualitative data are collected and analyzed. It is the results of the qualitative

FIGURE 4.7. *Two-phase mixed methods approach to provide a deeper explanation of a phenomenon.*

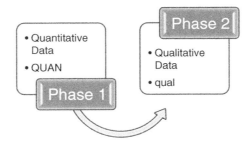

TABLE 4.4. Challenges with Using the Exploratory and Explanatory Sequential Designs for IRB

Exploratory designs	Explanatory designs
The nature of the study and the extended period required for the study	The nature of the study and the extended period required for the study.
The quantitative phase, which must be specified in advance of IRB approval	The qualitative phase must be specified in advance of IRB approval.
Requires two samples of the identified including a large sample in phase 2 to enhance generalization with both samples from the same population	The researcher must decide which results need to be explained.
Requiring the researcher to decide what to use from the qualitative study in the quantitative study	Since individuals from the first sample will be needed in the second phase, the researcher must decide whom to include.

Adapted from Creswell and Plano Clark (2018).

phase that leads to the development of the quantitative component. In the explanatory approach, since one study is dependent on the other, each component of the study cannot be fully described, and there are challenges with both designs in applying for IRB clearance for the research study (Table 4.4).

COMPLEX DESIGNS

Advanced frameworks achieve integration in multistage studies, intervention, case studies, and participatory research frameworks by incorporating more basic designs (Fetters et al., 2013). Multistage approaches include various approaches that may combine convergent, exploratory, and explanatory frameworks in a longitudinal research design. Intervention research incorporates qualitative data at the inception to understand the contextual factors that could affect the outcome and/or to explain the results when the mixed methods approach is used to support the development of the intervention.

In case study research both qualitative and quantitative data are used to help build a comprehensive understanding of the case in a single study that includes a relationship among the methods, the research questions, units of analysis, study samples, instrumentation, and data collection and analysis (Yin, 2006). The collected data depends on the nature of the research question. The qualitative data may include observations, semistructured interview, and journaling, whereas quantitative data may be collected using structured observations and survey approaches. See Case Study 4.1 in this module.

Mertens (2018) describes eight steps for the concurrent or sequential design that has the full engagement of community members in the transformative mixed methods design as applied to program evaluation. The steps are outlined in Figure 4.8.

In the transformative mixed methods model, phase 1 is the qualitative research, followed by phase 2, in which qualitative- and quantitative-style questions are developed for the survey. In the final phase, another qualitative study is conducted (Figure 4.9). The results were disseminated using multiple formats to ensure that there were follow-up actions to improve the program (Mertens, 2018).

In general, complex designs build on the basic structure of mixed methods by inserting them into large multi-investigator, intervention, or evaluation studies. Four examples of complex mixed methods design offered by Creswell and Plano (2018, p. 105) are:

- Experimental (intervention) design
- Mixed methods case study design
- Participatory social justice design
- Program evaluation design

Complex designs can incorporate convergent or sequential designs. They have multiple research phases, can be conducted over many years, have substantial amounts of funding, and include mixed methods as different phases of the research (Creswell and Plano Clark, 2018). In some cases, these conditions may not all be fulfilled, yet they may

FIGURE 4.8. *Mertens's (2018) steps for the concurrent or sequential design with community engagement (p. 328).*

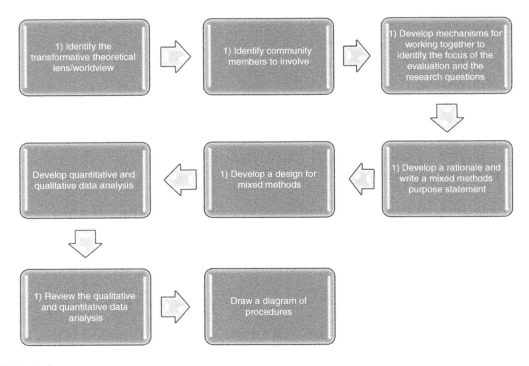

FIGURE 4.9. *Transformative mixed methods design.*

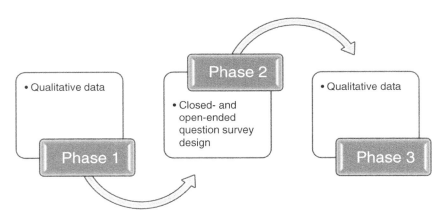

still be considered complex designs. Advancing the understanding of frameworks that may be considered as complex designs include work done by Plano Clark and Ivankova (2018):

- Embedding an additional qualitative or quantitative method within a research study design such as experimental design and case studies

- Inserting a mixed methods design within another research approach, such as a program evaluation, action research, social network analysis, and grounded theory studies

- Inserting a mixed methods design within a study's existing theoretical or philosophical framework such as social justice, participatory involvement, critical theory, and community-based participatory research that advance the needs of a population resulting in actions or change.

Additional components in a program evaluation conducted by one of the authors, with a focus on improving access to healthy foods, included both qualitative photographic/observation techniques (Figure 4.10) and incorporated GIS technology (Figure 4.11).

FIGURE 4.10. *Observation study within a program evaluation study.*

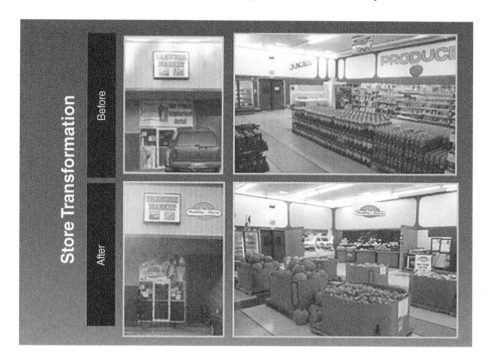

FIGURE 4.11. *GIS mapping study within a program evaluation study.*

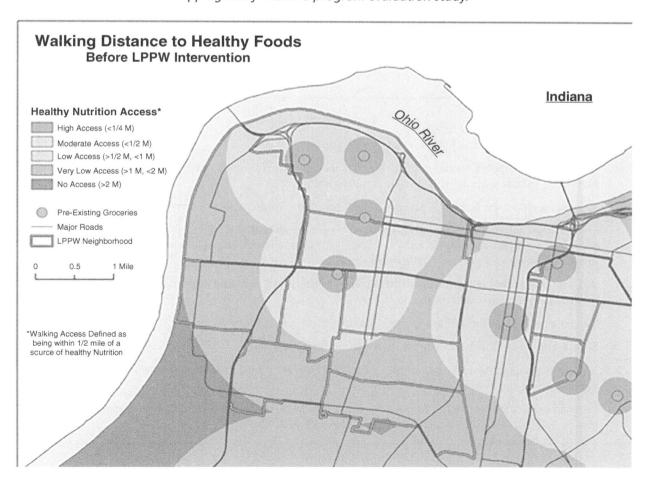

In conducting a mixed methods evaluation, Creswell and Plano Clark (2018) suggest the following steps:

- Conduct a needs assessment collecting both qualitative and quantitative data.
- Conduct a literature review to determine the evaluation approach.
- Locate measures and instruments to evaluate the program activities.
- Evaluate the program using the measures and instruments, including qualitative approaches
- Assess short- and long-term impacts of the program

In this model the evaluator would likely have been involved in the program from the start, so the measures and instruments used in the evaluation to assess short- and long-term outcomes would be integrated from the start and used for both the baseline and the outcome measures to demonstrate a change and therefore the effectiveness of the intervention (Figure 4.12).

FIGURE 4.12. *Evaluation design for improving health outcomes.*

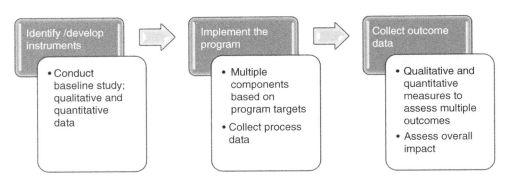

Case Study 4.2

The case study described earlier reached these conclusions:

- Providers were pleased overall with the services they provide; however, most were disappointed with the number of women entering PNC in their first trimester.
- Women identified the lack of awareness of their pregnancy as the primary barrier to seeking PNC early.
- Overall, staff and providers thought they understood patients' cultural beliefs related to PNC but expressed a concern over the diversity of cultural backgrounds and languages resulting in often less effective communication using interpreters.
- Almost half the respondents sought PNC services at this FQHC because of their satisfaction with the organization and the quality of the services.
- The women felt comfortable asking their provider questions.
- Scheduling conflicts may be barriers to women seeking early PNC.
- Women require additional educational material that includes information related to general health, contraception, and nutrition.
- Providers identified patient information needs as *when to start care, medications, self-care dos and don'ts, delivery information,* and *information about ultrasounds.*

Discuss Examples of Mixed Methods Approaches

1. Discuss mixed methods research you have been a part of and what that experience was like.

2. Identify two to three peer-reviewed articles that have used a mixed methods approach. Write a brief half-page summary of each article making sure that each summary reflects a different approach to mixed methods research. Discuss what you learned about each of the studies and how they differed from each other. Make sure to cite the references.

Advances in mixed methods research have led to alternative ways of conceptualizing mixed methods designs, and procedures include transforming qualitative data to quantitative data (quantitizing). Additional strategies include applying rapid assessments and analysis processes, strategies for sampling, the development of measures to assess implementation outcomes, and strategies for conducing random and purposive sampling (Palinkas et al., 2019). To provide a common notation for mixed methods research, Creswell and Plano (2018) proposed a range of notations for use in mixed methods research to represent and clarify the direction of the relationships between the variables (Table 4.5).

Validity in Mixed Methods Research Designs

The types of validity in quantitative research are statistical conclusion, internal, construct, and external. In qualitative research, validity is defined in terms of credibility, transferability, dependability, and confirmability (Onwuegbuzie and Johnson, 2006). Validity in mixed methods research includes the research, its parts, and its conclusions (Onwuegbuzie and Johnson, 2006). The validity in mixed methods is dependent on the validity of its components (qualitative quantitative approaches). Including respondents in the process and linking them to triangulation by adopting respondent validation approaches, the researcher incorporates democratic engagement and participation and facilitates the use of the data at the local level. Incorporating this process in mixed methods also recognizes a key validation measure of qualitative research, "member checking" alongside the traditional tools for validating quantitative research (Torrance, 2012).

TABLE 4.5. Notations and Their Uses in Mixed Methods Research

Notation	Use of the notation
→	A single arrow denoting the direction of the relationship
→ ←	Methods that are implemented in a recurring process QUAL → QUAN → QUAL → QUAN . . . . (continuing)
( )	When the mixed methods design is imbedded within a larger intervention
=	The intent for including a qualitative method is to explain the quantitative method QUAN → qual =

Mixed methods research can be conceptualized as combining qualitative and quantitative research in concurrent or sequential designs mixing primary and secondary research data in a shared empirical study. It incorporates a range of data, and a meta-inference incorporates the findings from both the quantitative and qualitative data, giving a more balanced perspective. However, Onwuegbuzie and Johnson (2006) question the appropriateness of comparing findings across a large random sample quantitative survey result when a small purposive sample was used for the qualitative study, especially if results are not consistent across both studies. Creswell and Plano Clark (2018) advance a list of principles to guide the consideration of validity in mixed methods designs and agree that the validity is dependent on the design. However, some are unique to the three basic mixed methods design shown in Table 4.6. For a complete list of the validity threats and strategies to minimize them, see Creswell and Plano Clark (2018, pp. 250–253).

TABLE 4.6. Threats to Validity in Mixed Methods Research and Strategies to Increase Validity

Type of design	Threat to validity	Strategies to minimize the threat
Convergent design	Not collecting the data at the same time (parallel concepts)	Create questions addressing the same concept.
	Unequal sample sizes	Use the same sample sizes or compare group means if more appropriate.
	Keeping results from the different databases separate	Use a joint display of the data from each or compare quantitative with qualitative analysis side by side.
Exploratory Sequential design	Not building the quantitative component on the qualitative data	Explain how each finding from the qualitative data is used to inform the development of the quantitative study.
	Quantitative study is weak	Use pretested and psychometrically sound instruments for quantitative study
	Selecting the same individuals for the quantitative study that are the same as individuals who participated in the qualitative study	Ensure that the samples are different.
Explanatory Sequential design	Failure to identify important results in the quantitative study to explain in the follow-up study	Incorporate all the findings and limit the follow-up study to only significant results.
	Not explaining difference in findings across the studies	Design the follow-up study to help explain any contradictory results in the quantitative study.
	Not connecting the two studies	Ensure that the follow-up sample is from the same sample as the previous study.

Creswell and Plano Clark (2018, pp. 251–252).

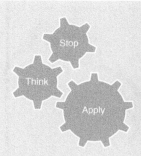

Identifying Mixed Methods Research

Describe the different formats for conducting a mixed methods research study. Look up at least two peer-reviewed journals specifying that mixed methods were used, and map out and name the design that was applied to the study. Compare the approaches and summarize the limitations of each study as described by the authors of the articles in the discussion or as a stand-alone limitations section of the article. Make sure to cite the references.

Data Analysis

Data analysis in a convergent cross-sectional study will be collected at one point in time; however, sequential data in a longitudinal design will be collected as appropriate at the beginning, middle, and end of the project design as specified by the plan. While mixed methods data are collected as and when required, Creswell and Plano Clark (2018) suggest that the meaningful integration of the data defines it as mixed methods research, allowing for a deeper understanding when qualitative research helps to explain findings in quantitative survey research. The level and type of integration will necessarily be defined by the design of the study. Creswell and Plano Clark (2018) provide a summary of the ways data can be linked (Table 4.7).

In convergent models, simultaneous integration of the data allows the researcher to collect, analyze, and integrate the results within the same time frame of the study. Creswell and Plano Clark (2018) suggest approaches to interpreting merged results that include:

- Summarize and interpret the results separately.
- Discuss to what extent and in what ways results from one study converge, diverge, or in other ways relate to each other.
- Explain divergence when it occurs and take steps to resolve it.
- Provide insight and answer the research question.

TABLE 4.7. Integration of Data for Each of the Three Mixed Methods Approaches

Core design	Intent of integration	Interpretation
Convergent	Simultaneous integration of data to develop integrated results and interpretation that validate and confirm results	Provide insight and answer the research question.
Exploratory	To provide building blocks to the development of the quantitative study	Provide contextual and culturally sensitive information for the design of the survey/data collection tool.
Explanatory	Connect the qualitative data and results to explain the quantitative results	Use the qualitative evidence to explain the quantitative results.

Adapted from Creswell and Plano Clark (2018, pp. 222–223).

Options for handling the data following collection include analyzing the data separately as described in other sections of this book or merging the data as described in the convergent approach.

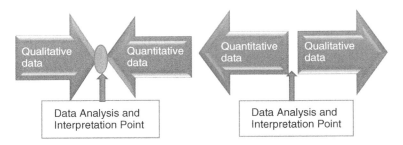

The data are analyzed first as prescribed by the methods, but the use of the data is determined by whether the approach is required for exploratory or explanatory purposes. Creswell and Plano Clark (2018) label data from both exploratory and explanatory mixed methods as *connected results*, which are interpreted in the following ways based on the order of the approaches:

- Summarize and interpret the quantitative results.
- Summarize and interpret the qualitative results.
- Discuss to what extent and in what ways the qualitative results help to explain the quantitative results and provide data to support the conclusions (Figure 4.13).

A key step in the analysis of exploratory sequential design data is building the connection between the qualitative analysis and the results for the development of the quantitative survey. The qualitative data are used to identify and develop the themes for the questionnaire items, and the survey that is developed from those results is used to assess the distribution of the variables across a large sample. The collection of qualitative data initially provides opportunities for cultural tailoring of the instrument. The subsequent data analysis can be represented in joint displays, with the qualitative data from the initial study, the quantitative variable from the survey, and the results and interpretation of the answer from the analysis of the research all represented in a table (Creswell and Plano Clark, 2018). The data integration can be seen in the following example from Watkins et al. (2015) in Creswell and Plano Clark (2018, p. 243): "Not only was it socially and culturally relevant, but it was also found to be statistically significant in the older church-going African American men in the study."

Similarly, the data from explanatory sequential designed mixed methods studies can be integrated since the purpose of the second study is to help explain the findings from the initial study, with the selection of the sample being determined by the characteristics of subgroups. Subgroups can include those who score at the extreme ends outside the mean and those who appear different in their responses (Creswell and Plano Clark, 2018). The procedure for integrating and interpreting the data involves:

- Analyzing the data from the quantitative study noting any results of concern
- Determining the sample required to help explain the results selected from the sample of those who participated in the initial study

FIGURE 4.13. *Data analysis and interpretation.*

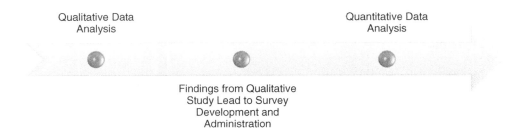

- Designing the qualitative study to obtain the information
- Collecting and analyzing the data
- Developing the display of the data
- Interpreting the data to report on the additional information gleaned as a result of the additional qualitative data

ETHICAL RESPONSIBILITIES

As in the conduct of other research approaches, mixed methods research requires researchers to consider the ethical responsibility they hold. A study may be considered unethical if it is scientifically unsound, breaches an individual or a community's confidentiality, or wastes resources. Culturally responsive research requires the researcher to continually reflect on their study population and how it might limit understanding of the issues in the study. In addition, it recognizes the importance of commitment to co-participants, ongoing consenting of the participants, and mutual respect and reciprocity (Chilisa, 2012). The fundamental principles of *respect for persons, beneficence,* and *justice* (Childress and Beauchamp, 2001) are maintained.

The inclusion of qualitative research, which consists of a range of approaches, will sometimes include observation studies and in-person methods in field research when ethical issues may not have been anticipated (Taylor et al., 2016). It is important to examine the potential ethical issues or unintended consequences of the research to minimize their occurrence by sometimes finding alternative approaches to collect the required data to answer the research question. In participatory and transformative research, these principles also include aspects of social justice that make the ethically responsible research one that focuses on the issues of power. The goal is to empower participants and to transform their situation. Using that philosophical lens, then, alternative approaches may also compromise the philosophical underpinnings of the study.

INFORMED CONSENT

The researcher must ensure that the document that individuals are asked to sign or approve is complete and must provide the potential participant a clear understanding of the risk and benefits of the study to them personally and to the larger population.

All research is required by an ethics review board in the country in which the research is being conducted. Universities will often require that their researchers obtain clearance both internally and from any other ethics review board in the jurisdiction of the research. A more complete description of the ethical responsibilities associated with research is described in other modules of this book.

CULTURAL RESPONSIVENESS

Culturally responsive methodologies allow for the conceptualization of research goals, the design of the study and the values of the stakeholders in the forefront of the design, and the implementation of the research study. Drawing on the principles of community-based participatory research, engaging the community to be part of the study throughout is a critical part of its philosophy. Culturally responsive research methodologies included in the design of mixed methods research intentionally incorporate cultural values and recognize the impact of the study on participation, retention, and trust in the process (Chilisa, 2012). Their underlying practice of engagement is one that could be incorporated in all research to increase the validity of its findings.

To improve the authenticity and validity of the research, researchers must strive to identify and incorporate those who provide a cultural bridge to the work. Torrance (2012) incorporates respondent validation as an aspect of triangulation with participants responding either to the data, transcripts of interviews, or observations to check them for accuracy and especially if the emergent themes are fair and a reasonable reflection of the research. Known as member checking (and a core construct in constructivist research), it has not been adopted as a core component of the whole study in mixed methods research even though the need to incorporate it remains the same (Torrance, 2012). It finds support in the transformative and pragmatist philosophies, which along with postpositivist and constructivism is one of the worldviews of mixed methods research (Creswell and Plano Clark, 2018).

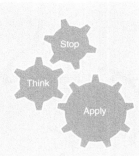

Ethical Issues in Mixed Methods Research

Ethical issues are an important component of any research study; however, in mixed methods research there are additional considerations for the respondents' participation and the methodology. Using the literature to support your response, what additional ethical issues must be considered in mixed methods research over and above quantitative and qualitative research?

 SUMMARY

Mixed methods research has been adopted across a variety of academic fields, and many find potential in using mixed methods approaches due to the ability of mixed methods designs to deal with complexity, flexibility, and transdisciplinary research.

There are a variety of uses of the term *mixed methods research* with the combination of qualitative and quantitative approaches for purposes of combining methods, philosophies, and theoretical frameworks. One reason to use mixed methods is that its focus is on the problem that needs to be solved. To facilitate the later analysis and interpretation of data from a mixed methods designs study, it is important that the intent for the approach is clearly defined.

There are three approaches for conducting a mixed methods research:-convergent, explanatory, and exploratory sequential designs—as well as the less common complex design. Embedding the standard mixed methods designs to make more complex designs can be achieved within an existing experimental intervention or evaluation study.

Validity in mixed methods research includes the research, its parts, and its conclusions and is based on the individual methodologies but including respondents in the process and linking them through triangulation by adopting respondent validation approaches such as member checking. In doing this, the researcher incorporates democratic engagement and participation and facilitates the use of the data at the local level.

Ethically responsible research in constructivist and postpositivist frameworks embraces the basic ethical principles of respect, beneficence, and justice; however, in participatory and transformative research, these principles also include aspects of social justice that make the ethically responsible research one that focuses on the issues of power. The goal is to empower participants and to transform their situation.

Now that I have reached the end this section, I am able to:

Course objective	Strongly agree	Somewhat agree	Neutral	Somewhat disagree	Strongly agree
Distinguish between the various philosophies that undergird mixed methods research					
Describe the different approaches to mixed methods research					
Discuss key features that distinguish mixed methods research from other research approaches					

SECTION 2: THE TWO PARADIGMS—MIXED METHODS RESEARCH DESIGNING THE RESEARCH STUDY

By the end of this section, learners will be able to:

- Describe how to conduct a mixed methods study
- Discuss the role of qualitative and qualitative research methods in mixed methods research
- Discuss practical approaches to mixed methods research

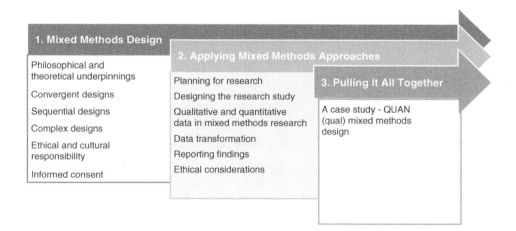

PLANNING FOR RESEARCH

The purpose of the convergent design is to obtain complete understanding from two approaches, and in most cases combining two or more philosophical approaches in the research study. In the convergent approach, the method and results corroborate each other, and the researcher can compare multiple levels of data within the same system. This approach is primarily used when there is a need to collect qualitative and quantitative data and there are appropriate resources to justify the collection of both. Another advantage convergent data have over sequential data is the shorter time frame required for data collection.

As in the previously described approaches to research, the best research is a planned systematic approach to answering the research question. Key considerations in planning research studies include asking and answering the following questions:

- Who will be engaged in the research study?
- Why is this study important to me, to the field of public health, and for whose benefit?
- What philosophical, ethical, and cultural underpinnings and what research design will be most appropriate to answer the research question?
- What will it take to collect, analyze, and report on valid and reliable data?

The planning process unfolds with identifying the answer to the first question: Who will be engaged in the research study? A researcher or a team of researchers generally initiates the process of identifying the need for the research, conceptualizing the study, and determining the research question. They collect, analyze, and interpret the results and report them to the larger population. The roles of the researchers are determined by the research team; however, their skill sets and experience with different data collection tools likely determine their activities within the team. In the case of mixed methods research, the team includes both qualitative and quantitative researchers answering the same research questions from different perspectives with the results of the analyses complementing each other. The approach to the research study will adopt the public health research study framework (Figure 4.14).

FIGURE 4.14. *Overview for designing a public health research study.*

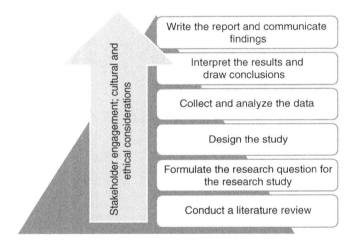

Culturally and ethically responsive research includes those who belong to the specific population about whom the research study will be focused and, as Terrance (2012) pointed out, will increase the validity of the study. The research team may include residents of the community in the research; colleagues across multiple professional areas; and organization, university, and agency staff. Given the mixed method approach, the team may contribute additional tools and frameworks. Ideally, stakeholders are involved in research throughout the process and have critical roles and responsibilities including giving voice to the study population. The first step in the research planning process is assembling the research team, followed by the steps that facilitate a systematic process for answering the research question.

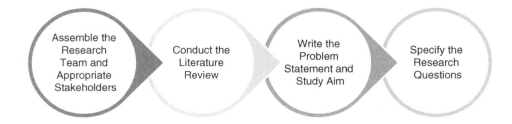

Assemble the Research Team

The terms of reference (ToR) for a research study is an explicit statement of personnel and resources for the project that includes roles, responsibilities, and processes the research team establishes at the outset. Researchers must recognize, however, that a ToR can serve as a contract or be perceived as such with positions on the team being organized in a hierarchical structure with those at the top seemingly having nothing to learn (Chilisa, 2012). It lays out the formal expectation of the project. Truly collaborative research teams would design the ToR together, clearly outlining:

- The purpose and goals of the research team
- The processes for conducting the research and accomplishing the research task
- Communication among and between the team and outside individuals and agencies
- Roles and responsibilities
- Confidentiality statements
- Milestones
- Publication agreements and authorship

The design of the mixed methods study may provide some additional considerations for the team, given that it will bring together a range of skill sets, some with expertise in qualitative research, some in quantitative research, and others in mixed methods design. The approach may also engender new stakeholders. For example, a complex mixed methods design requires collaboration with a possible ongoing project such as an evaluation or an intervention study that may utilize an experimental or quasi-experimental design. The more complicated the study, the more likely there will be stakeholders who have a varied interest in the study.

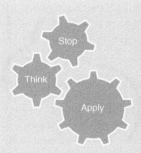

Identifying Stakeholders for Mixed Methods Research

As a researcher with a deep interest in understanding the factors that influence the high rates of diabetes, what data collection approaches would you propose for your mixed methods study? What philosophical underpinnings guide the selection of your methods? Who would you consider to be important stakeholders for your mixed methods research team? How would you go about recruiting them? What steps would you take to ensure buy-in from stakeholder groups?

Conduct the Literature Review

Determining the topic or question for the research requires completing the basic steps of a literature review the includes planning, conducting the review, and writing the report (Figure 4.15). The literature review in public health and for journal publications is best written as an integrative literature review. The integrative literature review provides a critical analysis of the literature that tells a story about the phenomenon with the goal of carefully identifying the components of the problem being researched by synthesizing the literature across multiple authors. A synthesis of the literature helps the researcher identify patterns that reflect new perspectives and a conceptual framework for the study and the research agenda (Torraco, 2005). It allows the researcher to identify gaps in the literature more readily as well as key contributions, strengths, weaknesses, and deficiencies (Torraco, 2005). The thematically organized review has

FIGURE 4.15. *Overview of the steps for conducting a literature review.*

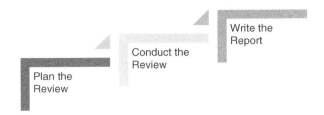

headings and subheadings that describe the independent variables in relationship to the dependent variable in the study with each combination of variables (independent and dependent) being compared across the literature. An important benefit of a thematic organization of the literature is that it reduces the risk of plagiarism.

Literature relevant to the research topic may cover two types of information: general and specific. The literature review begins with the general information and narrows down to the more specific information. It allows the researcher to review existing literature to understand what previous researchers have found and know about the topic of interest. By this step of the research process, the researchers have defined a broad topic area to focus the literature review.

Reviewing the Literature

- Provides an understanding of the theoretical frameworks across multiple disciplines that have guided the research of previous studies
- Clarifies ideas and establishes the basis for the research
- Helps to identify gaps in existing research and to conceptualize their research problem clearly
- Provides information about new research ideas and directions and references to new ideas and unanswered questions
- Provides insights into approaches and methodologies that have been used to answer similar research questions

Check List
- Organize information.
- Be succinct.
- Ensure references are complete.
- Capture only research findings.
- Examine each reference.
- Write the review.

The literature review provides the researcher with a clear justification for the study, situates it within the field as relevant and important and provides a firm foundation for posing the researcher's study question. When the study is based on previous research and built from identified gaps in the literature, it is of greater value to the field. There is always great value in conducting a well-developed literature review before embarking on a research project (Figure 4.16).

The literature review, which is covered in much more detail in Module 1 of this book, provides the foundation for the research study. Getting to the research question at the heart of the process requires four steps. First, a literature review is conducted to identify the gaps in the literature that lead to the development of the problem statement. Next, once the problem is identified, the researcher decides how the problem will be addressed by using the literature review as a backdrop and formulating the conceptual framework, which provides the specifics of the particular research project and in the third step, the researcher outlines the variables that will be included in the study and the direction that the research will take. Finally, the researcher can formulate the research questions. In mixed method research, the conceptual framework sets up how the studies will be combined to answer the questions and how the mixed method design will be incorporated in an evaluation or intervention design. The primary designs that will be considered are convergent, sequential, and complex.

The Problem Statement

The problem statement is developed from the literature review and provides the basis for moving forward into developing the conceptual framework for the study as it provides the justification and intent of the study. While the literature review provides the evidence, the problem statement is the result of the researcher stating the gap in the literature that

FIGURE 4.16. *Detailed plan for the three-stage literature review.*

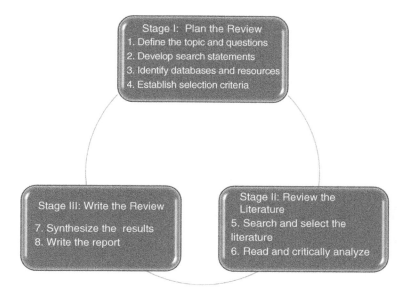

the study will address. It provides a clear indication of the significance of the problem. The components of the problem statement can be conceptualized in a summary statement as:

- What is already known about the specific problem?
- What major gaps were identified in the literature?
- What is the relevance of the present study in addressing the gap, and what benefits are there to understanding or resolving the problem?

Following the problem statement is the aim of the study. The researcher writes a statement such as, *The aim/purpose of this study is to determine/explore/understand/investigate/examine*.

It should include (a) the overall aim of the study, (b) the type of mixed methods design, (c) the types of data collection, (d) the data collection sites, and (e) the reason for collecting the data.

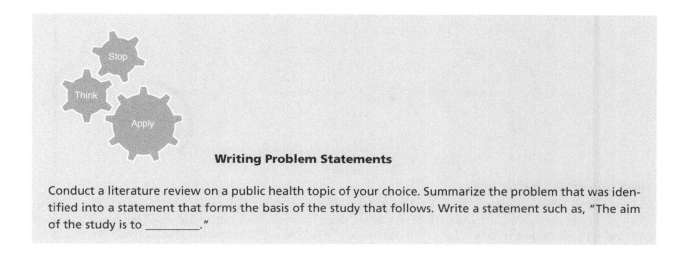

Writing Problem Statements

Conduct a literature review on a public health topic of your choice. Summarize the problem that was identified into a statement that forms the basis of the study that follows. Write a statement such as, "The aim of the study is to _____."

The Research Question in Mixed Methods Research

The research questions guide the conduct of the literature review and, later, the research study. When used at the beginning of the study, they help to narrow the literature around a particular theme or topic. Without a research question to guide the literature review, the researcher may spend too much time reading the literature without a focus. The initial research question that guides the study is one that provides a boundary for the reading and the resultant methodology. The question that gets answered in this section is about the relationship between various factors/constructs and the public health problem being investigated using a mixed methods research study approach, meaning the questions consider at least two integrated studies: quantitative and qualitative. Creswell and Plano Clark (2018, p. 169) propose the following examples of questions:

- To what extent do the quantitative results agree with the focus group findings on self-esteem for middle school boys?
- In what ways do the interview data reporting the views of middle school boys about their self-esteem help to explain the quantitative results about self-esteem reported on the surveys?
- Are the themes about self-esteem from middle school boys generalizable to a population of middle school boys?
- How are the profiles of cases based on qualitative descriptions and quantitative ratings of self-esteem both similar and different?
- How do the interview data with middle school boys and quantitative outcome results of the self-esteem program combine to challenge the school culture?

Once the research questions are chosen, the researcher then develops a conceptual framework. In mixed methods research, there is another step before the conceptual framework can be developed, in which the issue of how using a mixed methods approach will add value to the research study is addressed. Depending on the selected approach, one or more questions may need to be formulated, while the overarching question remains the same to allow for the integration of data in the analysis. The research questions guide the study design and the methodology, so make sure they are written to allow the researcher to fulfill the study aims. Questions need to be sufficiently comprehensive yet specific to give the researcher a road map and direction for the study. Research questions must be:

- Clear, concise, and specific
- Focused on the public health problem
- Feasible to answer given the time frame, financial resources, and access to the study population or data required to answer it
- Complex enough so that it requires thought and analysis
- Able to reflect the purpose of the study
- Relevant to the field of study and contributes to the development of research or practice

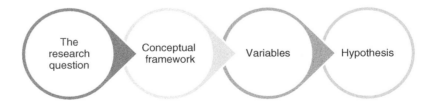

The Conceptual Framework

The conceptual framework provides the boundaries for the study in that it defines the focus of the research. Kumar (2014, p. 77) describes it as a "framework of reminders" since it represents the relationships of the variables to each other and reminds the researchers of important components to be covered. In researching the literature, the researcher identifies specific areas that are underresearched. In addition to exploring the research literature for purposes of getting to the research question, the researchers may engage cultural ambassadors to discuss local and cultural factors that influence the infection and prevention measures that were promoted and adopted. Engaging stakeholders during this process helps provide a cultural lens in developing the conceptual map to ensure the consideration of all possible elements and a fuller exploration of the literature. Community engagement is important for defining the research agenda (Chilisa, 2012), and considering social justice–based research examines the relationships and intersections and seeks to transform structural inequities and strive for critical engagement with communities, especially those of color and marginalized peoples (Jolivette, 2015). A conceptual map represents the framework for the proposed study and illustrates the relationships between the variables. It is a useful tool in the early stages of conceptualization of the research study.

> The conceptual framework builds from the gap in the literature that the research will address and focuses the methodology of the study.

It is critical to identify the literature that supports the assumed relationships to ensure that the study is fully conceptualized and to determine how the research study—and specifically the conceptual framework—is supported by the literature. One way to do this is to construct a table that summarizes all the relevant literature necessary to build the framework from the literature review (Table 4.8). Column 1 lists the construct, Column 2, theory associated with the construct (if known), Column 3 the reference, and Column 4 a brief summary of information that is relevant for the study—the relationship between the construct and the dependent–independent variable. This approach has three advantages for the researcher: it (1) provides a clear understanding of the underlying theoretical framework; (b) gives a quick reference to the reference and the relationship between the variable; and (c) reduces the risk of plagiarism.

One way to review the literature is to identify ways that mixed methods research has been used by other researchers, so identifying literature that is unique to this research methodology is important. Using mixed methods research as the only search term may not be helpful; however, not using the term may identify articles that while they have used a combination of qualitative and quantitative procedures have not been aligned with the philosophical or theoretical underpinnings of mixed methods research. In the present search, the term "mixed methods research" resulted in 598 articles and, combined in a search with "public health" (mixed methods research + public health) resulted in a search of 34 articles. Further refined for the search related to diabetes however, led to one article, "study protocol for investigating physician communication behaviors that link physician implicit racial bias and patient outcomes in Black patients with Type 2 diabetes using an exploratory sequential methods design" (Hagiwara et al., 2018).

The literature review provides the researcher with mixed methods designs in a variety of research approaches giving the researchers a way to think about their research study. The data may be combined with either qualitative data or quantitative being dominant (QUAL+quan or QUAN+qual) or where there is no distinction of dominance (QUAL+QUAN). This is the most familiar of the mixed methods designs and is used when the researcher believes that collecting addition data from an alternative source will enhance the validity of their study or explain the findings from the complementary study. In the study outlined in Table 4.8, the researchers compared the findings from a quantitative survey (HAT-QoL) with the findings from individual interviews of a population of persons living with HIV and AIDS. The 34-item Likert scale (quantitative) was administered following in-depth interviews (qualitative) of the participants.

Similarly, in another mixed methods study, Mauriën et al. (2019) adopted a mixed methods convergent parallel design in a cross-sectional study that included the use of three validated questionnaires about their psychological well-being and semistructured interviews using a phenomenological approach to interview 15 of the 90 parents who participated in total. A more complex design, however, was adopted in a multiphased cervical cancer screening using visual diagrams to communicate complex procedures. The approach involved 14 individual interviews supported by the lit-

TABLE 4.8. **Summarizing Findings in the Literature Review**

Construct	Theory	Reference	Summary
1	2	3	4
Quality of life	Not stated	Greeff et al. (2014)	Using a mixed methods convergent design study, the HIV/AIDS-targeted 34-item quality of life instrument (HAT-QoL) was used in conjunction with qualitative interview data to assess context specific, appropriateness and usefulness of the tool, in assessing QofL. The HAT-QofL was not sensitive to the life experiences of respondents in this Africa-based study of people living with HIV or AIDS.

erature review that led to the development of a survey instrument that was distributed to 424 women in two randomly assigned groups in a before-and-after design. The study was made up of three phases: (1) needs assessment and instrument development; (2) intervention development and implementation; and (3) program evaluation using an embedded mixed methods design (Hou and Fetters, 2018) (Figure 4.17).

In an alternative approach to the use of mixed methods, a sequential exploratory design (QUAL quan) was used to analyze and synthesize 22 peer-reviewed articles using the PRIMSA (Moher et al., 2009) framework with integrated qualitative and quantitative interpretation of the results, based on the following research questions: "What are the psychological factors related to human papillomavirus (HPV) testing in primary screening of cervical cancer?" and "What is the influence of these factors on women's acceptability of HPV testing in primary screening of cervical cancer?" (Tatar et al., 2018).

A case study design that included a QUAL core (individual face-to-face interviews, nonparticipant observations, and documentary data) of nurses' roles and practice was supported by three quantitative scales in a questionnaire component in a three-phased mixed methods design (Schadewaldt et al., 2016).

A community-based study in Ghana assessed the content of river and borehole use in a schistosomiasis-endemic community using urine samples from 800 students and 395 households that provided GPS coordinates matched to the children. A subsample of the participants was interviewed about water source preferences; data on water quality from the boreholes was collected, and laboratory testing was conducted for E. coli and coliform colonies; 13 focus group discussions of teenagers and adults participated in the study. While no explicit mention was made of the approach to mixed methods design, it appears to have been a convergent parallel design that incorporated laboratory testing and qualitative focus group data (Kosinski et al., 2016).

A two-phase exploratory sequential design was adopted by Bhuyan and Zhang (2020) to study children's play in urban environments using GIS-based special and statistical analysis following surveys and interviews to answer the following research questions demonstrating the range of questions that may be used to support a mixed methods design:

1. What are the constructions of children's play and play spaces in Dhaka from children's perspective?

2. How can we measure the configuration of urban and physical environments by taking children's outdoor play behavior into account?

3. Does configuration of urban physical environments affect children's location preferences for play, and if it does, to what extent?

In operationalizing the concept of transformative mixed methods, Camacho (2020) demonstrated how to actualize social justice with and for the academic immigrant population incorporated migrant identity and intersectionality frameworks using a critical theoretical reflectivity process to answer two primary question: "What workplace experiences and personal factors influence migrant identity formation for international postdoctoral scholars (IDPs) at the UC?" and "How do IPDs at UC think about and interpret experiences working within the United States relative to various identity influences and their immigrant status?" Qualitative data were used to contextualize the research findings from the survey in a thematic analysis (Figure 4.18).

FIGURE 4.17. *Mixed methods design of the components.*

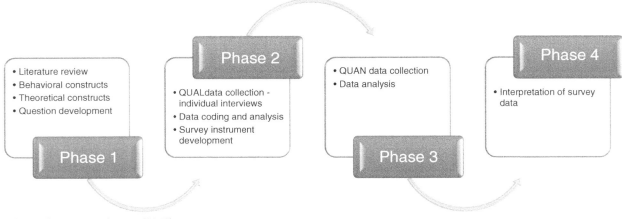

Adapted from Hou and Fettes (2018).

FIGURE 4.18. *Incorporating a transformative mixed methods philosophy.*

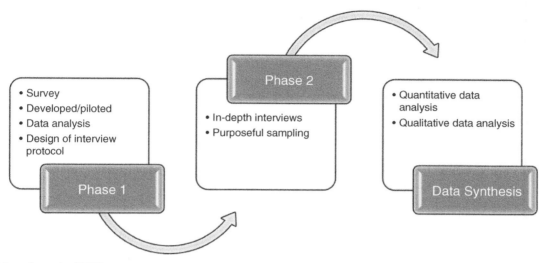

Adapted from Camacho (2020).

The design of the mixed methods study will be dependent on the purpose of combining qualitative and quantitative data. The approach will also determine the data collection approaches. In a QUAN dominant study when the quantitative research forms a major part of the study and the qualitative component being somewhat complementary, the goal of the researchers will be to ensure that the findings of the study are generalizable, therefore considering the approach to sampling for the study population and the sample size.

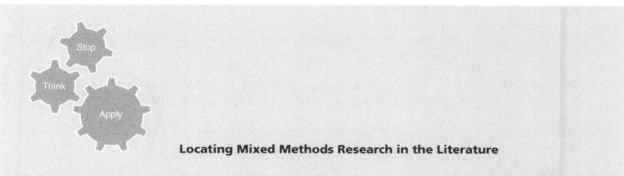

Locating Mixed Methods Research in the Literature

Search for and locate an article for a mixed methods design you would be interested in learning more about. Draw a diagram of the study's design and describe the philosophical underpinnings and procedures for collecting the data. Discuss how the results of the different qualitative and quantitative components were used to describe the findings from the study.

Sampling Schemes and Sample Size

In a mixed methods design, as in other research designs, the sample and the sample sizes are determined by the research question. However, an additional challenge in mixed methods research is the difference in sampling approaches for the variety of methods that might be used given that quantitative methods generally rely on probability sampling while qualitative research does not require probability sampling to assure validity. In a description of the approaches to combining qualitative and quantitative methods, after the convergent or sequential nature of the study is chosen, the decision can be made about how and at what point links with the other data will occur. In this way, the sample for the qualitative research component is drawn among those who responded to the survey as necessary (Fetters et al., 2013). Specifically, drawing on previous researchers, Creswell and Plano Clark (2018) identify multiple frameworks for sampling,

- Drawing on both probability and purposeful sampling incorporating stratified sampling as a substrategy
- Letting the first strand (phase) of data collection drive the second strand (phase) by using independent, related, or a single sample in a sequential mixed methods approach
- In a complex of multimethod approach, selecting different individuals from the same population for both the qualitative and quantitative arms; selecting individuals that are subsets of the larger sample; or using the same sample of individuals for each study; different individuals from different populations

Specifically, a variety of factors influence sampling and sample sizes that include:

- The data analysis is intended to compare or directly relate the data sets and the same sample
- Merging the data sets requires the samples to be roughly the same size
- Having parallel questions in the quantitative and qualitative arms of the study may require different studies
- Needing to explain one set of results with another
- Needing to explain a subset quantitative data with qualitative data depending on the results for the analysis
- Needing to have rigorous procedures in place to ensure external validity in a follow-up to an exploratory study
- The type of data being collected, each with a different expectation (e.g., focus groups, individual interview, and case studies)

Sampling approaches are described in detail in Module 2; however, the approaches are provided in Table 4.9. The sample sizes appropriate for quantitative data and qualitative data are markedly different, with surveys requiring at around 400 for a population sample—although much smaller samples may be appropriate. For example, a correlation analysis requires a minimum sample size of about 30.

TABLE 4.9. Summary of Sampling Approaches

Sampling approach	Description of approach
Cluster sampling	Intact groups are selected for the sample, and individuals within the sample and entered into the study
Convenience sampling	Choosing groups, individuals, or settings with no clearly defined strategy and the researcher relies on individual's willingness to participate
Heterogeneity/maximum variation sampling	Having a range of ideas from a cross section of persons who have differences in opinion
Homogenous sampling	Selecting units that share similar characteristics
Purposive/purposeful sampling	Selecting individuals to participate based on specific characteristics
Simple random sampling	Giving every individual has an equal chance of being included in the final sample for the study
Snowball sampling	Recruiting individuals into a study based on recommendations from others
Stratified sampling	Basing homogenous groups on one or more criteria and selecting a random sample from each stratus
Systematic sampling	Selecting individuals from a list or drawn in a systematic predetermined manner
Theoretical sampling	Selecting units (e.g., participants) individually, one at a time until theoretical saturation is reached

Unlike quantitative research, there is no formula for calculating the sample size in qualitative research. Participants, sites, documents, and activities are purposively sampled until data or thematic saturation is achieved, where subsequent data collection sessions (e.g., interviews, observations, document reviews) no longer produce new insights, where relationships between concepts and categories have been established, and where the research questions have been answered (Charmaz, 2014; Green and Thorogood, 2018). A qualitative study can adopt a single approach or a combination of sampling methods. The combination can involve a concurrent application of more than one sampling method in the convergence design or in a sequential combination of approaches where one sampling method is used to select the first level of the unit of analysis (e.g., study sites) and another sampling method is used to select the second level unit of analysis (e.g., participants within the selected study sites).

Data Collection

This section provides a summary of data collection approaches. More detailed accounts can be found in other modules in this book.

Data collection of quantitative data or qualitative data in mixed methods research adopts the same approaches as they would in a study that was not described as mixed methods research; however, the unique nature of mixed methods research requires additional thought to ensure appropriate timing of study samples, especially with regards to complex methods or indeed to follow the sequence in sequential designs and collect the data when it is required.

QUANTITATIVE DATA

In the selection of a mixed methods approach, there are just a couple of options for collecting or having quantitative data for analysis. Invariably, the design will incorporate the quantitative data in the form of a survey that occurs before or after the qualitative data collection phase in a phased study or concurrently in a concurrent study. Another option that some researchers adopt is quantitizing and qualitizing the data. In this approach, the data from a qualitative study are converted into numerical data and analyzed as such and vice versa. In addition, an observation study or a document review may provide opportunities to collect quantifiable data. In many cases a new instrument is developed, but researchers are well-advised to identify existing validated instruments when at all possible. They save time and a lot of effort, although if the population is different they may need to be validated again specifically for the study population. However, it is worth reminding readers that an existing instrument may not contain all the questions required for a particular study.

If a research study does have to adopt an instrument, there are three steps in determining if the existing instrument is appropriate:

1. Specify the purpose and the needs of the study
2. Explore existing measurement instruments that are appropriate for the study purpose.
3. Review the instrument and determine its suitability based on its psychometric properties; the comparability of the study population in characteristics such as gender, race/ethnicity, and education level; and its previous use from conducting a literature review.

Once the instrument is determined to be suitable for the existing study, the next steps are to pilot test it with the intended population. In mixed methods research a second phase of a sequential model could be using the data from a qualitative study to develop an instrument.

DeVellis (2012) in Creswell and Plano Clark (2018) outlines a general approach for moving from qualitative data to instrument development that includes:

- Determining from the qualitative data what needs to be measured and the theoretical framework that needs to be considered
- Generating an item pool with each question having only one theme/construct
- Determining the construction of the instrument
- Considering including validated items from other instruments

The additional components are outlined in Module 2 and summarized in Box 4.1.

> **BOX 4.1** Components of the Survey Development Process
>
> - Establish the purpose of the survey.
> - Conduct the literature review.
> - Specify the concepts.
> - Develop question items.
> - Consult a statistician to be sure the response categories are appropriate for the level of data analysis that is required to answer the research question.
> - Draft the survey and pretest the instrument.
> - Finalize the instrument and conduct validity and reliability tests.
> - Translate the instrument if necessary.
> - Pilot test.
> - Implement the survey with informed consent.

Developing an instrument takes time and a fair amount of effort and resources especially with regards to ensuring the items are designed to answer the research questions and the instrument is both reliable and valid for the population being studied. Using an existing instrument often seems attractive; however, it may not contain questions required for a particular study or that it was validated. Features of the instrument that would be worth considering in the design of a study include, the type of question, access to the study population and resources required for the study (Box 4.2).

> **BOX 4.2** Factors to Consider in Designing of a Survey Instrument
>
> - The type of questions
> - The most appropriate respondents and their characteristics
> - Access to the respondents
>   - Hard to reach populations (rare diseases, geographically, and socially marginalized)
> - How much time is needed to conduct the study?
> - What financial and material resources are available for the study?
>   - Incentives
>   - Access to telephones and other technology
>   - Access to lists of potential respondents
>   - Travel to reach populations of interest

In a mixed methods design with a transformatory/social justice philosophy, the data can be collected at the same time (concurrent/convergent) or sequentially. However, consideration is given to the philosophical underpinning of the methodology in addition to that of the responsiveness to the participants in the study, since participants are active participants throughout. Being culturally responsive allows the design of the study to keep the values of the stakeholders in the forefront of the process. Different from traditional postpositivist methodologies, this approach intentionally incorporates cultural values and recognizes their impact on study participation, retention, and trust in the process (Chilisa, 2012). In mixed methods research, this underlying practice of engagement is one that could be incorporated to increase the validity of its findings irrespective of the study design.

There are a number of different options for the delivery of surveys—whether they were based on existing surveys or are developed specifically for the present study—yet careful consideration needs to be given to a variety of factors that are likely to influence how the researcher gathers the data. In survey data collection, factors include the survey development and processing and survey distribution features. In the present internet era, prenotification by mail postcards or text messages increased responsiveness to survey completion (Keusch, 2015).

Face-to-face settings, by telephone or mail or electronically, via email or web browser approaches have advantages and disadvantages but have one feature in common: they each rely on the respondent providing answers to questions within the survey with often little opportunity for deviation from the pretested instrument. Data in a mixed methods designed study may also be collected through a semistructured format with a combination of closed and open-ended questions, adding another dimension to the difficulty in collecting the data. Even given all the limitation of these approaches they are likely to provide the most accurate responses to sensitive questions (Elliot, 2002), although many of the open-ended questions may have few if any responses.

Online and Web-Based Surveys Internet surveys have their limitations, the primary one being access to a computer for potential respondents. When they do, they may still not be able to complete the survey correctly due to their lack of computer skills. In addition, sampling errors arise with computer-based surveys when the intent is to extrapolate the findings to the larger population. Web-based surveys have the advantage of being delivered quickly and do not suffer from the delays that are inherent in mailed surveys. Web-based resources allow the researcher to use an existing template or develop their own template and send emails to respondents. One such platform is SurveyMonkey® that has features that include gathering responses via weblink, email, mobile chat, and social media, analyzing the results and then exporting the resulvts and the data to the researcher.

Case Study 4.3

Patients, Providers, and Staff Surveys

The team conducted a literature review on factors that influenced early entry into PNC prior to developing the survey. The team developed survey questions that reflected concepts related to this evaluation project from brainstorming activities and reviews of pertinent literature. The team assessed each question for relevance and selected those that were appropriate for each respondent category and research instrument. Three different but complementary instruments were developed for the study. Respondents were interviewed using a face-to-face approach with the use of translators where appropriate.

GIS MAPPING

GIS has the ability to provide visualization of both qualitative and quantitative data combining the postpositivist scientific approach to research with the qualitative, constructivist epistemology in an approach that allows social phenomena to be represented visually incorporating space into our thinking. In GIS visual representation of data, quantitative and qualitative take advantage of each other's strengths providing the researcher with the opportunity to be no less rigorous (Cope and Elwood, 2009). Harris et al. (2019) generated spatial maps from zip code data and patient demographic data to map the location of the federally qualified health clinics in relation to their patients (Figure 4.19).

QUALITATIVE RESEARCH

Qualitative data collection consists of interactive methods that involve (a) asking about and listening to people's accounts of their feelings, experiences, opinions, and knowledge related to a phenomenon; (b) gaining firsthand exposure to relevant behaviors, actions, processes, or activities; and (c) reviewing documents and other materials. Qualitative data in mixed methods research can include individual interviews, focus groups, observations, and document reviews.

INDIVIDUAL INTERVIEWS

Qualitative interviews are in-depth, purposeful, research-oriented conversations between a researcher and a participant to explore the participant's perspectives, experiences, behaviors, feelings, knowledge, and meanings related to a phenomenon of interest (Kvale, 1996; Kvale and Brinkmann, 2015; Patton, 2002). Unlike quantitative surveys, qualitative interviews primarily pose open-ended questions that do not limit response options but rather encourage

FIGURE 4.19. *Patients' residential zip codes and clinic locations.*

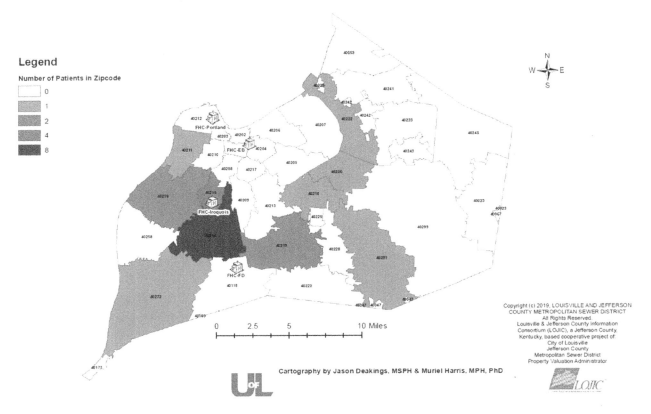

participants to provide elaborate responses. There are three types of qualitative interviews: structured, unstructured, and semistructured:

- A *structured interview* is a standardized interview that strictly adheres to a predetermined set of detailed questions in all interviews. It is not commonly used in qualitative research given its restrictive nature.

- An *unstructured interview* has no predetermined set of questions. The researcher poses a broad question to initiate the conversation, with the use of additional probing questions where necessary.

- A *semistructured interview* falls between the structured and unstructured formats and sometimes used in quantitative survey components to expand understanding from the closed-ended question.

Ideally, the qualitative interview guide should be uniquely developed (rather than adopted) and validated through expert review and feedback and pretesting in a subset of participants to ensure its relevance to the study, clarity, and suitability for the context. The interviews take place in mutually agreed upon locations and typically last 45–60 minutes depending on the complexity of the topic, although they can last longer. Interviews can be audio recorded with the participant's consent to preserve an accurate account for data analysis purposes. Any plans to audio record the interview must be specified in the research protocol and the consent document.

Focus Groups

Focus groups are researcher-facilitated group discussions that are designed to capture divergent and convergent views and experiences related to a phenomenon as participants interact with each other. Focus groups convene 6–12 purposively selected participants and generally last 90–120 minutes. The degree of homogeneity (similarity) or heterogeneity (diversity) of a focus group in terms of background and sociodemographic characteristics depends on the purpose of the study and of the focus group itself. Unlike individual interviews, focus groups are not appropriate for exploring sensitive topics due to potential breaches of confidentiality by other focus group participants. The researcher must consider the sociocultural context of their research, in addition to their research questions, when selecting data collection methods.

Observations

Observations enable the researcher to experience firsthand the physical setting, participants, behaviors, activities/processes, interactions, and less obvious factors (e.g., nonverbal cues) related to the phenomenon (Creswell, 2013; Merriam, 2009). Observations can be used as a stand-alone or primary data collection method when investigating observable issues for which a deep understanding cannot be developed through other data collection methods. Observations can also be used with other data collection methods to generate complementary or contextual data needed to achieve a holistic or in-depth understanding of the phenomenon. There are four major types of observations based on the researcher's disclosure (overt) or nondisclosure (covert) of their role as a researcher/observer and on the researcher's participation or nonparticipation in the event being observed. While covert observation methods reduce the effect of being watched or Hawthorne effect, they are subject to ethical issues when the privacy of the individuals is violated.

Case Study 4.4

Observations

In addition to semistructured interviews, an instrument was used to structure the team's observations of the patient flow, interactions, and PNC procedures within the sites. Questions for the observation instrument were developed based on the literature and comprised 11 dichotomous (yes/–no) items. Each item had a comment section, in which observers entered additional comments relevant to the visit. The final section of the instrument allowed the observer to record field notes.

Like qualitative interviews, observations can be unstructured, semistructured, or structured. Unstructured observations are not guided by an observation guide or protocol to naturally discover emergent issues related to the phenomenon. Structured observations are guided by an observation guide with detailed predetermined observation criteria (e.g., a checklist) to maintain consistency across observations or observers. A semistructured observation guide contains more general criteria or prompts, offering the flexibility to observe new criteria or elements within the criteria. During and immediately after observations, the researcher/observer takes (a) descriptive notes summarizing the process, setting, activities, interactions, and characteristics of participants being observed; and (b) reflective notes on their personal experience, reactions, and perceptions regarding the observation and their role as an observer. Researchers must interpret observation data with care since cultures are inherently different and cross-cultural research may result in misinterpretation of findings.

Document Review

In qualitative research, document review involves evaluating, analyzing, and interpreting various types of documents to shed light on a phenomenon of interest (Bowen, 2009). Document reviews are cost-efficient because documents are relatively easy to retrieve, inexpensive, unaltered by the research process, and faster to collect (Bowen, 2009; Merriam, 2009; Yin, 2009). They are particularly useful for the following circumstances: (a) when the phenomenon under study cannot be observed; (b) when participants cannot fully recall the details related to a phenomenon; (c) when the study aims to gather rich background and contextual information on the phenomenon; and (d) when it is necessary to identify relevant topics or concepts for further exploration through other data collection methods. Qualitative document review involves several types of documents within the following categories (Merriam, 2009): (a) public documents (e.g., governments or organizational reports); (b) personal/private documents (e.g., diaries, medical records); (c) physical objects or artifacts; and (d) audiovisual and digital documents.

Document review guides and worksheets can be developed to guide the evaluation of each document's characteristics and content. A limitation of this approach is that documents may not yield sufficient information to answer the research questions and some documents may be incomplete, missing, illegible, inaccurate, or inaccessible.

In a mixed methods research study, several documents could be considered for research purposes. Documents can comprise:

- Physical evidence: flyers, posters, training, and advertising material
- Personal artifacts: diaries, logs, reflections/journals, letters, and other documents containing person information and exchanges
- Public records and documents: newspapers, meeting notes, reports, and other publicly accessible information

These documents form part of the qualitative research component, although if there are counts involved, it could be considered a quantitative element.

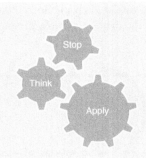

Designing A Mixed Methods Study

Part 1: Conduct a review of the literature to identify no fewer than six research articles that have used mixed methods convergent approaches in their study design. Compare their methodologies. Consider the appropriate research questions for your study.

Part 2: Design a mixed methods study of your own that is grounded in your preferences for mixed methods design (convergent, sequential, and complex) and the research questions that need to be answered. Develop a table to show the research question and the specific data collection strategies that will be required to answer the research question. Think creatively! Do another literature review to identify alternative approaches for collecting valid and reliable data.

Part 3: How would you collect the data? What sample size is required?

Analyze the Data

Mixed methods research data analysis and interpretation consists of analyzing qualitative or quantitative data that is determined by the specified approach. The purpose of using mixed methods designs is often to be able to triangulate the findings, a process that takes place at the interpretation stage of the data once the two sets of data have been analyzed.

Onwuegbuzie and Combs (2010) describe the approach to mixed methods analysis that is guided by a goal of being able to generalize the findings through external statistical generalizations, internal statistical generalizations, analytical generalizations, case-to-case transfer, and naturalistic generalization. The most integrated forms of mixed methods analysis involve some form of crossover analysis, where qualitative data are used to analyze quantitative data (Onwuegbuzie and Combs, 2010).

Other data analysis approaches used for mixed methods research data that Onwuegbuzie and Combs (2010) include (1) the rational for conducting the analyses; (2) philosophy underpinning the approach; (3) the time sequence of the analysis; (4) the priority of the analytical components given the mixed methods design that is selected; and (5) the phase of the research process when the analysis decisions are made.

Analyzing Qualitative and Quantitative Data

A discussion of approaches for analyzing qualitative and quantitative data is provided in other modules of this book and will not be covered here.

Case Study 4.5

Document Review

The team analyzed PNC reading materials provided to patients during their visits. If any reading material was available in Spanish, both versions were included in the analysis.

Print materials were analyzed for appearance, readability, and comprehension. The components of the tool were assembled primarily with the items from the Centers for Disease Control and Prevention (CDC) Clear Communication Index (Centers for Disease Control and Prevention, 2015), with additional items from the Patient Education Materials Assessment Tool (Agency for Healthcare Research and Quality, 2013). The tool assessed the layout of the material's main message, call to action, language, information design, behavioral recommendations, numbers used, and risks communicated. Additionally, researchers evaluated if material was available in Spanish.

To ensure consistency, the same evaluator assessed each individual print material using the same evaluation tool. Each aggregate score was divided by the number of possible answers to determine the overall value.

The convergent design—when data are collected and analyzed at the same time—brings together the results of the quantitative and qualitative data analysis so they are compared or combined, with the basic idea being to get a complete understanding of the problem and in some cases to validate one set of results against the other. The approach of using surveys with open-ended questions provides a mixed method design when a closed-ended question is followed immediately by an open-ended question that asks the respondent why, or to describe or explain their previous response. Another example would be a study in which a quantitative survey is conducted in the same sitting as an individual or group interview with qualitative data. Notations help to explain the relationships between methods and how qualitative and quantitative data approaches and findings are merged (Figure 4.20).

In the sequential mixed methods approach, the time sequence of the analysis refers to which data comes first in the sequence: the quantitative data or the qualitative data.

FIGURE 4.20. *Convergent design showing the potential merging of data in a mixed methods study.*

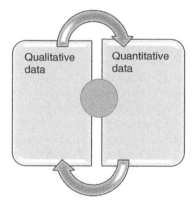

Strategies suggested for merging the two sets of results include:

- Identifying shared content in the two data sets and comparing, contrasting, or synthesizing the findings in a discussion or in a table
- Identifying differences and similarities within one set of data based on the other
- Creating a joint display of the data
- Transforming qualitative data to quantitative data and comparing the results with the existing quantitative data (Creswell and Plano Clark, 2018)

REPORT THE FINDINGS

In the traditional qualitative and qualitative approaches, the result of the data analysis is reported as described; however, in mixed methods research, how the results are reported is dependent on the approach that was used and the philosophy that underlined the study. Data analysis may occur at a single point or at multiple points in the process. In the traditional research studies, interpreting the data is done in each approach relative to the research questions, and in a mixed methods study the researchers look across the data for how jointly the findings from the qualitative and quantitative research studies complement (or not) each other to answer the research questions(s) (Creswell and Plano Clark, 2018). Data analysis in a convergent cross-sectional study will be collected at one point in time; however, sequential data in a longitudinal design will be collected as appropriate at the beginning, middle, and end of the project design as specified by the plan. While mixed methods data are collected as and when required, Creswell and Plano Clark (2018) suggest that the meaningful integration of the data defines it as mixed methods research allowing for a deeper understanding when qualitative research helps to explain findings in quantitative research (Table 4.10).

TABLE 4.10 Integration of Data the Convergent Mixed Methods Approach

Core design	Intent of integration	Interpretation
Convergent	Simultaneous integration of data to develop integrated results and interpretation that validate and confirm results	Provide insight and answer the research question.

Adapted from Creswell and Plano Clark (2018, pp. 222–223).

In convergent models' simultaneous integration of the data allows the researcher to collect, analyze, and integrate the results within the same time frame of the study. Creswell and Plano Clark (2018) suggest approaches to interpreting merged results that include:

- Summarizing and interpreting the results separately
- Discussing to what extent and in what ways results from one study converge, diverge or in other ways relate to each other
- Explaining divergence when it occurs and taking steps to resolve it
- Providing insight and answering the research question

Options for handling the data after they are collected include analyzing them separately as described in other sections of this book or merging them as described in the convergent approach. Figure 4.21 depicts the qualitative and quantitative data merging to provide research findings and recommendations as an oval between the two arrows in the image on the left; the image on the right depicts divergent data and findings.

A representation of the merged data can be achieved using table or graphs showing both the qualitative and quantitative data (Creswell and Plano Clark, 2018). The headings of the table could include the major topic, quantitative results, qualitative results, and a comparison of the methods. Once the table is set up, the researcher can then look for

FIGURE 4.21 *Potential data analysis interpretation points from a convergent design study.*

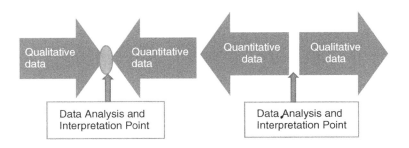

congruent or discrepant evidence across the data or consistencies, conflicts, contradictions, or complexities (Creswell and Plano Clark, 2018). Discrepancies in the findings may be addressed by repeating the study or identifying methodological challenges with one or other data, which can be noted in the limitations of the study.

> **BOX 4.3** A Convergent Parallel Mixed Methods Study
>
> The study design by Tomasi et al. (2018) had three primary objectives: (1) to characterize structured instances of information exchange with a primary focus on interdisciplinary bedside rounds and a secondary focus on within-discipline handover and peripheral information exchange activities; (2) to elucidate stakeholder perceptions of the current state of information exchange; and (3) to compare the current practices to those recommended by Lane et al.(2013) using a combination of qualitative and quantitative parallel data collection approaches. The setting for this study was the pediatric critical intensive care and the cardiac care units of the Hospital for Sick Children in Toronto, Ontario.
>
> In the interpretation of their findings, survey and interview data are compared with observational data to corroborate or contextualize the phenomena and to highlight discrepancies between the stakeholder impressions and objective third-party observations.
>
> Limitations of the study anticipated within the design process of the study were the voluntary nature of the study, the potential for being watched, potentially missing data in the capture of events, and recognition of the lack of external validity in the study of one unit within an institution.

DATA TRANSFORMATION

Over the years, various forms of data analysis have emerged in an effort to fully integrate two historically contradictory research paradigms, specifically the positivist/postpositivist paradigms underlying quantitative research and the interpretivist/constructivist paradigms underpinning qualitative research (Nzabonimpa, 2018). Data conversion or transformation (i.e., quantitizing and qualitizing) is an integrative or unifying analytic approach that has been increasingly utilized in mixed methods research and to some extent in both qualitative and quantitative research. Some analytical approaches in mixed methods research link both types of data while maintaining their diversity; however, data conversion or transformation merges the two types of data to form one data set, thus reducing or eliminating the diversity (Sandelowski et al., 2009). In mixed methods research, data conversion is performed to integrate and enhance the data so that the complex mixed methods research questions can be answered, thus enhancing the understanding of the phenomenon being investigated (Sandelowski et al., 2009). Data conversion involves two stages of data analysis: the data are (1) analyzed in their original form using the appropriate analytic approach (e.g., qualitative data analysis) and then (2) are transformed or converted into another type of data (e.g., qualitative to quantitative data), after which a second analysis is performed on the transformed data (e.g., quantitative data analysis).

Converting Qualitative data to Numerical Data

Quantitizing refers to the process of transforming or converting qualitative data into quantitative or numerical data. Essentially, the qualitative data are coded using qualitative data analysis approaches such as content analysis and the constant comparative method, after which the qualitative codes are then assigned numerical values and transformed into different types of quantitative variables. The qualitative codes can be converted into nominal variables by assigning numerical codes that indicate the presence or absence of a qualitative concept described by the code (e.g., 0-absence of feelings of grief, 1-presence of feelings of grief) or the nuances within the qualitative code or concept (e.g., 1 = accepting, 2 = denying, 3 = overcoming) (Nzabonimpa, 2018). Qualitative codes can also be transformed into ordinal variables that capture the increasing extent to which the concept described by the qualitative code is present or absent (e.g., 1 = not discernible, 2 = noted in passing, 3 = important, 4 = dominant) (Nzabonimpa, 2018; Sandelowski et al., 2009). Finally, while less common, interval variables can be created from qualitative codes and used in quantitative analysis (Sandelowski et al., 2009). Quantitizing is facilitated by qualitative and mixed methods data analysis software, most of which have the capacity to generate numerical values related to qualitative codes, which can be exported and converted into variables for statistical analysis.

Quantitizing facilitates the visualization or identification and verification of patterns in the qualitative data, thus enhancing the extraction of meaning and the interpretation of the data (Sandelowski et al., 2009). For instance, quantitizing can highlight important or influential codes within the data that are not otherwise easily visible using other approaches. Quantizing generates transformed qualitative data that can be merged/combined or compared with data originally derived from the quantitative strand, capturing additional themes or concepts that could not be captured by the original quantitative strand (Nzabonimpa, 2018; Sandelowski et al., 2009). While quantitizing has been reported to enrich quantitative data in a mixed methods approach, it has received criticism, particularly among qualitative researchers. It can result in a loss of meaning because it reduces the otherwise rich, thick, and complex qualitative data into numerical figures that do not adequately capture the complex nuances, meanings, and contexts in the original qualitative data. In addition, quantitizing can reduce the analytic power of the study, especially when using dichotomous variables that do not capture nuances in the data. As such, Sandelowski et al. (2009) suggest that the researcher should justify the unique value of this analytic approach in answering their research question or testing their hypothesis and explain how they intend to utilize quantitizing in their study.

Converting Numerical Data to Qualitative Data

Conversely, qualitizing refers to the transformation or conversion of quantitative data into qualitative data. Qualitizing entails grouping units (e.g., individuals or groups) into different clusters or categories based on their score on a scale, responses to a survey, or performance on some other quantitative measure, then generating descriptive labels or narrative profiles reflecting the shared characteristics of units within these clusters. These narrative profiles are then compared against or merged with the data derived from the original qualitative strand in further qualitative data analysis (Nzabonimpa, 2018). There are different types of narrative profile formation approaches used in qualitizing (Tashakkori & Teddlie, 1998). The *average profile* is the narrative description based on the mean attributes of the units within the cluster. The *modal profile* is a narrative description of the cluster based on the most frequent or most common attribute in the cluster. The *comparative profile* is a narrative profile that results from the comparison of the similarities and differences between one unit (e.g., individual or group) and another. The *normative profile* is based on the comparison of the individual or group against a standard (e.g., general population), rather than against another individual or group as with the comparative profile. Finally, the *holistic profile* is the narrative description of the cluster based on the researcher's general or overall impressions or inferences about the cluster. Qualitizing has been criticized for potentially overgeneralizing, misrepresenting, or oversimplifying the quantitative data (Teddlie and Tashakkori, 2009). To date, qualitizing is less commonly utilized and documented than quantitizing due to a combination of factors including the traditional positivist perceptions of the superiority of numerical data in terms of rigor and precision, the limitations of quantitative software, as well as the limited flexibility of numerical data in terms of being transformed into qualitative data (Nzabonimpa, 2018; Sandelowski et al., 2009).

ETHICAL CONSIDERATIONS

Oguegbuzie and Collins (2007) identified four ethical challenges that occur during mixed methods research: representation, legitimization, integration, and politics. These occur within both quantitative and qualitative aspects of the research and include the philosophical underpinning of the study, sample size related to under powering of a study, credibility of qualitative data, and the appropriate integration of data for data analysis (Table 4.11).

TABLE 4.11. **Challenges associated with Mixed Methods Research**

Ethical challenge	Research approach	
	Quantitative	Qualitative
Integration	Appropriate and adequate integration of the data	
Legitimization	Adequate internal and external validity	Data that are credible, transferable, dependable, and confirmable.
Politics	Challenges associated with the different philosophical approaches and preference	
Representation	When the sample size is too small for the research to have statistical power	There is difficulty in capturing lived experiences of the respondents.

SUMMARY

Once the research questions are confirmed, the researcher develops a conceptual framework, considers the underlying philosophy of the research approach, and determines the added value of using a mixed methods approach.

In a mixed methods design with a transformatory/social justice philosophy with active stakeholder participation throughout, the data are collected at the same time (concurrent/convergent) or sequentially.

The sample and the sample sizes are determined by the research question; however, an additional challenge in mixed methods research is the difference in sampling approaches given that quantitative methods generally rely on probability sampling while qualitative research does not require probability sampling to assure validity.

Mixed methods research requires that the data analysis and interpretation are determined by the usual approaches applied to qualitative and quantitive data. The purpose for using mixed methods designs is often to be able to triangulate the findings, a process that takes once the two sets of data have been analyzed separately. Mixed methods analysis is guided by a goal of being able to generalize the findings through external statistical generalizations, internal statistical generalizations, analytical generalizations, case-to-case transfer, and naturalistic generalization.

In mixed methods research, data analysis may occur at a single point or at multiple points in the process. Researchers look across the data for how the findings from the qualitative and quantitative research studies complement (or not) each other. The meaningful integration of the data defines it as mixed methods research.

Data conversion or transformation (i.e., quantitizing and qualitizing) is an integrative or unifying analytic approach merging the two types of data to form one data set.

Four ethical challenges that occur during mixed methods research include the philosophical underpinning of the study, sample size related to under powering of a study, credibility of qualitative data, and the appropriate integration of data for data analysis.

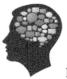

Now that I have reached the end this section, I am able to:

Course objective	Strongly agree	Somewhat agree	Neutral	Somewhat disagree	Strongly agree
Describe how to conduct a mixed methods study					
Discuss the role of qualitative and qualitative research methods in mixed methods research					
Discuss ethical principles as they relate specifically to mixed methods designs					

SECTION 3: CASE STUDY—EMBEDDED MIXED METHODS DESIGN

By the end of this section, learners will be able to:

- Describe the approach to conducting an embedded mixed methods research study
- Demonstrate the use of quantitative and qualitative research data in evaluation research
- Discuss a mixed methods approach to evaluation

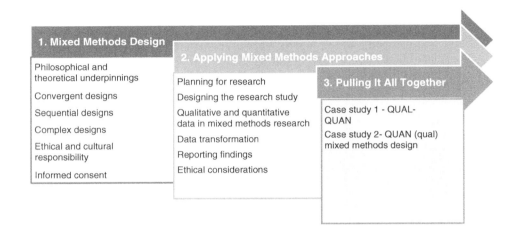

INTRODUCTION

The pragmatist draws on what works best to answer the research question(s), valuing both postpositivist and constructivist ways of knowing (Creswell and Plano Clark, 2018). This research study approach considers how quantitative and qualitative data are used to their best advantage. Researchers such as Teddlie and Tashakkori (2009) believe that pragmatism is the best philosophical basis for mixed methods designs, notwithstanding other perspectives in this debate. Mertens and Wilson (2012) extended the earlier work of Alkin and Christi (p. 14) to include four branches to evaluation theory: methods, use, theoretical approaches, and social justice. The 'methods' branch represents the positivist and postpositivist philosophies with the emphasis on research methods with a priority on experimental designs. The 'use' branch focuses on the application of the findings in constituent-building and decision-making. The 'values' branch focuses on the intervention/entity being evaluated with a focus on meaning or a focus on methodology. The addition of the 'social justice' branch provides opportunities for marginalized voices to be represented in the research and the research to address issues of power toward societal transformation (Mertens, 2018). This section of the module draws on these principles in two case studies evaluating community-based programs.

Case Study 4.6

Abstract

Title: Entry into Prenatal Care: An Evaluation of Federally Qualified Health Center's Process and Outcomes using a convergent mixed methods approach

Authors: Harris, M.J., Muvuka, B., Burton, C. & Advanced Evaluation Class, Spring 2019

Background: Early entry into PNC during the first trimester of pregnancy has been associated with positive maternal and infant health outcomes as it enables early detection and management of health issues and provides an opportunity to address behavioral and environmental factors that contribute to poor maternal and infant health (Luecken et al., 2009; Partridge et al., 2012; Taylor et al., 2005). In Kentucky, 79% of women entered PNC early, with women of color having the lowest early PNC entry rates (March of Dimes, 2019).

Methodology: This convergent case study evaluation considered women's entry into PNC and facilitators and barriers to utilization of services at a FQHC. It utilized in person survey interviews, document reviews, GIS mapping and observation techniques and reviewed educational materials provided to women.

Results: Providers were pleased overall, with the FQHC services they provide, although most were disappointed with the number of women entering PNC in their first trimester. Women identified the lack of awareness of their pregnancy as the primary barrier to early PNC. Overall, staff and providers thought they understood patients' cultural beliefs but expressed a concern over the diversity of cultural backgrounds and languages resulting in often less effective communication using interpreters. Almost half of the respondents sought PNC services at the FQHC because of their satisfaction with the quality of the services. The women felt very comfortable asking their provider questions. Scheduling conflicts may be barriers to women seeking early PNC. Women require additional educational material that included, *when to start care, medications, self-care dos and don'ts, delivery information, and ultrasounds*. GIS mapping showed that most women had easy access to one or more of the clinic sites with only 7% requiring the use of public transportation.

Conclusion: The study revealed a need for the FQHC to review some of its processes, although overall, patients, staff, and providers were satisfied with their services. In addition, women identified personal barriers to accessing care including the lack of awareness of the pregnancy in the first trimester, busy schedules, illness, and not wanting to be seen by a provider. There was a need to make more specific materials available both in content and language and make more onsite language services available. Study finding supported the need to provide women-centered care services and invest in preconception and reproductive health planning services with the goal of increasing access and utilization of PNC services in the first trimester of pregnancy.

LITERATURE REVIEW AND PROBLEM STATEMENT

Healthy People 2020 acknowledged the importance of early PNC by setting a goal that 77.6% of pregnant women initiate PNC within their first trimester of pregnancy (U.S. Department of Health and Human Services, 2019). In 2016, approximately 77% of women in the United States met the goal and began PNC in their first trimester of pregnancy as recommended, 19% entered late into their pregnancy (second or third trimester), and 2% did not receive PNC (Osterman and Martin, 2018). However, the same report suggests significant ($p < 0.05$) racial and ethnic disparities in early entry into PNC, with non-Hispanic White women being the most likely to enter PNC in their first trimester (82%) and Native Hawaiian and Other Pacific Islanders being the least likely. The first trimester PNC entry rates for Hispanic women were generally lower than those of non-Hispanic White and Asian women across all ages groups (Osterman and Martin, 2018). In 2014, Hispanic women were 70% more likely to receive late or no PNC compared with non-Hispanic White women (U.S. Department of Health and Human Services, Office of Minority Health, 2017).

In Kentucky, 79% of women entered PNC early, with Hispanic women having the lowest early PNC entry rates (66%) across all racial and ethnic groups (March of Dimes, 2019). During the same period in Jefferson County, early PNC entry was lowest among Black (70%) and Hispanic (74%) women and highest (86%) among non-Hispanic White women (March of Dimes, 2019).

The early entry into PNC (i.e., first trimester entry) has been associated with positive maternal and infant health outcomes as it enables early detection and management of health issues and provides an opportunity to address behavioral and environmental factors that contribute to poor maternal and infant health (Luecken et al., 2009; Partridge et al., 2012; Taylor et al., 2005). Understanding the many factors that influences entry into PNC requires an understanding of multiple level, which can be explored using the socioecological model.

The Socioecological Model (SEM)

The socioecological model (SEM) was utilized to explore the literature on factors that influence women's entry into PNC. The SEM is a theoretical framework for understanding the dynamic network of personal, social, and environmental factors that influence behaviors and health outcomes (McLeroy et al., 1988).

This model comprises the following levels of influence: individual/intrapersonal, interpersonal, organizational, community, and public policy (Figure 4.22). Research suggests that public health interventions should include strategies targeting all levels of influence to maximize program impact (McKenzie et al., 2017).

FIGURE 4.22. *Socioecological model.*

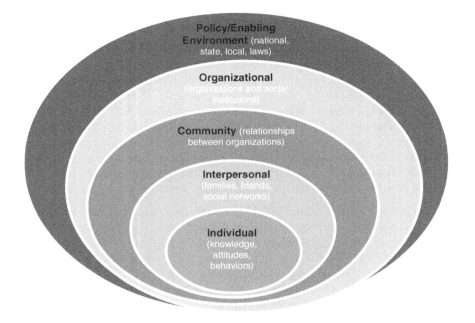

INDIVIDUAL FACTORS

The individual level of the SEM focuses on personal characteristics that influence health behaviors, such as knowledge, attitudes, and skills. Numerous individual-level factors influence women's early entry into PNC, one of which is a lack of knowledge of the pregnancy signs, symptoms, and status. Late pregnancy recognition is significantly associated with delayed PNC initiation (Selchau et al., 2017). In addition to knowledge of the pregnancy itself, inadequate knowledge of the recommended PNC timing can result in delayed PNC entry. Studies in Hispanic samples found that a larger proportion of women pregnant for the first time were not aware of their pregnancy until after the first trimester, and therefore initiated PNC later than multiparous women who had had multiple pregnancies (Daniels et al., 2006; Selchau et al., 2017). Selchau et al. (2017) found that especially younger Latina women had not received information from any source regarding when to start PNC.

Additionally, women with planned or desired pregnancies are more likely to seek early PNC than those with unintended pregnancies since the former are more likely to be physically, financially, mentally, and emotionally prepared (Luecken et al., 2009; Torres, 2005). Among Hispanic women with unintended pregnancies, fear, shame, and a lack of family or partner support delay their decisions to seek PNC (Luecken et al., 2009).

Financial barriers such as underinsurance or a lack insurance also delay entry into PNC, a situation that is particularly problematic in states lacking inclusive health insurance expansion policies (Selchau et al., 2017; Torres, 2005) and for undocumented immigrants who lack health insurance.

In addition, a considerable number of Hispanic women experience language barriers in accessing services (Selchau et al., 2017). While the use of an interpreter minimizes the language barrier, it does not eliminate this hurdle. A study by Shaffer (2002) found that even with interpreters, some patients found it much easier to explain their feelings and to ask questions directly without using an interpreter. Effective communication between health care providers and their patients is essential for quality care and the inability of health care providers to communicate effectively with their non–English-speaking clients renders their care inaccessible (National Research Council, 2006).

INTERPERSONAL FACTORS

Byrd et al. (1996) identified Hispanic women as being more family-oriented than their White American counterparts and that Hispanic women preferred their families to be involved throughout the pregnancy (Byrd et al., 1996). Social networks offer women both tangible (e.g., transportation, childcare, financial) and intangible (e.g., emotional support) benefits that encourage timely PNC utilization (Luecken et al., 2009). Some studies (e.g., Fitzgerald et al., 2015) suggest that without family involvement Hispanic women can develop feelings of isolation.

Psychological and material spousal or partner support during pregnancy is particularly critical as it has been positively correlated with early and adequate PNC (Luecken et al., 2009; Sangi-Haghpeykar et al., 2005). Even if the woman did not intend to get pregnant, the father's intention to have the child may increase the desirability of the pregnancy and the likelihood of PNC (Sangi-Haghpeykar et al., 2005). Studies have found that women are more likely to receive PNC within their first trimester when the father of the child is supportive or actively involved in the pregnancy (Martin et al., 2007; Sangi-Haghpeykar et al., 2005).

On the other hand, family influence can be a barrier to seeking PNC within the healthcare system. Family members' lack of trust in healthcare providers or the healthcare system may deter a woman from seeking PNC (Shaffer, 2002). In some cases, family members have been reported to encourage women to seek health services from elders within their family or to utilize home remedies rather than seek PNC services by skilled health professionals (Shaffer, 2002).

COMMUNITY FACTORS

The community dimension of the SEM focuses on relationships and informational networks between organizations and institutions. The elements of the community level include accessibility of specific locations within the community, transportation networks, the built environment, neighborhood associations, community leaders, and businesses (Healthy Campus, 2020, 2019). This dimension has not received sufficient attention in the literature as it relates to early PNC entry among Hispanic women. However, the lack of transportation has been identified as a major barrier to early PNC among Latinx women as it affects their ability to access PNC services (Bender et al., 2001; Shaffer, 2002). Transportation is a more significant issue among low-income women given their higher reliance on public transportation (Neutens, 2015).

ORGANIZATIONAL FACTORS

The most prominent organizational barriers related to women accessing PNC consist of both physical and social characteristics of the healthcare facility. Patient-provider interactions can be subdivided into social concordances and patient-centered care (PCC). Social concordances are social characteristics that are shared between patients and their healthcare providers. These include, but are not limited to race, gender, age, language, and education. These characteristics can influence patients' perceptions of providers and are linked to treatment adherence, decision making, patient satisfaction (Johnson-Thornton et al., 2011) and healthcare service utilization by Hispanic patients (Agency for Healthcare Research and Quality, 2006). Increased numbers of shared characteristics between patients and providers create an opportunity for improved communication and increased perceptions of health care (Johnson-Thornton et al., 2011).

PCC recognizes patients' individual experiences and the role that the context and identities play in their illness experience (Vanderford et al., 1997). Hispanic women seeking PNC do not always receive PCC due to language and cultural incompatibilities (Perez-Escamilla, 2010). In a 2013 study exploring PCC expectations of Hispanic women seeking PNC in the United States, the most important were a friendly relationship with providers, effective medical care, and the availability of Spanish speakers (Bergman and Connaughton, 2013). In addition to patient-provider communication, the lack of cultural sensitivity among providers emerged as a barrier to quality PNC among women of color (Coley et al., 2018). Studies suggest that health care providers' attitudes and insensitivities hinder non–English-speaking, low-income women from seeking adequate and timely PNC (Fitzgerald, Cronin, and Boccella, 2015). Studies examining the perspectives of Hispanic women's satisfaction with PNC suggested that physicians were not spending adequate time answering patients' questions (Byrd et al., 1996), while others noted that some providers did not attempt to clarify possible misunderstandings that arose from language barriers (Fitzgerald et al., 2015).

Structural barriers that women face in receiving PNC include the location of the healthcare facility, parking availability, the hours of clinic operation, appointment availability, and associated costs for uninsured women (Phillippi, 2010). The organizational level is essential to service delivery and ensuring individuals are able to access the services effectively.

POLICY FACTORS

The policy level focuses on local, state, national, and global laws and policies that influence behavior. Many policy factors, such as access to healthcare and immigration, affect a woman's decision to seek PNC. For insured women, Medicaid expansion correlated with an increased likelihood that women would seek medical care during pregnancy (Wherry, 2018). However, it is also important to note that women who are eligible for pregnancy-related Medicaid experience delays in accessing PNC due to delayed pregnancy recognition and late insurance enrollment (Daw and Sommers, 2018; Torres, 2016).

Undocumented women, however, are the least likely to access PNC (Korinek & Smith 2011) due to the ineligibility of undocumented immigrants to receive healthcare coverage from the majority of policies. In addition, undocumented Hispanic women may avoid using health services from hospitals or clinics due to a lack of trust in government and medical institutions, fear of deportation for themselves or family members, a lack of required documentation, interactions with law enforcement personnel, and racial profiling (Korinek and Smith, 2011; Rhodes et al., 2015). This fear also leads undocumented Hispanic women to withhold information from health care providers (Rhodes et al., 2015). Korinek and Smith (2011) believed that implementing appropriate immigration policies can help reduce the overall healthcare costs associated with preterm birth and pregnancy complications from not receiving the recommended PNC.

In Kentucky, under the Medicaid expansion rule, undocumented pregnant women may qualify for *presumptive eligibility* (Kentucky Cabinet for Health and Family Services, 2019). Presumptive eligibility (PE) enables pregnant women to receive PNC through Medicaid for up to 60 days while their eligibility for full Medicaid benefits is determined. This status is designed to improve pregnant women's access to outpatient PNC services. Enrolled providers and their office staff complete an application to determine whether a pregnant woman qualifies for *Presumptive Eligibility* for Medicaid. Providers are assured payment for early PNC services, and help women obtain pharmacy and other prenatal benefits immediately. These services may include primary care services offered by family practitioners, general practitioners, obstetricians/gynecologists, advanced registered nurse practitioners, nurse midwives, and physician assistants. It also includes any service provided by primary care centers, rural health clinics, local health departments, laboratory services, X-ray services (including ultrasounds), dental services, emergency room services, prescription drugs, and transportation (Kentucky Cabinet for Health and Family Services, 2019). However, it is not clear how PE status has helped Hispanic mothers seek PNC.

Ideally, all levels of influence should be considered in health program planning and implementation. The social, economic, political, or physical environments that shape and constrain Hispanic women's early entry into PNC are multifaceted and require a multifaceted evidence-based approach to achieve greater impact.

BEST PRACTICES IN PRENATAL CARE

PNC programs should be grounded in evidence-based practice and theoretical frameworks (Chedid and Phillips, 2019). To increase patient reach, organizations must have adequately trained staff who provide accessible, culturally sensitive, and inclusive care. Organizations that utilize a woman-centered approach to care are more likely to have successful PNC programs (Gennaro et al., 2016). A woman-centered approach relies heavily on shared decision-making and respect for the patient's autonomy, including the opportunity to choose their PNC provider rather than being assigned one (Kirkham et al., 2005). Gennaro et al. (2016) acknowledged that two-thirds of minority women access PNC within the first trimester, however, this did not seem to improve birth outcomes.

Research suggests that early entry into PNC is best achieved by investing in preconception and reproductive care planning (Atrash et al., 2006). Though this seems to be an innovative approach for successful PNC, Tuomainen et al. (2013), suggested that talking about family planning and conception may be abstract to women who are not planning for the near future. For women who are planning a pregnancy, the period between planning and conception tends to be "secretive" which may influence the patient's willingness to discuss plans with her provider. Tuomainen et al. (2013) also suggested that preconception planning should be discussed with both male and female patients.

The purpose of this evaluation was to assess the factors that influence women's early entry into PNC. This process evaluation considered women in general but specifically Hispanic women's facilitators and barriers to their utilization of PNC at the FQHC. In addition, this study reviewed pregnancy related educational materials provided to women.

Evaluation Research Questions

a. What are the experiences of patients, providers, and staff with PNC at the FQHC?

b. What are the barriers to the implementation and utilization of PNC services?

c. What are the information/education needs of patients who attend PNC at the FQHC?

EVALUATION DESIGN

This study adopted a case study design allowing researchers to study a complex phenomenon within the natural contexts in which it exists while drawing from multiple data sources (Baxter and Jack, 2008). This design allowed the researcher to consider how and why questions and the context of the phenomenon being studied (Yin, 2003). The advantage of utilizing a case study design is the ability to consider the research questions and the case. This methodology is useful and effective in evaluating programs (Yin, 2003). The focus of this study is the low first trimester PNC participation rates across multiple clinic sites with PNC services. The single case embedded units design allowed the evaluators to explore the case while also considering specific attributes of the various sites. This mixed methods design allowed investigators to collect and incorporate quantitative survey data as well as qualitative data providing a more holistic view and understanding (Baxter and Jack, 2008).

THE STUDY SETTING

The setting for this study was an FQHC that provides adult and children's health services to residents of Jefferson County. The executive director and senior staff oversee four sites that offer PNC clinic-based services.

The clinics follow the American College of Obstetricians and Gynecologists (ACOG) guidelines for PNC. The first PNC visit generally consists of a full physical exam, blood tests, calculation of the duration of the pregnancy, and the expected date of birth. However, FHC requires the first visit to be a confirmation of the pregnancy. FHC monitors the fetal heart rate using a fetal Doppler starting around 12 weeks of pregnancy and refers patients to the local hospital for delivery care services at 36 weeks.

The research team used key informants and relevant program documents to develop a logic model of PNC program (Figure 4.23).

FIGURE 4.23. *Prenatal Program Logic Model*

Inputs	Activities	Outcomes	
		Short / Medium	Long
Trained FHC health care providers and staff	Pregnancy testing	Increased access to information presented in Spanish • Website • Social media • Print materials	Reduced risk of poor health outcomes for mother and child
Information on best pregnancy practices	Scheduled prenatal care appointments		
	Prenatal care services		
Website/social media outreach	Distribution of prenatal care print materials (English and Spanish)	Decreased time between pregnancy test and first doctor's visit	
Coordination with family planning/ women's health centers	Referrals for high-risk patients to University of Louisville Hospital	Increased attendance at prenatal care appointment in first trimester	
	Patient referrals for delivery		
Transportation options for patients	Language training for providers and staff		
Interpretation services			

Assumptions	External Factors
Participation in prenatal care will reduce the risk of poor health outcomes; factors that influence participation in early prenatal care can be mitigated through addressing organizational culture and increasing information in Spanish	Bus routes and schedules Work schedules of patients

METHODOLOGY

This evaluation case study utilized multiple data collection methods in a *convergent mixed methods design* (QUAL-QUAN) that included an analysis of the clinics database, surveys, observations, document reviews, and GIS mapping to answer the research questions.

REVIEW OF EXISTING DATABASES

Existing databases for all FHC locations provided by the Family Health Centers were reviewed. Statistical software SPSS® and Microsoft Excel® were utilized to summarize the data. Two researchers conducted the review of the PNC patients. Frequencies, crosstabs, Chi-Square tests and symmetric measures were used to summarize the data.

PATIENTS, PROVIDERS, AND STAFF SURVEYS (QUANT)

The team developed survey questions that reflected concepts related to this evaluation project from brainstorming activities and reviews of pertinent literature. The team assessed each question for relevance and selected those that were appropriate for each respondent category and research instrument. Three different but complementary instruments were developed for the study.

Patient Survey

A 26-item patient survey assessed patient experiences with PNC services using a face-to-face approach for data collection given the large proportion of non–English speakers. The tool comprised a combination of open-ended, closed ended (Yes/No), and Likert scale questions that were organized into the following sections:

1. General experience and satisfaction with services: This section contained questions about how the patient found out about the PNC services, their satisfaction levels, and experience with scheduling appointments.

2. Experience during provider visit: This section contained questions about their comfort levels asking the provider questions, general appointment experiences, and information provided to the patient.

3. Beliefs and values regarding PNC: This section contained questions about the importance of PNC.

4. Actual and perceived barriers to receiving care from FHC: This section contained questions about FHC's hours of operation and transportation.

5. Demographics: This section contained questions about age, race/ethnicity, health insurance, partner support, zip code of residence, and country of origin

Staff and Provider Surveys

Staff and provider surveys assessed their perceptions and experiences with providing PNC services, as well as their interactions with PNC patients. In addition, both groups were asked for recommendations to improve PNC.

The 29-item staff survey had four sections: (1) women's perceptions of entering PNC; (2) perceptions of patients' experiences; (3) provision of PNC-related information; and (4) demographics. The survey utilized a mixture of dichotomous, multiple-choice, Likert-scale, and open-ended questions.

The 26-item provider survey comprised the following four sections: (a) perceptions of PNC services (b) provider interaction with patients, (c) information provided to patients, and (d) demographics. The demographic section elicited information on the provider's race/ethnicity, role in the clinic, clinic location, and number of years they had worked with the FQHC. This survey consisted of a mixture of dichotomous, multiple choice, Likert-Scale, and open-ended questions.

Administrative staff reviewed the interviews and provided feedback. The research team incorporated their feedback and refined the instruments. All three instruments underwent multiple rounds of review. All research team members completed the Human Subjects Training (CITI) in preparation for the study and signed confidentiality statements provided by the FQHC. The team participated in a training prior to data collection, that included role-plays for administering the informed consent and the survey.

OBSERVATIONS (QUAL)

In addition to semistructured interviews, an instrument was used to structure the team's observations of the patient flow, interactions, and PNC procedures within the sites. Questions for the observation instrument were developed based on the literature and comprised 11 dichotomous (yes–nNo) items. Each item had a comment section, in which observers entered additional comments relevant to the visit. The final section of the instrument allowed the observer to record field notes.

DOCUMENT REVIEW (QUAL)

The team analyzed PNC reading materials provided to patients during their visits. If any reading material was available in Spanish, both versions were included in the analysis. Print materials were analyzed for appearance, readability, and comprehension. The components of the tool were assembled primarily with the items from the CDC Clear Communication Index (Centers for Disease Control and Prevention, 2015), with additional items from the Patient Education Materials Assessment Tool (Agency for Healthcare Research and Quality, 2013). The tool assessed the material's layout of its main message, call to action, language, information design, behavioral recommendations, numbers used, and risks communicated. Additionally, researchers evaluated if material was available in Spanish. To ensure consistency, the same evaluator assessed each individual print material using the same evaluation tool. Each aggregate score was divided by the number of possible answers to determine the overall value.

GIS MAPPING (QUAL)

This study employed GIS to map the location of PNC patients in relation to the four clinics. Arc GIS software was used to generate spatial maps from zip codes and the FHC clinic database and data from the demographic section on the patient surveys. The analysis resulted in a map of the study population density in relation to the PNC clinics.

DATA ANALYSIS

The quantitative data from the surveys and observation data were entered into a Microsoft Excel® and then imported into SPSS® for analysis. Descriptive statistics consisting of frequencies, proportions, and measures of central tendency were generated in SPSS®. The qualitative data from the interviews and observations were coded in Microsoft Word® to identify emergent and recurrent themes across the data.

RESULTS

Demographic Profile of the Sample

A total of 47 individuals participated in the study: 27 patients, 13 staff members, and 7 PNC providers. Of the 27 PNC patients surveyed, 18.5% ($n = 5$) were in their first trimester of pregnancy on the interview date (Table 4.12). The patient sample had a mean age of 27 years old, with a range of 20–42 years old.

TABLE 4.12. Distribution of Patient Survey Respondents by Pregnancy Trimester

Trimester	Frequency	Valid percent
First trimester (0–13 weeks)	5	18.5
Second trimester (14–27 weeks)	11	40.7
Third trimester (28+ weeks)	11	40.7
Total	27	100

FIGURE 4.24. *Race/ethnicity distribution of patient survey responses.*

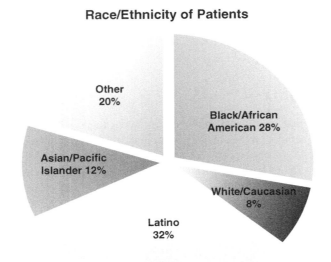

The patients were predominantly Latinx (32%), and 28% were African American. The most represented countries of origin were the United States (15%), Mexico (12%), Honduras (9%), and Somalia (9%). Over half (56%) of the patients who utilized interpreting services during the interviews were Spanish speaking (Figure 4.24).

Just over half (52%) of respondents were single, 33% were married, and 8% were divorced or separated. With respect to social support, 89% of respondents reported receiving partner support during the pregnancy, while 71% received support from family and friends. About 41% of respondents reported having an unplanned pregnancy, while 35% indicated that it was planned. Nearly half (48%) of the patients were insured, while the rest were uninsured.

Most (93%) had a personal vehicle or went to the clinic in a family member's vehicle, while 7% utilized public transportation. Most patients were recruited from zip codes that were mapped to each of the four clinic locations (Figure 4.25).

Staff and Provider Demographics

A total of 13 FHC staff were surveyed: 10 medical assistants, 2 front desk clerks, and 1 unidentified. Additionally, seven different providers completed the survey from all clinic locations: five nurse practitioners and two physicians. All seven providers identified as White. None of the providers self-reported being fluent in any language other than English.

Experiences with Prenatal Care Services

Patients' Experiences with PNC The patient survey revealed that word of mouth was the most common referral source for PNC. More specifically, 59% of respondents of the Latinx respondents heard about the PNC services through friends or family members. Overall, only 11% ($n = 5$) of respondents were referred to the PNC services from other services or locations.

Care Seeking at FHC Forty-one percent (41%) of participants sought PNC based on the overall quality of the services offered by the FQHC, while others (19%) liked the accessibility of the locations.

Operations at FHC Fifty-five percent ($n = 14$) of respondents reported an "easy" scheduling process and did not encounter any issues. However, three respondents described their scheduling experience as "long" or "hard." The majority (96.3%) of the women were satisfied with the operating hours of their location. Similarly, participants

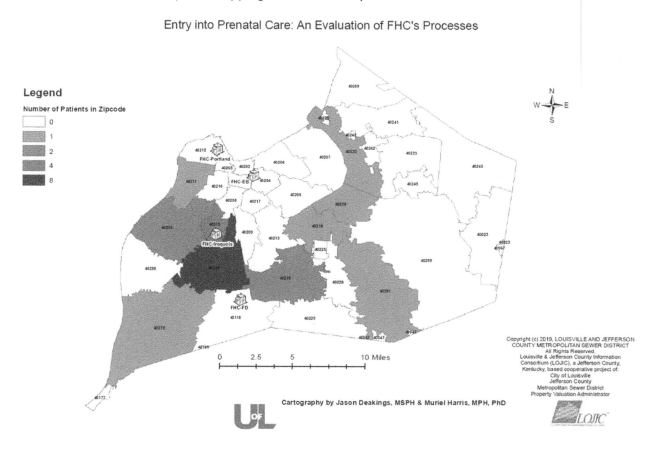

FIGURE 4.25. *GIS spatial mapping of residential zip codes and clinic locations.*

expressed general satisfaction with their first PNC appointment, with 78% describing it as "good" or "very good." All participants were comfortable asking their provider questions related to their pregnancy during a PNC visit, with 92.6% of respondents feeling *very comfortable* and 7.4% feeling *comfortable or somewhat comfortable.*

Staff's Experiences and Perceptions of PNC Services When asked if PNC had dedicated staff on site, approximately 92% said yes, which was corroborated by the research team through their observations. Half of the staff members interviewed estimated an average wait time of 15 minutes or less for a patient to be seen by a provider. This was consistent with direct observations by the research team, which found that patients waited an average of 11 minutes.

Over 75% of staff felt comfortable working with Hispanic women despite 66% reporting that they had not received any cultural competency training. Two out of the four staff members who received cultural competency training reported receiving their training from the Louisville Metro Department of Public Health and Wellness.

Provider Perceptions and Experiences of PNC The researchers found that 72% of providers spent 15 minutes or less with each patient at each visit (Table 4.13). Direct observations by the research team revealed that the entire PNC visit lasted on average 28 minutes, inclusive of the time spent outside of the provider's examination room.

The majority (72%) of providers reported being often or very often satisfied with the PNC services at FHC (Table 4.14). However, 71% of providers were not satisfied with the number of women entering PNC in their first trimester of pregnancy. They noted that these numbers are lower than desired, and they would like to see an increase in the early entry into PNC.

When asked if they understand their patients' cultural beliefs related to PNC, 57% ($n = 4$) of providers reported that they do, while 43% ($n = 3$) mentioned that they do not fully understand their patients and are constantly learning. One provider specifically mentioned that it is difficult to understand beliefs surrounding PNC given the number of patients from diverse cultural backgrounds with a diversity of beliefs surrounding PNC.

TABLE 4.13. Observed Time Spent by Providers with Patients

Time (min)	Count	Percentage (%)
<10	2	29
<15	3	43
<30	1	14
>60	1	14

TABLE 4.14. Providers' Satisfaction with Prenatal Care at Family Health Centers

Answer	Count	Percentage (%)
Occasionally	1	14.3
Somewhat often	1	14.3
Often	3	42.9
Very often	2	28.6

Barriers to Early Prenatal Care Entry

Patient, staff, and provider surveys elicited perceptions of barriers to women's early entry into PNC. These findings are discussed following.

Patient-Perceived Barriers Women identified several barriers to early PNC. The lack of awareness of the pregnancy was the primary barrier identified by about a third (38%) of respondents. More specifically, six of the eight (75%) Latinx women surveyed reported that they were unaware of their pregnancy in the first trimester. Other barriers to early PNC identified by patients included busy schedules (15%), illness (12%), not wanting to be seen by a provider, or frustrations that patients were not being seen right away following a positive pregnancy test.

Staff-Perceived Barriers Staff identified language and culture as major barriers to early entry into PNC, particularly among Hispanic women. Additional barriers included health insurance coverage, education, and scheduling or availability issues (Figure 4.26). Some staff members observed that many patients feel insecure and/or unsure about their health insurance coverage and costs, while others experience conflicting schedules or availability issues and are not able to follow through with their appointment. A few staff members ($n = 3$) also pointed to transportation issues as among the reasons for late PNC or no-shows.

Provider-Perceived Barriers Providers' perceived barriers to the early entry into PNC corroborated reports from patients and staff members. Consistent with patients' self-reports, the majority (86%) of the providers also suggested that most of their patients had unintended pregnancies, which they believed to affect their timing of entry into PNC. Additionally, providers highlighted that the following issues delay women's entry into PNC: transportation issues, the costs of care for uninsured women, language barriers, scheduling issues, a lack of awareness of the pregnancy, and a lack of knowledge of the need for and timing of PNC. While this study revealed that all providers have access to an interpreter, the lack of privacy and poor telephone reception hindered the effective use of interpreters in the clinical setting.

FIGURE 4.26. *Barriers to prenatal care as perceived by family health centers' staff.*

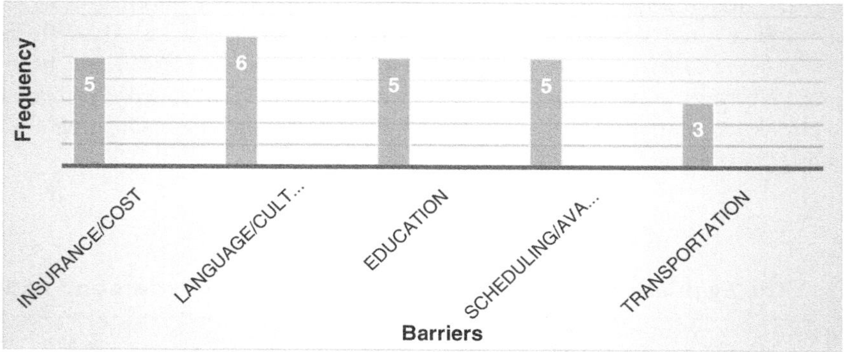

Information Needs of Prenatal Care Patients

All women interviewed believed in the importance of PNC in promoting maternal and child health, many of whom highlighted the importance of complying with the providers' recommendations or orders. When asked about the type of preconception information they would have wished to receive prior to their pregnancy, about half (56%) of the women in the study indicated that they did not need any additional information, while a third (33%) indicated the need for additional information on general health (22%), contraception (7.4%), and nutrition (3.7%).

Providers' Perceptions of Patient Information Needs

All providers reported raising awareness of the importance of first trimester PNC entry to their patients during the preconception period, particularly among patients attending family planning services. Most providers reported providing nutritional information related to the importance of folic acid or prenatal vitamins in their diet. However, they identified the following common information needs among PNC patients: when to start care, medication, self-care dos and don'ts, delivery information, and ultrasounds. In addition to patient and provider perceptions of the information needs of PNC patients, the document review of PNC materials indicated additional health information needs for patients.

A REVIEW OF FAMILY HEALTH CENTERS' PRENATAL CARE MATERIALS AND WEBSITE

Forty-two items were sorted into three categories and analyzed: (1) resource materials; (2) educational materials on pregnancy-related health conditions and situations; and (3) materials with clinical information (Table 4.15). Four of the materials had Spanish versions.

A higher score indicated a more beneficial and understandable piece of material, while a score below 0.80 indicated some deficits in content and the need for revision. Most (84%) materials scored above 0.80 (Table 4.16), suggesting effective presentation of the information provided. The items that scored lowest were not necessarily materials produced for health information or education purposes but rather for commercial use. Materials were sorted based on primary aspect/purpose of the material. While all materials in the clinical category had Spanish translations, only 31.8% of the resource materials and 30.7% of the educational materials had Spanish versions. This means that while

TABLE 4.15. Prenatal Care Materials Evaluated

Materials sorted and categorized	Resource materials	22
	Educational materials on pregnancy-related conditions	13
	Clinical information	7

Spanish-speaking patients may know what to do during pregnancy, they may have difficulty understanding other aspects of this experience and may not know all the resources available to them (Table 4.16).

Additionally, a review of the organization's website revealed that it contains information of services offered, locations, transportation, resources, and personal medical information for current patients. The website is available in both English and Spanish. However, there were two critical missing components. First, the website does not contain a specific tab or page for PNC services, which are only referenced in information related to primary care and clinic locations. Second, the website does not contain educational information for patients, indicating a need for electronic or downloadable versions of educational materials on the website.

TABLE 4.16. **The Evaluation Scores of FHC's Prenatal Care Materials and Patient Handouts**

Material	Score	Spanish translation
	Resources	
Arts in healing	1.00	
Beautiful beginnings	0.94	
Breastfeeding help	0.88	X
Community resources	0.91	X
Congratulations!	1.00	
Covered by KY Medicaid	0.93	
Family playgroup	0.92	
Hands	0.93	
Health education programs	0.92	
How to get to FHC Portland	1.00	X
Kentucky Medicaid	0.93	
Mommy Xpress	0.91	
Options for pregnancy	0.75[a]	X
Pregnant?	1.00	X
Prenatal and family programs	0.87	X
Program promotes benefits of breastfeeding	0.59	

(Continued)

TABLE 4.16. (Continued)

Material	Score	Spanish translation
She's one smart mom	0.83	
UofL medical complex map	1.00	
Where can I go for help with:	1.00	
WIC clinics	1.00	X
WIC growing healthy families	1.00	
WIC helps	0.88	
Education		
I don't feel like myself	0.90	
Lead poisoning	0.86	
Parents are Latina	0.35	X
Reasons to be proud	0.82	
Td or Tdap	0.87	X
UofL center for women and infants	0.71	
Vaccine information statement	0.91	
Choosing good foods	1.00	X
Congratulations on your new baby	0.95	
Great expectations	0.96	X
What you should know about HIV/AIDS	0.78	
What you should know about newborn circumcision	0.90	X
When labor begins	0.91	
Your weight and weight gain	0.95	

(Continued)

TABLE 4.16. (Continued)

Material	Score	Spanish translation
	Clinical	
My 9 Months	1.00	X
Pregnancy	0.77	X
Six-week postdelivery planner	0.85	X
Pregnancy Guidebook First Trimester	0.95	X
Pregnancy Guidebook Second Trimester	0.95	X
Pregnancy Guidebook Third Trimester	0.95	X

Note: Blue highlights reflect scores less than 0.8.

PROVIDER AND STAFF RECOMMENDATIONS TO INCREASE EARLY ENTRY INTO PNC

As a part of the study, participants provided recommendations to increase first-trimester entry into PNC. Both provider and staff surveys highlighted three main recommendations. First, to address language barriers, 62% ($n = 8$) of staff and 86% ($n = 6$) of providers recommended developing patient education materials in multiple languages. Second, to improve the accessibility and availability of PNC-related information, 61.5% ($n = 8$) of staff and 71% ($n = 5$) of providers recommended uploading PNC-related patient education materials on the website. Third, 69% ($n = 9$) of staff and 42% ($n = 3$) providers recommended scheduling the initial PNC appointment within seven days of a positive home pregnancy test. Some providers recommended hiring more in-person interpreters (Table 4.17).

TABLE 4.17. Interventions to Improve Entry into Prenatal Care

Intervention suggestion	Provider ($n = 7$)	Staff ($n = 12$)	Total
Develop patient education materials in multiple languages	6	8	14
Develop website to provide detailed prenatal care information	5	8	13
Schedule OB appointment for patients within 7 days of a positive home pregnancy test	3	9	12
Offering OB appointments on evenings	5	5	10
Offering pregnancy test and OB visit same day	4	5	9
Offering pregnancy test and scheduling OB visit within 7 days	3	6	9
Offering OB appointments on Saturdays	4	5	9
Dedicated prenatal care clinic	3	5	8

DISCUSSION

This study examined the factors influencing women's participation in PNC services during the first trimester of pregnancy using a convergent mixed methods case study design, including both qualitative and quantitative data. It yielded several important findings. Although providers were pleased overall with the PNC services they provided, most were disappointed with the number of women entering PNC in their first trimester of pregnancy. Similar to findings in the literature (Daniels et al., 2006; Selchau et al., 2017), this study found that women often did not know they were pregnant and therefore did not seek care, affecting the timing of their entry into PNC. One third of women in the study identified the lack of awareness of pregnancy as the primary barrier to seeking PNC early, with six women reporting that they themselves were unaware of their pregnancy in the first trimester. The study by Selchau et al. (2017) also found that women lacked knowledge of pregnancy signs and symptoms. In addition, 41% of women in this study reported having an unplanned pregnancy that could also have influenced their knowledge of the pregnancy and their subsequent response.

Additionally, staff identified language and culture as major barriers to early entry into PNC; however, this study was unable to determine specific cultural barriers. Overall, staff and providers thought they understood patients' cultural beliefs related to PNC, but providers expressed a concern over the diversity of cultural backgrounds of their patients. While interpreters are available, when necessary, the diversity of languages also meant that patients did not always have an interpreter in the room, often resulting in less effective communication. A lack of understanding of the diverse cultural backgrounds of patients and their belief systems regarding the health system suggests that racial/ethnic minorities, specifically Latinx women, may be at a disproportionate risk of receiving less than ideal health care services. In this study, most staff felt comfortable working with Latinx women, although over half said they had not received any specific cultural competency training.

In this study, almost half of the respondents sought PNC services at FHC based on the quality of the services and their satisfaction with their first encounters. Nearly all women felt very comfortable asking their provider questions. In their study, Johnson-Thornton et al. (2011) linked treatment adherence, decision-making, and patient satisfaction to patient–provider interactions. Despite the reports of positive scheduling experiences and patient–provider interactions by most patients, results suggest that the lack of health insurance coverage and the limited understanding of PNC could affect women's early entry into PNC. While most patients spent an average of 15 minutes during each visit, a few patients stayed longer as they waited for an interpreter.

This study also assessed patient education needs and found that half of the women said they did not need any additional information. However, those who identified the need for additional educational material indicated that they mostly needed information related to *general health, contraception,* and *nutrition*. In addition, providers also perceived that the patients needed information about *when to start care, medications, self-care dos and don'ts, delivery information,* and *ultrasounds*. A review of existing materials confirmed the gap in general educational resources provided to women during their pregnancy, especially for those who do not speak English. This gap is even more evident on the website, which only provides information related to primary care and clinic locations. This is a missed opportunity for reaching and educating women in need of PNC services.

The findings in this study support the use of a women centered approach (Gennaro et al., 2016) which posits that early entry into PNC is best achieved by investing in preconception and reproductive health planning (Atrash et al., 2006). There are barriers to adopting preconception planning since women often view planning and conception as secretive. However, implementing this approach may ensure that women who seek primary care services and services related to family planning and sexually transmitted infections (STIs) are provided educational resources. Ideally, information should be provided in print, in person, and electronically. Given the diversity of the population that is served by FHC, it is important that these educational materials are produced in multiple languages.

Limitations of This Study

This study had several limitations. First, the study had a small sample size given its short duration. Second, there were language barriers between the respondents and the researchers as most patients interviewed were non–English speaking. When interpreters were used, and particularly via telephone, the researchers were unable to validate participants' responses. Last, researchers were unable to accurately decipher and/or capture race/ethnicity.

RECOMMENDATIONS

Based on the gaps identified in this study, the following are recommendations to improve women's early entry into PNC at FHC:

- Promotion and Marketing
  - Improve the FHC website by adding a specific page or tab for PNC services. This PNC tab should contain general information on the PNC services offered, including the sites/locations, operating hours, providers, and downloadable education materials in multiple languages.
  - Promote more active referrals of women to women's health from other FHC services.
- Preconception counseling in women's health
  - Improve patient access to in-person, print, and electronic health information related to pregnancy and PNC.
  - Utilize culturally sensitive approaches to material development with the active engagement of community members in their development, evaluation, and refinement.
- Provide cultural competency training to staff and providers to improve the quality of their interactions with patients from diverse cultural and linguistic backgrounds.

The Case Study 4.7

Abstract

Title: An embedded multimethod evaluation study of a community-based intervention to improve access to opportunities for healthy eating and safe physical activity

Authors: CPPW Evaluation Research Team

Background: Physical activity and healthy nutrition are critical for preventing the onset of noncommunicable diseases (NCD) such as heart disease, high blood pressure and diabetes among the top six causes of death globally. Multipronged interventions with systems, environmental, and policy changes are critical for ensuring safe and healthy environments. Disenfranchised communities are often without opportunities for healthy eating and safe physical activity hence carry a heavier burden of disease and disability.

Methods: Thirty-six interventions in five disenfranchised low-income neighborhoods (population 80,204) included nutrition and physical activity in school and community settings. This embedded mixed methods evaluation assessed the impact of the multipronged intervention on individuals using the Behavioral Risk Factor System Survey (BRFSS), 500 pretest–posttest semistructured surveys and 38 family interviews.

Results: In the follow-up study 18 months later, the intervention was successful in decreasing calories consumed ($p<0.01$) and increasing consumption of fruits and vegetables ($p<0.01$). However, respondents did not increase their physical activity, although the perception of safety did. Most believed that it was important to improve conditions through policy change (80%, $p<0.01$) and it should be easier for people to get healthy foods (90%, $p<0.01$), and those who strongly agreed that it should be easier to walk, bike and play in their neighborhoods increased ($p<0.01$).

Conclusion: To address high rates of NCD, systems and environments must address the dire need. Policies must be enacted and enforced to ensure equitable distribution of resources to redress many years of neglect through underfunding and abandonment of what have become low-income communities.

THE LITERATURE REVIEW AND PROBLEM STATEMENT

Overweight is associated with an increased body mass index (BMI): overweight (25–29.9%); obesity (> 30%). A normal BMI is 19.5–24.9%. Obesity carries an increased risk of many diseases and health conditions National Institute of Diabetes and Digestive and Kidney Diseases (2019) (Table 4.18). Globally, heart disease, stroke, and diabetes make up

TABLE 4.18. Diseases Associated with Individuals Being Overweight

Diseases with increased risk associated individuals being overweight	
Type 2 diabetes	Fatty liver disease
High blood pressure	Kidney disease
Heart disease and stroke	Pregnancy-related high blood pressure, increased blood sugar, increased risk of have a caesarian section
Sleep Apnea	Certain cancers (endometrial, breast, ovarian, prostate, liver, gallbladder, and colon)

the top 10 of the deadliest diseases worldwide. Worldwide obesity has nearly tripled since 1975 with 1.9 billion adults (13% of the world's population) and 340 million children 5–19 years being overweight in 2016 (WHO, 2021). In addition, children in low-income and diverse communities were found to be overweight or obese (40%), with 50% being Black and 39.4% being Hispanic (Ohri-Vachaspati et al., 2015). In addition, 54% of the children living within a quarter of a mile of corner stores were overweight or obese (Ohri-Vachaspati et al., 2015) since rather than healthy food options, corner stores sell mostly snacks.

One of the most familiar of the non-communicable diseases (NCD) is type 2 diabetes, also known as diabetes mellitus. Apart from being a disease, it is a risk factor for cardiovascular disease. Like heart disease and high blood pressure, it is thought to be associated with environmental factors and influenced by diet and lifestyle. In their study of 692 individuals, Rose et al. (2019) found that being overweight, poor diet, lack of physical activity, the environment, and genetics were causes of type 2 diabetes. While genetics and family history will not be affected through prevention interventions, diabetes, heart disease, and high blood pressure can be prevented by activities at multiple levels of the socioecological model.

The most often used approach to reduce obesity and improve quality of life is health education. Individuals are asked to increase physical activity and consumption of fruits and vegetables. Modifying diets and increasing physical activity need to be culturally appropriate and sensitive to the needs of different population groups (Robinson, 2008). Diets high in fruits and vegetables have benefits for decreasing morbidity and mortality associated with chronic disease, hypertension, and stroke (Robinson, 2008). However, in many communities, and especially in minority communities, there is a dearth of healthy food choices in what have come to be known as food deserts. In addition, these same communities have limited access to environmental structures, systems, and supports for individuals to be physically active. The World Health Organization (WHO, 2018) identified four levels of activities that operate in a synergistic and systems approach to ensure the creation of healthy environments:

- Changing social norms and attitudes
- Creating health environments through healthy spaces and places
- Programs and opportunities
- Systems change through governance and policy enablers

The community-based intervention in this evaluation addressed all aspects of changing the environment primarily to improve opportunities for healthy lifestyles for those who have been disenfranchised and live in low neighborhoods with limited access to healthy spaces for physical activity and healthy foods in recognition of the importance of changing the environment to improve the quality of life for low-income individuals by adopting the socioecological model as the guiding framework.

Evaluation Research Questions

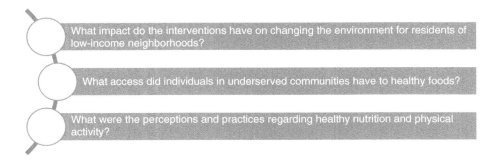

The Evaluation Design

The evaluation study adopted a convergent mixed methods design. The before and after survey assessed the processes that led to changes in the social and physical environment intended to improve access to physical activity and healthy foods, depicted in the logic model (Figure 4.27). This single-sample longitudinal time series study focuses on changes that occurred in the short- and medium-term of this three-year intervention. The intervention contained a total of 36 strategies that included:

- School-based nutrition
- School-based physical activity and health education
- School-based strategies to change policies and governance
- Community-based strategies to improve nutrition
- Community-based strategies to improve access to healthy foods
- Community-based strategies to improve access to physical activity
- Social marketing strategies to change social norms around physical activity and healthy nutrition to improve heart health and reduce the rates of obesity

Survey questions on a five-point Likert scale of strongly agree to strongly disagree included:

1. I think it's easy to find good quality fruits and vegetables in my neighborhood.
2. I think it's easy to find affordable fruits and vegetables in my neighborhood.
3. Most people I know think it is important to eat several servings of fruits and vegetables each day.
4. Most people I know use local parks and walking or bike trails for exercise or physical activity.

In addition, the process monitoring monthly reports assessed the levels of project implementation including the following: (a) barriers faced in the previous 30 days; (b) strategies to overcome the barriers; and (c) support or technical assistance needed or used to achieve specified milestones. The study incorporated a formative assessment of media activity with subsequent changes in the promotion of healthy foods through community mounted billboards and other media. Ethical clearance for this study was obtained from the local IRB/ethics center.

A mixed methods evaluation design systematically integrates two or more methods drawing on both qualitative and quantitative approaches. In addition to mixed methods designs being helpful for answering a range of different research questions, incorporating different methods increasing validity and reliability of the results, and using one method to design the next phase of the study, mixed methods may also be helpful when the researcher wants to achieve a deeper understanding of the effects of the intervention or get multiple perspectives. A transformative approach would provide additional opportunities for stakeholders to be involved and ensure community engagement and support (Mertens, 2018). This study adopted the embedded mixed methods design for the evaluation with a dominant quantitative component and a less dominant qualitative component (QUAN qual) in a pretest–posttest evaluation research design (Figure 4.28).

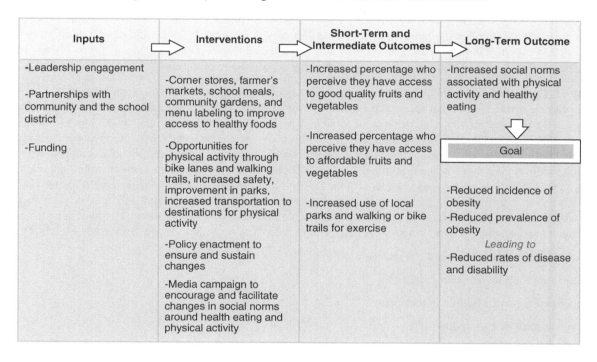

FIGURE 4.27. *Logic model representing intervention activities and outcomes.*

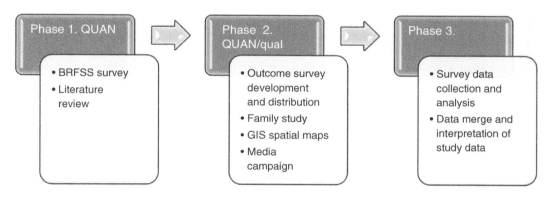

FIGURE 4.28. *Multiphased evaluation mixed methods study.*

Baseline and Pretest–Posttest Data (QUAN) The BRFSS with a sample size of 1,511 was used in conjunction with the outcomes study survey at the start of the intervention to assess the study population characteristics and to monitor the intervention. A pretest–posttest outcomes survey of 500 individuals was randomly selected from a population of approximately 80,204 to measure the impact of the interventions on participants' attitude, perceptions and intended behavior. The sample was selected from among residents within a preselected geographical area that was predominantly African American (70%), but the sample population was 58% African American. Individual who participated in the study were 18 years and over. A random digit dial (RDD) frame was obtained from a marketing company to reach land lines and cellular phones were used in a telephone interview to administer the survey. A CATI system was used to capture the responses. A minimum of 10% of the complete interviews were validated. The sample was selected by using a stratified sampling approach by both geography and demographics while maintaining statistical representation of the five neighborhoods that formed part of the study based on their population size. Sample selection within the household adopted the Hagan Collier (Rizzo et al., 2004) technique requiring the person within the household to be rotated to ensure an appropriate distribution of demographic characteristics within the sample. Calls were made on three weekdays at varied times selecting time slots from the morning, afternoon and evening. All interviewers were trained prior to the interviews in using a predesigned survey instrument. Pretests were conducted to ensure that any difficulties in delivering the survey were addressed. Spanish speaking individuals were interviewed by Spanish speaking interviewers. Interviews were conducted on weekdays and weekends at varying times with up to five calls per interview for a total of 15,614 calls with 1,813 refusals. Data was collected by an established research organization with a track record of collecting public health–related data as was required for this evaluation in addition to having demonstrated expertise in the market. The organization was selected from a pool of applicants following an open call for proposals that described the needs of the project and the expectations for the study.

Family Study (qual) A semistructured interview guide was developed by the evaluation team to conduct this exploratory qualitative research study that assessed the extent to which the interventions that had been implemented influenced changes in the physical activity or nutrition at the family level. Based on the first five initial "pilot" interviews, the semistructured interview guide was fine-tuned and modified. This more open-ended qualitative interview structure provided the opportunity for a deeper understanding of the socioecological context as it influenced physical activity and nutrition, from the family perspective. The socioecological model of health was used to create the semistructured interview guide (Casey et al., 2009). Interviews were conducted at the family's home in their natural environment. While provision was made to conduct interviews in other safe spaces, this was not necessary. A team of trained interviewers conducted the interviews that included nuclear and extended families. Each family interview was moderated by two trained interviewers. Training sessions for all interviewers were held prior to field work on a range of pertinent issues including:

- Administering the semistructured interview tool
- Using appropriate question probes
- Interviewing with children in the room
- Sociocultural sensitivity training
- Navigating challenging interview situations, and
- Postinterview memo writing[1]

Data coding and analysis took place using the constant comparative method (Strauss and Corbin, 1998). This iterative process of simultaneous data collection and analysis involved ongoing comparing data within and between interviews as core themes, concepts, patterns, metaphors, and categories were identified and developed. Identifying concepts and theoretical relationships derived from the data continued until theoretical saturation (Strauss and Corbin, 1998) occurred and no new information was emerging. The NVivo® qualitative data software program was used to facilitate the coding and aid the systematic analysis of interview data. Additional data from neighborhood maps and photographs were collected to expand understanding.

Participant Eligibility

- Residents in one of the five selected neighborhoods for at least six months
- Family with at least one school-age child (ages 7–18 years) currently living in the home
- Consent for participation from every family member in the home. Assent forms were completed by family members younger than 18 years of age
- Willingness to participate in an interview that lasted 1 ½–2 hours.

Each family received $100 as compensation for their time. Initial coding to develop the code book had two project staff independently code and compare 10% of the transcripts. A goal of greater than 90% interrater reliability was set and achieved before further transcripts were coded. The coding framework was used for the remaining transcripts. After every 10 transcripts, coders' transcripts were compared, coding discrepancies were reconciled, and the codebook was updated to reflect any changes in definitions or additions. Other qualitative data from standardized logs and observation tools were recorded and analyzed appropriately. The sample size for this study was 40 families selected from the five intervention neighborhoods that met the criteria for inclusion.

GIS mapping (qual) GIS mapping was used to provide visualization of both qualitative and quantitative data combining to allow social phenomena to be represented visually within the study neighborhoods. The GIS visual represen-

---

[1] Memos, or field notes, are brief documents written after an interview. They include additional research insights, observations, reflections, and information about any challenges encountered during the research process.

tation of quantitative and qualitative data took advantage of the opportunity to be no less rigorous (Cope and Elwood, 2009). The GIS maps that were drawn used locally collected population level census data and combined it with data from the local health department that depicted the existence of healthy food before and after the interventions to increase access to healthy foods. Maps also displayed the distribution of health risk factors for disease across the geographic landscape. The maps revealed patterns and relationships between population distribution, population size, and access indicators.

Media Campaign (qual) A social marketing media campaign to promote healthy living was composed of three campaigns of three components to increase awareness of and support for the various initiatives combating obesity: (1) healthy eating; (2) breastfeeding; and (3) physical activity. The campaign sought to highlight the policy and environmental changes brought about by the partners who participated in the initiatives to make the *healthy choice, the easy choice* by changing systems, environments, and policy. Radio ads, graphics on bus shelters, billboards, print ads, and a Facebook account supported the campaign.

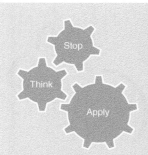

Choosing an Alternative Mixed Methods Design

Search the literature for an evaluation of a program on any area of public health of your choice. Describe the approach to the evaluation. Would you have done the evaluation differently? If so, what? What mixed methods design would you adopt? What methods would you incorporate?

Study Findings and Conclusions

The BRFSS was used in conjunction with the outcomes study survey at the start of the intervention to assess the study population. The BRFSS sample was 1,511 in the larger metropolitan area, while the intervention neighborhoods sample was 515 and similar to the random sample used in the outcomes study. Some differences in the characteristics of the samples were noted. For example, the sample for the outcomes study sample was 71% Black compared with the BRFSS sample of 58%, and the proportion of college graduates was 20% compared to 11% (Table 4.19).

TABLE 4.19. Distribution of the Population in the Larger Metropolitan Area Compared with the Study Site

Demographic or clinical characteristic	BRFSS data ($n = 1,511$) (%)	BRFSS Data study site ($n = 515$) (%)	Baseline study data ($n = 500$) (%)
Age			
18–24	NA	12	13
25–34	21	26	16
35–44	18	24	22
45–54	20	19	19
55–64	14	8	12
65+	18	11	19

TABLE 4.19. (Continued)

Demographic or clinical characteristic	BRFSS data (n = 1,511) (%)	BRFSS Data study site (n = 515) (%)	Baseline study data (n = 500) (%)
Race			
Black	70	58	71
White	27	40	26
Gender			
Female	53	46	54
Male	47	54	46
Education			
High school or less	43	55	49
Some college or technical school	31	34	31
College graduate	26	11	20
Household income			
Less than 10,000 –$19,999	47	59	42
$21,000–34,999	28	24	27
$35,000–54,999	—	—16	18
$55,000 or more	25		14

TABLE 4.20. Self-Reported Prevalence of Noncommunicable Diseases (BRFSS data)

Prevalent disease	Total (n = 1,501)	Study site (n = 515)	Metro area (n = 986)	p-value
Myocardial infarction	5.43	3.93	5.66	0.3192
Angina/CHD	5.19	2.56	5.59	0.0121[a]
Stroke	2.72	2.54	2.75	0.8676
Diabetes	12.18	20.48	10.92	0.0777

a p<0.05.

The importance of healthy eating among residents is reflected in the rates of chronic lifestyle related diseases. Diabetes is the most prevalent disease (12%); however, approximately 5% of residents also report heart disease (BRFSS, 2010). The prevalence of congestive heart disease (CHD) is higher in the study site ($p < 0.05$), while the prevalence of diabetes is higher in the study sites compared with the metro area—although the difference does not

TABLE 4.21. Body Mass Index of Study and Metro residents (BRFSS data)

Body mass index	Total (n = 1,501)	IDN (n = 515)	Non-IDN (n = 986)
Normal	29.88	23.53	30.82
Overweight	38.29	40.62	37.95
Obese	29.33	35.03	28.49

reach significance ($p = 0.07$) (Table 4.20). In addition, the BMI of individuals is similar between the study site and the metro area (Table 4.21).

Respondents in the family study, which was a subset of the larger sample of individuals from the intervention-focused neighborhoods, were predominantly African American, aged 20–40 years, female, and had competed one to three years of college. The mean household income of participants in the family study was $35,000 (Table 4.22), which was higher than the mean household income of $22,250 for the population at the heart of this study.

The GIS maps were used to assess changes in access within the study neighborhoods and showed the ratio of grocery stores to residents was 1:25,000 at baseline. As a result of the intervention, access to health foods increased for 57,479 residents, exceeding the target of 50,000 through several strategies that included six *Healthy in a Hurry* corner stores, a mobile market, and two greenhouses relocated to community gardens, nutrition and health education, and increased access to financial resources for low-income participants through the use of EBT machines at farmer's markets (Figure 4.29).

One of the goals of the intervention was to change individuals' perceptions and to change social norms using a multiple strategy approach including social media. The social media campaign produced 35 million impressions online, in print, through television, radio, transit, and outdoor signage, which almost certainly influenced 80–90% of adults who believed that systems and policy changes were important to support physical activity and healthier nutrition. Responses in the outcomes survey were supported by qualitative data from open-ended questions that included:

- *I believe that policy change is important to improve conditions for physical activity and healthy eating in my neighborhood.*

- *My community should do more to make it easier for people to get healthy foods and for people to walk, bike, and play.*

- *My community should do more to make to easier for children to get healthy foods in schools.*

TABLE 4.22. Characteristics of the Family Study Participants

Characteristic	Percent (n = 38) (%)
African American	83
Age range 20–40 years	84
Female	81
1–3 years of college	88
Household income < $35,000	90

FIGURE 4.29. *Before and after GIS-spatial maps showing change in access to healthy foods.*

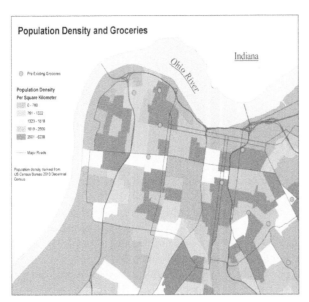
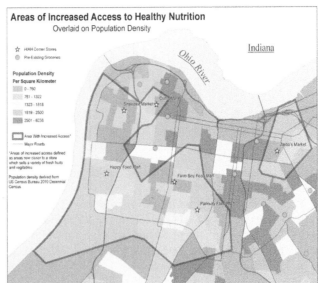

The consumption of adequate amounts of fruits and vegetables has been promoted as important for addressing the high rates of obesity, and BRFSS survey asked respondents whether they ate five or more servings of fruits or vegetables per day. In this study at the baseline, only 18% reported their consumption to be five or more per day. Females were more likely to have consumed more daily servings (22% vs.14%) and getting five or more servings became more common with greater education and higher income. While 14.3% of those with an income of $75,000 or greater reported consuming five or more servings of fruits or vegetables per day, only 6.3% of those with an income of less than $15,000 were doing so, showing a clear dispiriting in healthy eating. While the intergroup differences may be noteworthy, the overriding concern is that less than one in five adults consumed the minimum recommended servings of fruits or vegetables each day.

In the outcomes study, overall, 67% of respondents reported eating at least two servings of vegetables in the day preceding the interview, and 56% reported consuming a half cup or less fruit servings the previous day. The BRFSS asked about the consumption of five or more, but given that experience, in the development of the outcomes study, the evaluators were more interested in knowing consumption at a lower level for the study population. The consumption therefore of two servings of vegetables was at least encouraging although the servings of fruit were lower than expected. When asked about the consumption patterns, 19% of study participants identified limited access to stores selling produce and not liking produce as reasons for not consuming more. However, the family study showed that for some families cost was also a barrier to obtaining healthy food. For example, consider the following excerpt from a participant about buying fruit at a corner store.

I probably wouldn't buy it [fruit from corner store] when I could get a whole bushel of bananas for the same cost [the corner store] might charge me for one. I think it's ridiculous. You go to a corner store for something, the cost of one apple [female].

On the other hand, 52% reported eating foods high in fat (e.g., chips, fried foods, desserts, snacks) three or more time in the previous week. Almost half said they had decreased their calorie intake, and of those who had not decreased their calorie intake 35% said they were actively making plans to do so in next 30 days. Families also commented on the value of the menu labeling that was another intervention within the overall project.

I think that's good. . .to know what we eat, sometimes I may not even eat the whole thing, cause I'm like, do I want to eat all this fat? [male]

When participants were asked if they had seen or heard any advertisements that encouraged the consumption of healthy food and beverages, findings differed somewhat across zip codes. A total of 77% of respondents in one neighborhood of 95% African Americans had seen or heard the advertisements, whereas only 55.6% of those from a neighborhood that was only 55.6% African American. Three quarters of respondents reported seeing the messages on television and 22% said they had seen them reading the newspapers. Most had not heard or seen anything on billboards or listening to the radio. One participant remembered the following message:

> *You should eat at least five servings of fruit and vegetables, drink plenty of water and include fiber and grains in your diet.-*

Most had seen messages about choosing healthier foods like fruits and vegetables or just eating healthier (Table 4.23).

A total of 36% said that the messages had a positive impact on them. Recalling the messages, respondents said, *It will affect my grandchildren, flavored drinks are not good for you,* and *[I am] growing some of my own vegetables.*

In the outcomes study, individuals in the intervention neighborhoods were asked if they thought their streets and sidewalks were safe for walking—even at night—and 54% disagreed. Some residents felt less safe than others depending on where they lived, although up to 65% felt unsafe across the study site. It is unclear if the question was being interpreted the same way by all participants since perception of safety is an important concept in the individual's physical activity and may serve as a deterrent to outdoor activities like walking, jogging, and biking. The study found that nearly 60% of respondents agreed or strongly agreed that they felt unsafe walking in the streets and on sidewalk in their neighborhood, even at night. In the family study families favored walking, and often the park was their destination. However, abandoned and neglected buildings, broken glass, garbage, unleashed dogs, uneven sidewalks, overgrown bushes and grass and broken or nonexistent lighting were all noted as deterrents to neighborhood physical activity (Figure 4.30).

TABLE 4.23. **Respondents Describing What They Saw, Heard, or Read in Advertising**

Media message	Reported (%)
Eat healthier	25
Eat fruit and vegetables/drink juice	12
Avoid sugar/fat/high calories	12
Healthier fast food restaurants	9
Avoid sugar sweetened beverages	8

FIGURE 4.30. *Photographs representing the state of the neighborhood where this study was conducted.*

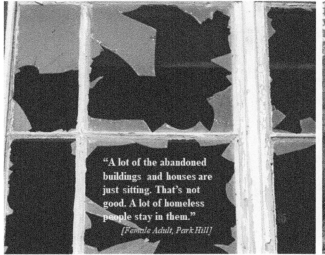
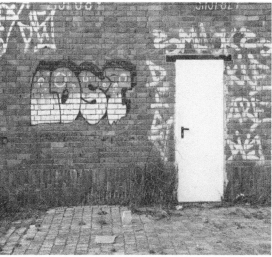

In the words of one respondent:

If you walk outside, you see a neighborhood trashy and stuff like that. It's not going to make you want to get active or help your neighborhood. . .If you walk out and you see flowers planted and its clean, the grass is cut, it's going to make you walk out in the neighborhood, everybody else is doing it too, kind of bandwagon [female]

Two respondents talking about neighborhood crime represented the sentiments of many of those who were interviewed:

I try to stay safe because there's so much going on now. . .times are not like they used to be when we were coming up. . .it's a lot more crime going on at nighttime. . .I don't really do too much after dark [female]

Physical activity and being healthy could be positioned as fun and playful, rather than as work. In the words of two participants: "*It has to be fun. . .if it is a chore, nobody will do it.*" "*Make it cool to be healthy!*"

In the follow-up study about 18 months later, overall the intervention was successful in decreasing the number of calories consumed as well as an increase in consumption of fruits and vegetables (Table 4.24). In assessing the changes in social norms around food consumption, physical activity, and the relevance and importance of policy, the proportion of respondents who strongly agreed with each item increased significantly from baseline to the posttest ($p<0.01$). This was the case for all the variables that the researchers believed would be impacted by the intervention (Table 4.25).

TABLE 4.24. Pretest–Posttest Results of the Outcome Survey

Survey item	Pretest (%)	Posttest (%)	*p*-value
Decreased the amount of calories consumed on most days	31	39	$p<0.1$
Increased the amount of fruits and vegetables eaten most days	32	39	$p<0.1$

TABLE 4.25. Pretest–Posttest Results of the Outcome Survey

Survey item (Likert scale)	Pretest (%) (strongly agree)	Posttest (%) (strongly agree)	*p*-value
Most people I know think it's important to eat several servings of fruit and vegetables each day.	25	38	$p<0.01$
Most people I know use local parks and walking and biking trails for exercise or physical activity.	10	20	$p<0.01$
I think it is easy to find good quality fruits and vegetables in my neighborhood.	10	21	$p<0.01$
I think it's easy to find affordable fruits and vegetables in my neighborhood.	5	15	$p<0.01$
I think the streets and sidewalk in my neighborhood are safe for walking, even at night.	4	10	$p<0.01$
I believe that policy change is important to improve conditions for physical activity and health eating in my neighborhood.	15	16	$p<0.01$
My community should do more to make it easier for people to get healthy foods.	15	22	$p<0.01$
My community should do more to make it easier for people to walk, bike, and play.	9	24	$p<0.01$

It is important to pay attention to the cultural and social factors that influence the behavior. Many in this community felt that efforts to change the norms associated with healthy eating and being active would be more successful if:

- Messages are positioned as doing it for others. Examples include *for the sake of their children and grandchildren; wanting to be around to see their kids grow up*
- Goal setting in small increments is a part of motivating individuals
- Controlling or preventing a chronic condition (diabetes, high blood pressure) is the focus of direct messaging
- Health providers make the recommendation (for healthy eating and physical activity) and give prescriptions to help motivate individuals
- Multimedia provides information that is direct yet culturally sensitive and appropriate

CONCLUSIONS

- Those who lived in the study neighborhoods compared with those who lived in the metropolitan area had on average less education ($p = 0.02$) and earned less ($p < 0.001$), demonstrating the need to direct initiatives intended to narrow the health equity gap to this population in an effort to improve health outcomes.
- A variety of approaches is required to address the myriad socioeconomic, cultural, and situational factors that influence the health disparities created by this gap in health equity. These approaches must be at the individual, institutional, community, and policy levels embracing an ecological approach.
- The focus of this intervention was addressing environmental, systems, and policy changes. In this initiative, however, the policy changes occurred primarily at the institutional level.

STUDY LIMITATIONS

The sample for the pretest–posttest was not exactly the same, although a comparison of the demographic profiles showed that the differences in the sample were not significant ($p > 0.05$) for all but the average income of individuals ($22,250 vs. $25,000). The strength of the study, however, was its use of quantitative and qualitative measures to support the other's findings in a convergent design of this mixed methods approach to evaluating a multipronged intervention. The results provided an opportunity to understand many of the challenges faced by families who are represented in this study from both quantitative and qualitative data.

ACKNOWLEDGMENT

With special thanks to the CPPW Evaluation team that collected and analyzed the data from the many studies that were embedded within this evaluation.

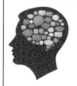

Now that I have reached the end this section, I am able to:					
Course objective	**Strongly agree**	**Somewhat agree**	**Neutral**	**Somewhat disagree**	**Strongly agree**
Describe the approach to conducting an embedded mixed methods research study					
Demonstrate the use of quantitative and qualitative research data in evaluation research					
Discuss a mixed methods approach to evaluation					

REFERENCES

Agency for Healthcare Research and Quality (2013, October). The Patient Education Materials Assessment Tool (PEMAT) and User's Guide. Retrieved from Agency for Healthcare Research and Quality Website: https://www.ahrq.gov/professionals/prevention-chronic-care/improve/self-mgmt/pemat/pemat-p.html

Arnon, S., & Reichel, N. (2009). Closed and open-ended question tools in a telephone survey about "the good teacher.". *Journal of Mixed Methods Research, 3*(2), 172–196.

Atrash, H. K., Johnson, K., Adams, M., Cordero, J. F., & Howse, J. (2006). Preconception care for improving perinatal outcomes: The time to act. *Maternal and Child Health Journal,* 3–11.

Bartholomew, T. T., & Lockard, A. J. (2018). Mixed methods in psychotherapy research: A review of method(ology) integration in psychotherapy science. *Journal of Clinical Psychology, 74,* 1687–1709.

Baxter, P., and Jack, S. (2008). Qualitative case study methodology: Study design and implementation for novice researchers. The Qualtiative Report. https://nsuworks.nova.edu/cgi/viewcontent.cgi?article=1573&context=tqr

Behavioral Risk Factor Surveillance System Survey Data and Documentation. Centers for Disease Control and Prevention (CDC). U.S. Department of Health and Human Services, Centers for Disease Control and Prevention, Atlanta, Georgia: 2010, 2018. https://www.cdc.gov/brfss/data_documentation/index.htm.

Bender, D. E., Harbour, C., Thorp, J., & Morris, P. (2001). Tell me what you mean by "si" : Perceptions of quality of prenatal care among immigrant Latina women. *Qualitative Health Research,* 780–794.

Bergman, A. A., & Connaughton, S. L. (2013). What is Patient-Centered Care Really? Voices of Hispanic Prenatal Patients. *Health Communications,* 789–799.

Bergman, M. M. (2018). The century of migration and the contribution of mixed methods research. *Journal of Mixed Methods Research, 12*(4), 371–373.

Beauchamp, T. L., & Childress, J. F. (2001). Principles of biomedical ethics, Oxford Press.

Bhuyan, M. R., & Zhang, Y. (2020). A mixed methods research strategy to study children's play and urban physical environments in Dhaka. *Journal of Mixed Methods Research, 14*(3), 258–278.

Bowen, G. A. (2009). Document analysis as a qualitative research method. *Qualitative Research Journal, 9*(2), 27–40. https://doi.org/10.3316/QRJ0902027

Byrd, T. L., Mullen, P. D., Selwyn, B. J., & Lorimor, R. (1996). Initation of prenatal care by low-income Hispanic women in Houston. *Public Health Reports,* 536–540.

Camacho, S. (2020). From theory to practice: Operationalizing transformative mixed methods with and for the studied population. *Journal of Mixed Methods Research, 14*(3), 305–335.

Casey, M. M., Eime, R., Payne, W., & Jarvey, J. (2009). Using a socioecological approach to examine participation in sport and physical activity among adolescent girls. *Qualitative Health Research, 19*(7), 881–893.

Centers for Disease Control and Prevention. (2015, November 10). The CDC Clear Communication Index. https://www.cdc.gov/ccindex/

Charmaz, K. (2014). *Constructing grounded theory* (2nd ed.). Sage.

Chedid, R. A., & Phillips, K. P. (2019). Best practices for the design, implementation and evaluation of prenatal health programs. *Maternal and Child Health Journal,* 109–119.

Chilisa, B. (2012). *Indigenous research methodologies.* Sage.

Coley, S. L., Zapata, J. Y., Schwei, R. J., Milalovic, G. E., Matabele, M. N., Jacobs, E. A., & Anderson, C. K. (2018). More Than a "Number": Perspective of Prenatal Care Quality from Mothers of Color and Providers. Women's Health Issues , 158–164.

Cope, M., & Elwood, S. (2009). *Qualitative GIS. mixed methods approach.* Sage.

Creswell, J. W. (2013). *Qualitative inquiry and research design: Choosing among five approaches* (3rd ed.). SAGE Publications.

Creswell, J. W., & Creswell, J. D. (2018). *Research design qualitative, quantitative, and mixed methods approaches.* Sage.

Creswell, J. W., & Plano Clark, V. L. (2011). *Designing and conducting mixed methods research* (2nd ed.). Sage.

Creswell, J. W., & Plano Clark, V. L. (2018). *Designing and conducting mixed methods research* (3rd ed.). Thousand Oaks: SAGE. (Not 2017)

Daniels, P., Noe, G. F., & Mayberry, R. (2006). Barriers to prenatal care among Black women of low socioeconomic status. *American Journal of Health Behavior,* 188–198.

Daw, J. R., & Sommers, B. D. (2018). Association of the affordable care act dependent coverage provision with prenatal care use and birth outcomes. *Journal of the American Medical Association (JAMA),* 579–587.

Demir, S. B., & Pismek, N. (2018). A convergent parallel mixed-methods study of controversial issues in social studies classes: A clash of ideologies. *Education Sciences: Theory & Practice, 18*(1), 119–149.

Denzin, N. (1989). *The research act* (3rd ed.). Prentice Hall.

DeVellis, R. F. (2012, 2018). In J. W. Creswell & V. L. P. Clark (Eds.), *Designing and conducting mixed methods research.* Sage.

Elliott, M. (2002). Conducting research surveys via e-mail and the web. *RAND.*.

Fetters, M. D., Curry, L. A., & Creswell, J. W. (2013). Achieving integration in mixed methods designs—principles and practices. *Health Services Research, 48,* 6.

Fitzgerald, E. M., Cronin, S. N., & Boccella, S. H. (2015). Anguish, yearning, and identity: Toward a better understanding of the pregnant Hispanic woman's prenatal care experience. *Journal of Transcultural Nursing,* 1–7.

Flick, U. (2017). Mantras and myths: The disenchantment of mixed-methods research and revising triangulation as a perspective. *Qualitative Inquiry, 23*(1), 46–57.

Frels, J. G., Frels, R. K., & Onwuegbuzie, A. J. (2011). Geographic information systems: A mixed methods spataial approach in business and management research and beyond. *International Journal of Multiple Research Approaches, 5,* 367–386.

Gennaro, S., Melnyk, B. M., O'Connor, C., Gibeau, A. M., & Nadel, E. (2016). Improving prenatal care for minority women. *The American Journal of Maternal Child Nursing,* 147–153.

Greeff, M., Chepuka, L. M., Chilemba, W., Chimwaza, A. F., Kululanga, L., Kgositau, M., Manyedi, E., Shaibu, S., & Wright, S. C. D. (2014). Using an innovative mixed method methodology to investigate the appropriateness of a quantitative instrument in an African context: Antiretroviral treatment and quality of life. *AIDS Care, 26*(7), 817–820.

Green, J. (2007). *Mixed methods in social inquiry*. Jossey-Bass.

Green, J., & Thorogood, N. (2018). *Qualitative methods for health research* (4th ed.). SAGE.

Hagiwara, N., Mezuk, B., Lafata, J. E., Vrana, S. R., & Fetters, M. D. (2018). Study protocol for investigating physician communication behaviors that link physician implicit racial bias and patient outcomes in Black patients with type 2 diabetes using an exploratory sequential mixed methods design. *BMJ Open, 8*, e022623. https://doi.org/10.1136/bmjopen-2018-022623

Healthy Campus 2020. (2019, April 5). Ecological model. https://www.acha.org/healthycampus/healthycampus/ecological_model.aspx

Hood, S., Irby-Shasanmi, A., de Groot, M., Martin, E., & LaJoie, A. S. (2018). Understanding diabetes-related distress characteristics and psychological support preferences of urban African American adults living with type 2 diabetes: A mixed-methods study. *The Diabetes Educator, 44*(2), 144–157.

Johnson, R. B., & Stefurak, T. (2013). Considering the evidence-and-credibility discussion in evaluation through the lens of dialectical pluralism. *New Directions for Evaluation, 138*, 137–148.

Johnson-Thornton, R. L., Powe, N. R., Roter, D., & Cooper, L. A. (2011). Patient-physican social concordance, medical visit communication and patients' perceptions of health care quality. *Patient Education and Counseling*, 201–208.

Jolivetté, A. J. (2015). In A. J. Jolivetté (Ed.), *Research justice methodologies for social change*. Policy Press.

Kentucky Cabinet for Health and Family Services. (2019, March 25). Presumptive eligibility for pregnant women. https://chfs.ky.gov/agencies/dms/dpo/epb/Pages/presumptive-eligibility.aspx

Keusch, F. (2015). Why do people participate in Web surveys? Applying survey participation theory to internet survey data collection. *Management Review Quarterly, 65*, 183–216.

Kirkham, C., Harris, S., & Grzybowski, S. (2005, April 1). Evidence-based prenatal care: Part I. General prenatal care and counseling issues. *American Academy of Family Physician*. pp. 1307-13-1316. https://www.aafp.org/afp/2005/0401/p1307.pdf

Korinek, K., & Smith, K. R. (2011). Prenatal care among immigrant and racial-ethnic minority women in a new immigrant destination: Exploring the impact of immigrant legal status. *Social Science & Medicine*, 1695–1703.

Kosinski, K. C., Kulinkina, A. V., Abrah, A. F. A., Adjei, M. N., Breen, K. M., Chaudhry, M. H., Nevin, P. E., Warner, S. H., & Tendulkar, S. A. (2016). A mixed-methods approach to understanding water use and water infrastructure in a schistosomiasis-endemic community: Case study of Asamama, Ghana. *BMC Public Health, 16*(322), 1–10.

Kumar, R. (2014). *Research methodology, a step-by-step guide for beginners*. Sage.

Kvale, S. (1996). *InterViews: An introduction to qualitative research interviewing*. Sage Publications.

Kvale, S., & Brinkmann, S. (2015). *InterViews : learning the craft of qualitative research interviewing* (3rd ed.). Sage Publications.

Luecken, L. J., Purdom, C. L., & Howe, R. (2009). Prenatal care initiation in low-income Hispanic women: Risk and protective factors. *American Journal of Health Behavior*, 264–275.

March of Dimes. (2019, March 21). Peristats: Kentucky, Jefferson. https://www.marchofdimes.org/Peristats/ViewSubtopic.aspx?reg=21111&top=5&stop=24&lev=1&slev=6&obj=1

Martin, L. T., McNamara, M. J., Milot, A. S., Halle, T., & Hair, E. C. (2007). The effects of father involvement during pregnancy on receipt of prenatal care and maternal smoking. *Maternal and Child Health Journal*, 595–602.

Mauriën, K., Van de Casteele, E., & Nadjmi, N. (2019). Psychological well-being and medical guidance of parents of children with cleft in Belgium during feeding problems of the child: a mixed method study. *Journal of Pediatric Nursing, 48*, e56–e66.

Maxwell, J. A., & Mittapalli, K. (2010). Realism as a stance for mixed methods research. In A. Tashakkori & C. Teddlie (Eds.), *Sage handbook of mixed methods in social and behavioral research* (2nd ed., pp. 145–167). Sage.

McKenzie, J. F., Neiger, B. L., & Thackeray, R. (2017). *Planning, Implementing and Evaluating Health Promotion Programs: A Primer* (7th ed.). PEARSON.

McLeroy, K. R., Bibeau, D., Steckler, A., & Glanz, K. (1988). An ecological perspective on health promotion programs. *Health Education Quarterly*, 351–377.

Merriam, S. B. (2009). *Qualitative research: A guide to design and implementation*. Jossey-Bass.

Mertens, D. M. (2010). Transformative mixed methods research. *Qualitative Inquiry, 16*, 469–474.

Mertens, D. M. (2018). *Mixed methods design in evaluation (evaluation in practice series)*. Sage.

Modell, S. (2009). In defense of triangulation: A critical realist approach to mixed methods research in management accounting. *Management Accounting Research, 20*, 208–221.

Morgan, D. L. (2007). Paradigms lost and pragmatism regained: Methodological implications of combining qualitative and quantitative methods. *Journal of Mixed Methods Research, 1*(1), 48–76.

Morse, J. (1991). Approaches to qualitative-quantitative methodological triangulation. *Nursing Research, 40*(2), 120–123.

National Research Council. (2006). *Hispanics and the future of America*. National Academies Press.

Neutens, T. (2015). Accessibility, equity and health care: review and research directions for transport geographers. *Journal of Transport Geography*, 14–27.

Nzabonimpa, J. P. (2018). Quantitizing and qualitizing (im-)possibilities in mixed methods research. *Methodological Innovations, 11*(2), 2059799118789021. https://doi.org/10.1177/2059799118789021

Ohri-Vachaspati, P., DeLia, D., DeWeese, R. S., Crespo, N. C., Todd, M., Yedidia, M., & J. (2015). The relative contribution of layers of the Social Ecological Model to childhood obesity. *Public Health Nutrition, 18*(11), 2055–2066.

Onwuegbuzie, A. J., & Collins, K. M. T. (2007). A typology of mixed methods sampling designs in social science research. *Qualitative Report, 12*(2), 281–316. https://nsuworks.nova.edu/tqr/vol12/iss2/9

Onwuegbuzie, A. J., & Combs, J. P. (2010). Data analysis in mixed research: A primer. *International Journal of Education, 3*(1), E13.

Onwuegbuzie, A. J., & Johnson, R. B. (2006). The validity issue in mixed research. *Research in the Schools, 13*(1), 48–63.

Osterman, M.J., and Martin, J.A. (2018). Timing and adequacy of prenatal care in the United States, 2016. U.S. Deparment of Health and Human Services; Centers for Disease Control and Prevention; National Center of Health Statistics; National Vital Statistics System.

Palinkas, L. A., Aarons, G. A., Horwitz, S., Chamberlain, P., Hurlburt, M., & Landsverk, J. (2011). Mixed method designs in implementation research. *Administration and Policy in Mental Health, 38*, 44–53.

Palinkas, L. A., Mendon, S. J., Sapna, J., & Hamilton, A. B. (2019). Innovations in mixed methods evaluations. *Annual Review of Public Health, 40*, 423–442.

Rhodes, S., Mann, L., Siman, F. M., Song, E., Alonzo, J., Downs, M., . . . Hall, M. A. (2015). The Impact of Local Immigrantion Enforcement Policies on the Health of Immigrant Hispanic/Latinos in the United States. *American Journal of Public Health*, 329–337.

Rizzo, L., Brick, J. M., & Park, I. (2004). A minimally intrusive method for sampling persons in random digit dial surveys. *Public Opinion Quarterly*, *68*(2), 267–274.

Robinson, T. (2008). Applying the socio-ecological model to improving fruit and vegetable intake among low income African Americans. *Journal of Community Health*, *33*, 395–406.

Sandelowski, M., Voils, C. I., & Knafl, G. (2009). On quantitizing. *Journal of Mixed Methods Research*, *3*(3), 208–222. https://doi.org/10.1177/1558689809334210

Schadewaldt, V., McInnes, E., Hiller, J. E., & Gardner, A. (2016). Experiences of nurse practitioners and medical practitioners working in collaborative practice models in primary health care in Australia—multiple case study using mixed methods. *BMC Family Practice*, *17*, 99.

Schoonenboom, J., & Johnson, R. B. (2017). How to construct a mixed methods research design. *Kölner Zeitschrift für Soziologie*, *69*(Suppl 2), 107–131.

Shannon-Baker, P. (2016). Making paradigms meaningful in mixed methods research. *Journal of Mixed Methods Research*, *10*(4), 319–334.

Silverman, D. (2001). *Interpreting qualitative data*. Sage.

Tashakkori, A., & Teddlie, C. (1998). *Mixed methodology: combining qualitative and quantitative approaches*. Sage.

Tatar, O., Thompson, E., Naz, A., Perez, S., Shapiro, G. K., Wade, K., Zimet, G., Gilca, V., Janda, M., Kahn, J., Daley, E., & Rosberger, Z. (2018). Factors associated with human papillomavirus (HPV) test acceptability in primary screening for cervical cancer: A mixed methods research synthesis. *Preventive Medicine*, *116*, 40–50.

Taylor, S. J., Bogdan, R., & DeVault, M. (2016). *Introduction to qualitative research methods: a guidebook and resource* (4th ed.). John Wiley & Sons Inc.

Teddlie, C., & Tashakkori, A. (2009). *Foundations of mixed methods research : integrating quantitative and qualitative approaches in the social and behavioral sciences*. SAGE.

Tomasi, J., Warren, C., Kolodzey, L., et al. (2018). Convergent parallel mixed-methods study to understand information exchange in pediatric critical care and inform the development of safety enhancing interventions: a protocol study. *BMJ Open*. https://doi.org/10.1136/bmjopen-2018-023691

Torraco, R. J. (2005). Writing integrative literature reviews: guidelines and examples. *Human Resource Development Review*, *4*(3), 356–367.

Torrance, H. (2012). Triangulation, respondent validation, and democratic participation in mixed methods research. *Journal of Mixed Methods Research*, *6*(2), 111–123.

World Health Organization (WHO). (2018). Global action plan on physical activity 2018–2030: more active people in a healthier world. Accessed August 21, 2020, from https://www.who.int/ncds/prevention/physical-activity/global-action-plan-2018-2030/en/

Yin, R. K. (2006). Mixed methods research: are the methods genuinely integrated or merely parallel. *Research in the Schools*, *13*(1), 41–47.

Yin, R. K. (2009). *Case study research: design and methods* (4th ed.). Sage Publications.

Watkins, D. C., Wharton, T., Mitchell, J. A., Matusko, N., & Khales, H. C. (2015, 2018). In J. W. Creswell & V. L. P. Clark (Eds.), *Designing and conducting mixed methods research* (3rd ed.). Sage.

Patton, M. Q. (2002). *Qualitative research & evaluation methods: Integrating theory and practice* (3rd ed.). Sage Publications.

Partridge, S., Balayla, J., Holcroft, C. A., & Abenhaim, H. A. (2012). Inadequate prenatal care utilization and risks of infant mortality and poor birth outcome: A retrospective analysis of 28, 729, 765 U.S. deliveries over 8 years. *American Journal of Perinatology*, 787–794.

Taylor, C., Alexander, G. R., & Hepworth, J. T. (2005). Clustering of U.S. women receiving no prenatal care: Differences in pregnancy outcomes and implications for targeting interventions. *Maternal and Child Health Journal*, 125–133.

U.S. Department of Health and Human Services. (2019, March 21). Maternal, infant, and child health. https://www.healthypeople.gov/2020/leading-health-indicators/2020-lhi-topics/Maternal-Infant-and-Child-Health

U.S. Department of Health and Human Services, Office of Minority Health. (2017, October 6). Infant mortality and Hispanic Americans. https://minorityhealth.hhs.gov/omh/browse.aspx?lvl=4&lvlid=68

Shaffer, C. F. (2002). Factors influencing the access to prenatal care by Hispanic pregnant women. *Journal of the American Academy of Nurse Practitioners*, 93–96.

Sangi-Haghpeykar, H., Mehta, M., Posner, S., & Poindexter, A. N. (2005). Paternal influences on the timing of prenatal care among Hispanics. *Maternal and Child Health Journal*, 159–163.

Selchau, K., Babuca, M., Bower, K., Castro, Y., Coakley, E., Flores, A., . . . Shattuck, L. (2017). First Trimester Prenatal Care Initiation Among Hispanic Women Along the U.S.-Mexico Border. Maternal and Child Health Journal, 11–18.

Vanderford, M. L., Jenks, E. B., & Sharf, B. F. (1997). Exploring patients' experiences as a primary source of meaning. *Journal of Health Communication*, 13–26.

Perez-Escamilla, R. (2010). Health care access among Latinos: Implications for social and health care reforms. *Journal of Hispanic Higher Education*, 43–60.

Phillippi, J. C. (2010). Women's perceptions of access to prenatal care in the United States: A literature review. *Journal of Midwifery & Women's Health*, 219–225.

Wherry, L. R. (2018). State Medicaid expansions for parents led to increased coverage and prenatal care utilization among pregnant mothers. *Health Services Research*, 3569–3591.

Torres, R. (2005). Latina Perceptions of Prenatal Care. Hispanic Health Care International, 153–159.

Torres, R. (2016). Access barriers to prenatal care in emerging adult Latinas. *Hispanic Health Care International*, 10–16.

Tuomainen, H., Cross-Bardell, L., Bhoday, M., Qureshi, N., & Kai, J. (2013). Opportunities and challenges for enhancing preconception health in primary care: Qualitative study with women from ethnically diverse communities. *BMJ Open*, 1–9.

Yin, R. K. (2003). *Case study research: Design and methods* (3rd ed.). Sage.

World Health Organization (WHO). (2021). Obesity and overweight key facts. https://www.who.int/news-room/fact-sheets/detail/obesity-and-overweight

Rose, M. K., Costabile, K. A., Boland, S. E., Cohen, R. W., & Persky, S. (2019). *BMJ Open Diabetes Research & Care*, *7*, e000708. https://doi.org/10.1136/bmjdrc-2019-000708

Strauss, A., & Corbin, J. (1998). *Basics of qualitative research: techniques and procedures for developing grounded theory*. Sage Publications.

CHAPTER 5

MODULE 5: WRITING AND DISSEMINATING THE RESEARCH FINDINGS

Once the research study is completed, a report is developed and disseminated to intended audiences using appropriate formats and channels. Researchers have historically focused on disseminating findings to academic (i.e., research) audiences with less attention to nonacademic (i.e., nonresearch) audiences, creating research-practice translation gaps. This focus on academic audiences can be attributed to several factors including institutional reporting requirements, the value placed on academic platforms for professional career advancement, resource constraints, and the desire to contribute to the scholarly debate on the topic. This module provides an overview of the structure and contents of a scientific research report, followed by a discussion of specific methods and tools for disseminating research findings to both academic and nonacademic audiences. This module also discusses the peer-review process and ethical concerns related to reporting and disseminating research findings.

By the end of this module, learners will be able to:

- Discuss the structure and components of a scientific research report

- Critically evaluate the quality of a peer-reviewed research report and conference abstract

- Describe methods for disseminating research findings to academic and nonacademic audiences

Module 5: Writing and Disseminating the Research Findings

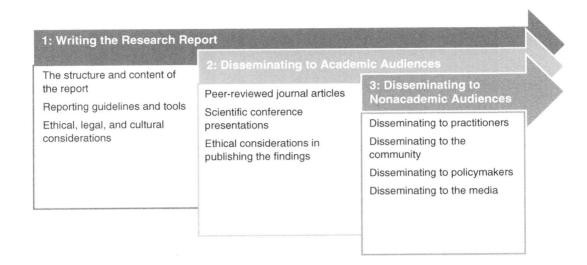

SECTION 1: WRITING THE RESEARCH REPORT

By the end of this section, learners will be able to:

- Describe the components of a research report
- Discuss ethical, legal, and cultural and considerations in writing a research report
- Describe different forms of plagiarism

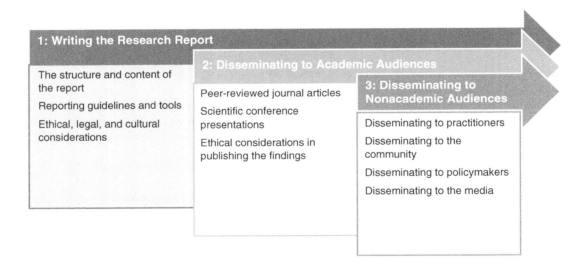

INTRODUCTION

As discussed in the previous modules, a research study is designed to contribute new knowledge toward addressing a specific problem or knowledge gap. Researchers therefore have a professional and ethical obligation of reporting and disseminating their findings to diverse audiences, including those who commissioned or funded the study, those affected by the issue, and those with the capacity to act on the issue. A written research report is often the primary deliverable produced by the end of the research process. This report forms the basis for designing appropriate dissemination products and tools to reach diverse academic (Section 2) and nonacademic audiences (Section 3). The process

FIGURE 5.1. *The process for writing a research report.*

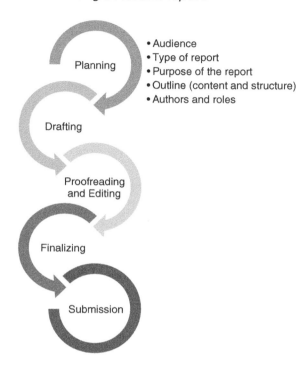

of writing a research report can create mixed emotions, including excitement about reporting the findings and frustration related to deciding the amount of information to include, framing and writing mechanics (i.e., grammar, spelling, syntax), structure and coherence, and the attribution of sources. Producing a quality research report is an iterative process that requires careful planning about its audience, content, and structure, combined with multiple rounds of drafting, proofreading, and editing (Figure 5.1).

THE STRUCTURE AND CONTENT OF THE REPORT

Structure and content are critical elements of a research report that must be strategically selected to maximize its readability, visibility, and potential impact. The content is the meat of the report, while the structure makes up its skeleton. The structure and content of a scientific research report generally depend on the research approach or study design (e.g., quantitative, qualitative, mixed methods), the specific type of report (Table 5.1), and the institution's requirements. However, the report should always be written with the reader or audience in mind; the reader should be able to understand the purpose, methods, results, significance, and implications of the study. It is therefore important to balance institutional reporting requirements with the intended audience's information needs and communication preferences. For instance, a research report developed for the community or general audience is less technical and more creative than a scientific report intended for academic and professional audiences. The first two sections of this module are focused on preparing scientific research reports, while Section 3 presents various formats for reporting to nonacademic or nonresearch audiences.

The standard structure of a scientific research report follows the AIM(RaD)C acronym, with additional components or slight variations across types of scientific reports: <u>A</u>bstract, (<u>I</u>ntroduction, (<u>M</u>ethods, <u>R</u>esults, <u>D</u>iscussion, and <u>C</u>onclusion. The research report can be broadly divided into three main sections: the front matter, body, and end matter.

Front Matter of the Report

The front matter is the preliminary section of the report, which provides a preview of its contents and structure to introduce the readers to the body of the report. The front matter may include the title page, dedications, acknowledgements,

TABLE 5.1. Common Types of Scientific and Technical Research Reports

Terms	Description	Audience
Thesis or dissertation	A scholarly project conducted by a student as a culmination of an academic degree program	Academics/researchers, practitioners (less)
A term paper	An independent or collaborative scholarly research paper submitted by students to meet the course requirements	Academics
Journal article	A short scholarly article that presents new knowledge from original research or the critical synthesis of existing evidence. It undergoes a peer-review process, where it is critically evaluated by other scholars (peers) and is published in a scientific peer-reviewed journal if accepted	Academics/researchers, practitioners, other stakeholders (less)
Technical report	A report that presents the research processes, findings, and practical implications to sponsors or funding agencies	Practitioners, funders, academics/researchers, and other stakeholders (e.g., policymakers or community)
Evaluation report	A report of an evaluation study that is commissioned by an organization to assess, judge, or improve a policy or program's processes and outcomes	Practitioners, funders, academics/researchers, and other stakeholders (e.g., policymakers or community)

table of contents, abstract, or executive summary. It is usually the last to be written despite it being the first section of the report.

The *title page* is the reader's first introduction to the study (Omar, 2014). It often contains the title of the study, the authors' names, credentials, affiliations, date submitted or prepared, and organization to whom the report is submitted. The title of the study should accurately reflect the focus and nature of the study. It must also be attractive to the prospective reader (Sullivan, 2012) because readers first review the title to evaluate a report's relevance. For the title to be selected from a list of references, an online database, or a journal's table of contents, its key words must provide an instant connection to the content of the article and the reader's interest. Ideally, a title should indicate the research topic, the specific focus (e.g., setting, sample), and the study design. The following are examples of titles of research studies:

- A Rapid Mixed Methods Assessment of the Impacts of Gold Mining on Community Health and Quality of Life in Ashanti Region, Ghana
- "This is a Lifelong Kinda Thing": A Phenomenological Study of Healing and Recovery among Refugee Survivors of Torture Resettled in the United States

The *acknowledgments* section recognizes those who have been instrumental and supportive in the research study but do not meet the requirements of authorship. This can include the study participants or key informants (general mention only), stakeholders or advisory group, local gatekeepers or community leadership, funding organizations, support staff, and mentors or advisors. For funded research, the grant title and number can be included in this section to acknowledge the financial support received from the funding agency. Acknowledgements should not be confused with *dedications*, which is commonly found in dissertation and thesis reports. *Dedications* is a statement of tribute to individuals or groups that inspired the work or are affected by the research problem. Researchers often dedicate their work to family members, friends, significant others, or the priority population, as exemplified by the following statement: "To all victims and survivors of torture who inspired this work."

The *table of contents* and the *list of tables and figures* provide a comprehensive overview of the structure and contents of the report, linked with their specific locations in the document. While the table of contents generally features the main themes or headings of the report, some reports (e.g., dissertations or theses) also include a separate list of tables and figures after the table of contents. Both the table of contents and list of tables and figures are developed after the report is completed to reflect its final structure.

The *abstract* provides a summary of the entire report in 150–500 words depending on the organization or publisher's specific guidelines. An abstract can be structured or unstructured. An unstructured abstract is written in paragraph form without any section headings while a structured abstract organizes this information under the following section headings that mirror those of the full report: Introduction/Background, Methods, Results, and Conclusions. Structured abstracts are the preferred format by many publishers of health and public health research. The abstract should align with the full text and should not present new information that is not included in the report (Cook and Bordage, 2016). In fact, an abstract is written after the full report has been completed, using excerpts from the full report. Unlike the abstract, the *executive summary* provides a more detailed synopsis or overview of the entire report, with a focus on the results and recommendations. An executive summary should stand alone and provide sufficient detail to draw the reader's attention to the full report or relevant sections of the report. It is commonly found in technical or evaluation reports.

Body of the Report

The body of the report is the heart of the report as it presents a detailed discussion of its main content. The body of a scholarly research report is generally structured around the standard IMRADC format (Introduction, Methods, Results, Discussion, and Conclusion), but it can also include additional sections such as the literature review, theoretical and conceptual framework, and philosophical underpinnings. The researcher writes the initial sections of the body of the report such as the introduction, literature review, and the methods as part of the research proposal completed earlier in the research process. It is highly recommended to begin writing these initial sections of the body as the study progresses rather than waiting until the completion of the research study. Doing so enables the researcher to allocate sufficient time to writing the remaining sections, proofreading, and refining the report. If sections of the research proposal are used in the final report, the researcher must make necessary updates such as changing the tense from future to past tense to indicate that the activities have been completed.

The *introduction* is the first section or chapter (for dissertations and theses) of the body. It describes the scope and significance of the problem, justifies the need for the study, and communicates the purpose and focus of the study. More specifically, the introduction section provides an overview of the problem within its context (i.e., what, why, when, where, how many/how much?). It clearly points to the gap, controversy, or debate in research, theory, or practice that the study aims to investigate (i.e., the problem). In addition, it declares the purpose and study objectives, which directly lead to the specific research questions and/or hypothesis that the study sets out to investigate.

The *literature review* critically analyzes and synthesizes the current empirical and theoretical literature on the topic and provides a detailed account of the research gaps that inspired the research questions. In some types of reports, the literature review is incorporated into the introduction section, in which case it is a concise account of the comprehensive literature review conducted in the early stages of the research process (Module 1). In traditional dissertation or thesis reports, the literature review is a stand-alone chapter of the report and a more comprehensive account of the literature. The literature review section often concludes with a discussion of the theoretical and conceptual frameworks of the study, both of which naturally set the stage for the methodology section. Alternatively, the theoretical and conceptual frameworks can be discussed in the methodology section.

The *methodology* explains the methods, procedures, and materials that are used to answer the research questions and/or test the hypothesis. Sullivan (2012) describes the methods section as a recipe that clearly outlines the steps and procedures so that they can be reproduced or replicated by others. This section describes the following: study setting, research design, philosophical underpinnings, sampling strategy, sample size, recruitment and selection procedures, the intervention (if any), unit of analysis, variables or measures, data collection methods and tools, equipment and materials, data management and analysis procedures, researcher's role/positionality statement (qualitative), strategies for ensuring reliability and validity (quantitative research) or trustworthiness (qualitative research), as well as the ethical protections of participants and their data as specified by the ethics or institutional review board. The methodology section receives the most scrutiny by research advisors and committees, ethics committees, and peer reviewers. As such, it is very important to get the methodology right both in writing as well as in actual practice when implementing the research procedures. A flawed methodology leads to flawed results and once the study has been completed, the methodology cannot be refined or improved—it is what it is.

The *results/findings* present the answers to the research questions and/or hypothesis. This section essentially presents the findings derived from the data collection, analysis, and interpretation. The results should be an accurate and detailed reflection of the data collected. In both quantitative and qualitative studies, the results section starts with a description of the sample size and characteristics using descriptive statistics (e.g., frequencies, proportions). This description is then followed by the research findings in response to the research questions or hypothesis. Quantitative findings primarily take a numerical or statistical form, while qualitative findings are primarily textual narratives supported by selected verbatim quotes from participants. In both research approaches, the results section is primarily written in narrative format, with graphics or visuals (e.g., charts, graphs, figures, diagrams) taking a secondary or supportive role to supplement the narrative, emphasize important results, or condense detailed information. The extent to which graphics are utilized in the report varies by research approach. Visuals are more frequently used in quantitative research reports to portray statistical information and less in qualitative research to illustrate relationships between concepts or themes.

All visuals should be preceded by a concise narrative that introduces their content and should be properly labeled with descriptive titles, captions, legends, or footnotes so they can be self-explanatory or stand-alone (Duquia et al., 2014; Fah and Aziz, 2006). The results should not be duplicated in both textual and visual format; rather, the narrative should provide only an overview or highlight only the most important content presented in visual form. Visuals are not needed for each research finding. The researcher must decide which results require support of visuals to enhance the reader's understanding or draw their attention to the finding. In addition to deciding which information to present visually, the researcher should select the visuals that best communicate this information. For instance, tables are best suited for presenting precise numerical values and for condensing larger volumes of data, while charts and graphs are best for presenting proportions and trends (Fah and Aziz, 2006; In and Lee, 2017). Bar graphs and pie charts are specifically appropriate for displaying categorical data, while histograms and line graphs are used to display continuous data. Measures of central tendency (e.g., mean, standard deviation) can be reported using visuals (e.g., bar graphs with error bars, box plots) but are best reported in text and tables to provide the precise values (Fah and Aziz, 2006; In and Lee, 2017). Statistical information should be presented in a way that makes them understandable to a wide audience yet with sufficient detail for expert audiences. For instance, the exact p-value and confidence intervals should be reported in addition to stating their statistical significance. P-values less than 0.001 are often written as $p<0.001$ rather than $p = 0.00001$ for example.

The *discussion* section presents an interpretation and explanation of the underlying meaning and significance of the results (i.e., making sense of the results) in light of the evidence from previous research, theories, and practice (i.e., the literature review). The discussion links the study's findings to the research questions and is often structured around the research questions, hypothesis, or the main themes from the study. The literature review conducted earlier in the research process plays an important role in interpreting and contextualizing the findings in the discussion section. While the literature review flows from a broader research topic area to more specific literature that informs the specific research questions, the discussion section relates the study's specific findings with the broader literature on the topic (Figure 5.2).

The discussion section specifically includes the following components:

- *A reiteration of the overall purpose of the study*

- *A summary of the main findings* in response to each research question, indicating whether and how they are answered. These should be presented in order of most to least important. This should not be a duplication of what was written in the results section but should be an interpretive or reflective account of the main findings.

FIGURE 5.2. *The relationship between the literature review and the discussion section.*

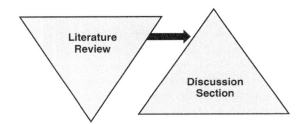

- *An interpretation of the meaning and significance of the results through comparisons with the literature.* The literature is used to (a) discuss any agreements or contradictions between the research findings and the existing evidence, (b) explore possible or alternative explanations of conflicting, unexpected, or inconclusive findings, and (c) highlight the theoretical, empirical, or conceptual contribution of the study. In quantitative research, the researcher's interpretation of the findings is reserved for the discussion section. However, this is not always the case for qualitative research due to its interpretivist underpinnings and the concurrent data collection, analysis, and interpretation of the findings. The results section of a qualitative research report often integrates the researcher's interpretation or co-construction that is grounded in the data. However, the more thorough interpretation of the qualitative findings within the context of the existing literature is placed in the discussion section.

- *An acknowledgment of the limitations and strengths of the study.* The limitations of the study highlight the anticipated or unanticipated methodological or design-related shortcomings that influence the internal and external validity or trustworthiness of the research findings. The limitations also discuss the extent to which the results may have been influenced by shortcomings in sampling, study design, data collection, analysis, and interpretation. Each study has limitations, some of which are delimitations or boundaries set by the researcher to focus and enhance the feasibility of the study while others are unexpected or beyond the researcher's immediate control. Researchers must be transparent in acknowledging the limitations of their study to guide the reader's evaluation of the research findings and their decisions about the relevance, generalizability, applicability, or utility of the findings. Examples of limitations that can affect the validity of the findings include the sample size (for quantitative studies), biases (e.g., social desirability bias, selection bias), poor data quality, resource constraints (e.g., time and finances), and data collection limitations. It is important to conclude the limitations section on a positive note. This can include a statement of the main strengths of the study.

- *Discussion of the implications and recommendations for practice, policy, and research.* Both implications and recommendations are discussed based on the findings and the literature, with consideration of the study's limitations. The implications refer to the impact or consequences of the results on policy, practice, and research—essentially how the results influence or shape policy, practice, and future research on the issue. On the other hand, the recommendations propose specific and concrete practice, policy, or research actions, steps, or measures that should be implemented to address the issue. The recommendations for future research are usually formulated around the new questions raised by the research study, the relevant gaps identified during the review of related literature, and the limitations of the study. These recommendations for future research should be very specific in identifying additional research needed to expand the evidence on the issue.

- The *conclusion* section concisely synthesizes the purpose, main findings, and significance of the study, leaving the reader with a takeaway message. It starts by restating the purpose or aim of the study, followed by a synthesis of the major findings in response to the research questions. This section then emphasizes the significance or unique contribution of the study to the literature, leaving the reader with a clear understanding of the study's addition to the scholarly debate on the topic. The conclusion then reiterates the key recommendations for policy, practice, and future research. The conclusion should not include new information that has not been discussed elsewhere in the report. In some reports, the conclusion is incorporated into the discussion section.

End Matter of the Report

The end matter contains supplemental materials to support the body of the report. It typically includes the references and appendices. The *references* section provides a list of the sources that were cited within the report. A reference list is different from a bibliography, the latter of which is a comprehensive list of all sources consulted in writing the report whether or not they were cited. The references should be cited using the appropriate citation or referencing style based on the style guide adopted by the organization or discipline as discussed subsequently. The references can be formatted manually or electronically using novel digital tools. For instance, a reference management software stores the sources into electronic folders and generates automatic in-text citations linked with end-of text references in different citation styles. There is a wide variety of reference management tools some of which require individual or institutional subscriptions. Some common reference management software includes Zotero (free), Mendeley (free), Papers, EndNote, and RefWorks. The majority of electronic bibliographic databases (Module 1) provide options to save, email, or export retrieved sources to a reference management software for automatic citations (Efron and Ravid, 2019).

Finally, the *appendices* contain supplementary or supportive materials that are referenced but not included in the main body of the report because of their length or volume. This can include copies of the data collection instruments, consent forms, recruitment materials, authorization letters, and memorandums of understanding or data use agreements.

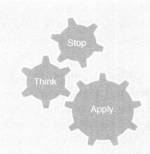

Comparing and Contrasting Types of Reports

Conduct an online search for reports that fall into each of the categories described in Table 5.1. Write a one-page summary highlighting the similarities and differences between the types of reports, focusing on their structure and content. Include in-text citations and a reference list (at least four references) at the end of the paper using any citation format utilized within your field or organization (e.g., American Psychological Association [APA] or American Medical Association [AMA]).

REPORTING GUIDELINES AND TOOLS

Several tools have been developed to help researchers meet the reporting and formatting standards established by institutions, disciplines, or publishers. Such tools include reporting guidelines, style guides or manuals, and the reference management software discussed earlier. Reporting guidelines provide a set of standards or criteria for writing research reports for different research designs. These guidelines are developed by expert panels of researchers, methodologists, and editors based on the evidence and on their collective experiences. Some widely utilized and validated guidelines have been adopted or adapted by various organizations and journals to provide guidance for writing and evaluating scientific reports.

There are several reporting guidelines for quantitative research. For instance, the STROBE tool (Strengthening the Reporting of Observational studies in Epidemiology) is a quantitative reporting tool for observational study designs such as cohort, case–control, and cross-sectional studies. It describes several items that must be included in a research report, including the study design, setting, participants (inclusion and exclusion criteria), the variables, sample size (including power calculations), and statistical methods (Stroup et al., 2017). While still limited, there is a growing body of literature focused on developing reporting guidelines for qualitative and mixed methods studies. COREQ (Standards for Consolidated Criteria for Reporting Qualitative Research) is an example of a qualitative research reporting tool for studies involving interviews and focus groups. COREQ is a 32-item checklist that requires authors to report on the researchers' characteristics, study context, sampling strategy, ethics protections, data collection methods, unit of study, data processing and analysis as well as the strategies used to enhance the trustworthiness of findings (Tong et al., 2007). For mixed methods studies, the GRAMMS (Good Reporting of a Mixed Methods) a commonly applied reporting tool which requires the following information: the rationale for using a mixed methods approach, the weight given to each method, the weight or priority and sequencing of both methods, sampling, data collection, and analysis procedures for each arm of the study, where and how integration occurs, and limitations, among other criteria (O'Cathain et al., 2008). Finally, most systematic reviews and meta-analyses are reported based on the Preferred Reporting Items for Systematic reviews and Meta-Analysis (PRISMA) statement (Moher et al., 2009). This 27-item checklist helps ensure a systematic reporting of the literature review process and findings. The Equator (Enhancing the QUAlity and Transparency Of health Research) network provides a comprehensive searchable database of reporting guidelines for different study designs, some of which are summarized in Table 5.2.

In addition to reporting guidelines, style manuals offer standard discipline-specific guidelines for writing technical or scientific reports. These guidelines provide specific instructions related to the following topics: formatting

TABLE 5.2. Reporting Guidelines for Different Study Designs

Type of study	Reporting guideline	References
Case reports	CARE	Gagnier et al. (2013)
Health economic evaluations	CHEERS	Husereau et al. (2022)
Mixed methods	GRAMMS	O'Cathain et al. (2008)
Observational studies (cohort, case–control studies, cross-sectional studies)	STROBE	von Elm et al. (2014)
Qualitative research	SRQR	O'Brien et al. (2014)
Qualitative research	COREQ	Tong et al. (2007)
Randomized controlled trials	CONSORT	Schulz et al. (2010)
Systematic reviews and meta-analyses	PRISMA	Page et al. (2021)
Rapid reviews	PRISMA-RR	Steven et al. (2018) *PRISMA-RR was under development at the time of writing
Scoping reviews	PRISMA-ScR	Tricco et al. (2018)
Overviews of reviews	PRIOR	Pollock et al. (2019)

EQUATOR Network. (n.d.). Library for health research reporting. Retrieved July 24 from https://www.equator-network.org/library

in-text citations and end-of text references, formatting headings and subheadings, manuscript structure, writing mechanics, displaying results, and labeling tables and figures. Institutional reporting requirements are often adapted from style manuals. Table 5.3 provides a list of common style manuals and the disciplines in which they are used. The APA and American Medical Association (AMA) styles are the most utilized in public health research.

TABLE 5.3. Common Style Guides and Manuals

Style guide/manual	Discipline
American Psychological Association (APA) Source: *Publication Manual of the American Psychological Association* (7th ed.) https://apastyle.apa.org/products/publication-manual-7th-edition	Psychology, history, education, social sciences, and some allied health sciences (including Public Health)
American Medical Association (AMA) Source: *AMA Manual of Style: A Guide for Authors and Editors* (11th ed.) https://www.amamanualofstyle.com	Medicine and related disciplines (including Public Health)
Modern Language Association (MLA) Source: *MLA Handbook* (8th ed.) https://www.mla.org/Publications/Bookstore/Nonseries/MLA-Handbook-Eighth-Edition	English, modern languages, art, literature, and the humanities

(Continued)

TABLE 5.3. (Continued)

Style guide/manual	Discipline
American Sociological Association (ASA) Source: *ASA Style Guide* (6th ed.) https://www.asanet.org/asa-style-guide-sixth-edition	Sociology
Chicago Manual of Style Source: *Chicago Manual of Style* (17th ed.) https://www.chicagomanualofstyle.org/home.html	Humanities, arts, history, business, other disciplines
American Political Science Association (APSA) Source: Style Manual for Political Science (2018 ed.) https://connect.apsanet.org/stylemanual	Political science and related disciplines

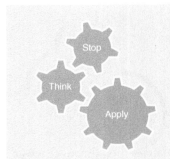

Citing References in Different Citation Styles

Retrieve one peer-reviewed article on a topic of interest to you and cite this article using APA, AMA, and one additional style of choice from Table 5.3.

ETHICAL, LEGAL, AND CULTURAL CONSIDERATIONS IN WRITING A RESEARCH REPORT

In addition to ensuring the integrity of the research process, researchers are also professionally obligated to report their research findings in a legally, ethically, and culturally appropriate manner.

Intellectual Property and Ownership

The proper attribution of work produced by others is an important legal and ethical consideration when writing a research report since the ownership of such materials is often governed by intellectual property laws including copyright, patent, or trademark (WIPO, n.d.). Copyright laws offer exclusive rights for creators, owners, or authors over their original intellectual and creative work such as books, research instruments, images, figures, music, and computer programs (WIPO, n.d.). The holder of the copyright has the rights to use or reproduce, distribute, modify, receive credits, benefit from their work, and authorize the use of their work under specific conditions. Sponsored research, research produced for administrative or managerial purposes, and publications are often subject to special agreements related to intellectual property. In these cases, while the author or creator maintains the moral right to their intellectual property, the legal and economic right is often transferred to the organization or publisher by signing a copyright transfer agreement between the author/creator and the organization (University of Cambridge, n.d.; WIPO, n.d.). With this agreement in place, the publisher or organization becomes the legal holder of the copyright and can use, reproduce, or authorize the use of the work.

A copyright can be identified by the "©" symbol followed by the year the material was produced, the name of the individual or organization owning the rights, and the types of rights (e.g., © 2023 by Muriel Harris and Baraka Muvuka All rights reserved). Using copyrighted material often requires securing permission from the owner to use their work for free or for a fee unless they are in the public domain or designated as fair use. Materials in the public domain are not protected by copyright laws, thus can be used by anyone for free and for any purpose. On the other hand, fair use is a legal limitation to the copyright that enables the use of copyrighted work for selected purposes or circumstances (e.g., education, teaching, research) without permission from the copyright holder (US Copyright Office, n.d.).

Securing permission to use copyrighted materials can be a long, complex, or expensive process. However, settling a copyright infringement due to the unauthorized or unlicensed use of copyrighted materials involves legal processes that are even more time-consuming, complex, expensive, and potentially harmful to one's career. If the use of a copyrighted material is deemed necessary for research or reporting purposes, we recommend securing written permission by contacting the owner and properly acknowledging the source once granted (e.g., reprinted with permission from). Some websites or sources have standard fillable forms for requesting permission to use copyrighted materials. In many cases, the author can send an email or a letter containing the following information: name, role, and affiliation of the researcher requesting the material, the title, author, and location of the desired copyrighted material (e.g., page, link), the purpose and nature of the use, and the number of copies of the material needed (if applicable). Where a license must be purchased to use the copyrighted material, this can be done by paying the required fee online or by mail.

Representation of Research Findings

The research report should be framed and presented in an ethical and culturally sensitive manner. Chilisa (2012) puts the onus on researchers to build ethically responsible research partnerships that respect participants' rights to decide what is written about them as well as how the research results are reported and disseminated. The researcher is responsible for ensuring that individuals and communities are not stigmatized or stereotyped by the report and that the publication of the results benefits the community and society. For instance, Achkar and Macklin (2009) discuss the ethical concerns surrounding the publication of research results using the example of tuberculosis (TB) in the United States. They discuss that research on TB, a reportable health condition in the United States, is conducted to support public health programming (i.e., TB control), yet TB reports and research studies have the potential to reinforce the stigmatization and discrimination of undocumented foreign-born persons who experience a higher burden of TB in the United States.

When the report does not comply with the ethical codes of respect for persons and when findings are incorrectly generalized to larger communities, community members may feel disrespected and stigmatized (Chilisa, 2012). Insensitive reporting can result in psychological and social harm to communities. The balance between telling and not telling is often a dilemma in public health. For instance, the COVID-19 pandemic triggered some soul searching by public health officials worldwide as they struggled with the benefits of providing information to the public for surveillance and educational purposes versus the potential stigmatization of individuals who had acquired COVID-19. The Centers for Disease Control and Prevention (2019) identified the following groups at risk for stigmatization as a result of the discriminatory language used in some COVID-19–related public communications:

- Certain racial and ethnic minority groups including Asian Americans, Pacific Islanders, and African Americans
- People who tested positive for COVID-19, have recovered, or were released from quarantine
- Emergency responders or health-care providers
- Other frontline workers
- People with disabilities, developmental, or behavioral disorders, who have difficulty following recommendations
- People with underlying health conditions that cause a cough
- People living in group settings such as people experiencing homelessness

Oftentimes, the question is not *whether* to report the research findings related to sensitive or stigmatized topics but rather *how* to frame or report such findings so as not to further stigmatize affected communities. Language and words are powerful tools that should be carefully chosen when reporting the research findings. Negative reporting can potentially stigmatize the affected community regardless of the nature of the topic or the findings by reinforcing existing stereotypes or preconceived notions about the community (Centers for Disease Control and Prevention, 2019). Using community-engaged and participatory approaches throughout the research process enables the development of community-centered and culturally appropriate research dissemination strategies. At the minimum, the researcher should proactively seek feedback from community stakeholders, peers, and advisors prior to disseminating the research findings. During the HIV and COVID-19 pandemics, the World Health Organization (WHO) and partners promoted the use of people-first language, which is inclusive and less stigmatizing. Table 5.4 presents examples of less stigmatizing terms related to HIV and COVID-19.

TABLE 5.4. Examples of Stigmatizing and Less Stigmatizing Reporting

Terms to avoid	Preferred terms
COVID-19 suspects; cases; victims	People who may have; are being treated for; died after contracting COVID-19
Drug user/ Intravenous drug user	Person who uses drugs or substances/Person who injects drugs or substances
High risk group	Key population at high risk
HIV-infected, AIDS victim	Person living with HIV, HIV-positive person, person with HIV-related illness or disease
People spreading, infecting, transmitting COVID-19 to others (these terms assign blame)	People acquiring or contracting COVID-19
Prostitution	For adults, use: sex work, transactional sex, commercial sex For children, use: commercial sexual exploitation of children
Wuhan virus, Chinese virus	COVID-19 (Coronavirus Disease-19)

(1) UNAIDS. (2015). *UNAIDS Terminology Guidelines*. Geneva, Switzerland: UNAIDS. Retrieved June 24, 2020 from https://www.unaids.org/sites/default/files/media_asset/2015_terminology_guidelines_en.pdf.(2) IFRC, UNICEF, & WHO. (2020). *Social stigma associated with COVID-19: A guide to preventing and addressing social stigma*. Retrieved June 24, 2020 from https://www.who.int/docs/default-source/coronaviruse/covid19-stigma-guide.pdf?sfvrsn = 226180f4_2.

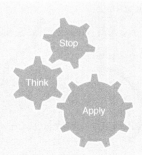

Minimizing Stigma in Reporting Research Findings

Think about a situation in which you felt stigmatized based on a characteristic over which you have no control. What memories come from being ignored, stigmatized, or labeled in a way that made you feel less valued? How did you feel? After about five minutes of individual reflection about this situation, share your experience with a peer, colleague, or classmate. What were the similarities and differences in your experiences? Based on the similarities, write down two best practices to avoid or minimize stigma in reporting research findings.

Plagiarism

Plagiarism is the act of copying another individual's intellectual property or published and unpublished ideas, words, or work and presenting them as ones' own original work by not properly acknowledging or crediting the original source. The Committee on Public Ethics (COPE Council, 2017) suggests that plagiarism is not only limited to the writing or publication phase but also can occur at any phase of the research process. Plagiarism can be broadly classified as intentional or unintentional and it can take several forms (iThenticate, 2013; Kumar et al., 2014):

- *Direct or verbatim plagiarism:* copying sections or excerpts of another source verbatim or word-for-word without enclosing the borrowed excerpt in quotation marks nor proper attribution of the original source. It also includes paraphrasing without crediting the original source and passing someone else's entire work as one's own (also known as global or complete plagiarism).

- *Self-plagiarism or auto-plagiarism:* duplicating, recycling, or reusing one's own published or submitted work without reference to the original work. Examples of self-plagiarism include submitting the same assignment to meet the requirements of a different course without prior permission from the instructor, submitting previously published work to another journal, or submitting the same manuscript to multiple publishers at the same time.

- *Mosaic/patchwork plagiarism:* includes sporadically replacing a few words from the original source with synonyms while retaining the same sentence structure and main idea and not crediting the original source. Another form of mosaic plagiarism involves copying and rearranging texts or ideas taken from multiple sources to create one's own work with or without citing the original sources.

- *Accidental plagiarism:* an unintentional form of plagiarism that often results from neglect or poor attention to detail. This includes instances where an author unintentionally omits a citation or direct quotations, misquotes a source, accidentally fails to paraphrase a direct quote, unintentionally cites the wrong author/source, or neglects to cite the source properly.

- *Inaccurate authorship/misleading attribution*: an individual is not given credit as an author despite their contribution to the work or the contrary, where an individual is credited or cited for work to which they did not contribute.

- *Unethical collaboration:* Failing to disclose the collaborative nature of one's work and taking credit for all the work produced.

- *Secondary source plagiarism:* Taking ideas from a secondary source (e.g., systematic review) but only citing the primary sources cited by the secondary source, without acknowledging the secondary source from which the idea was taken.

There is no acceptable excuse for plagiarism. Any form of plagiarism is an academic or scientific misconduct or dishonesty, with serious academic (e.g., expulsion), professional (e.g., retraction of published work, termination), and legal consequences (e.g., criminal charges). For instance, in academic institutions, plagiarism is an offense worthy of dismissal from a program as indicated in academic honesty policies. Similarly, an individual can face legal challenges surrounding copyright infringement. Many students or professionals do not fully understand the concept of plagiarism nor its consequences, thus may inadvertently commit acts of plagiarism and still suffer the legal and professional repercussions. As such it is best to take proactive measures for preventing plagiarism (Figure 5.3).

Quoting involves enclosing any verbatim passage taken from a source within quotation marks, followed by an appropriate citation of the source. Direct quotes should be used sparingly throughout the document and should be reserved for emphasizing pertinent or unique information. A commonly used method in scientific writing is paraphrasing, which involves rewriting passages taken from another source in one's own words while maintaining the original meaning, followed by an appropriate citation of the source. Note that simply replacing a few words with synonyms is considered plagiarism. One practical way of avoiding plagiarism when paraphrasing, is to read the entire passage within its context and immediately synthesize or rewrite the information in one's own words without looking at the source. Overall, any work or information that is not common or general knowledge should be properly cited or attributed to the author using the appropriate citation style. The general rule is to cite or ask an advisor, mentor, or instructor when in doubt.

While plagiarism is difficult to detect manually, electronic plagiarism detection tools or anti-plagiarism software such as SafeAssign and TurnitIn facilitate the detection of plagiarism by screening and comparing an electronic

FIGURE 5.3. *Strategies for avoiding plagiarism.*

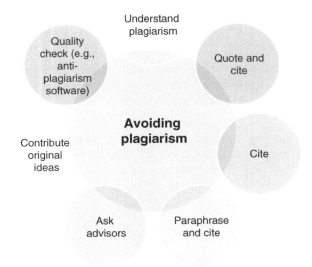

document with other documents (e.g., peer-reviewed articles, scholarly papers) within its comprehensive databases. The similarities in the documents are highlighted for further review by the author or the entity to which the report is submitted. Each phrase or section that is highlighted by the software must be reviewed against the document with which it shares the phrase or section prior to drawing conclusions of plagiarism. Such software can also flag self-plagiarism. It often takes students by surprise when they are told that their paper contains plagiarized sections. For instance, an anti-plagiarism software detected an incident in which a student attempted to use a research topic and methodology from a published paper without referencing the paper. A keyword search quickly found the original paper and identified the plagiarized sections. Academic institutions generally purchase software to assist faculty and students in detecting plagiarism. Students are also encouraged to scan their papers before submitting them for final review. Peer-reviewed journals and other publishers also make use of similar software for screening work submitted to them.

 SUMMARY

Researchers have a professional and ethical obligation of reporting and disseminating their findings to the sponsor organization and the wider community using appropriate platforms. A research report is the primary deliverable of the research process, which can be reproduced in various formats for various audiences. A research report generally comprises an abstract, introduction, methods, results, discussion, and conclusion section, with some variations by study type.

Researchers are professionally obligated to report their research findings in a legally, ethically, and culturally appropriate manner. Researchers must refrain from using stigmatizing terminology and incorrect generalizations in their reports so as not to stigmatize and disrespect individuals and communities.

The proper attribution of work produced by others is an important legal and ethical consideration when writing a research report since the ownership of such materials is often governed by intellectual property laws. Plagiarism is the act of copying another individual's published or unpublished work and presenting it as ones' own original work by not properly acknowledging or crediting the original source. Plagiarism can be broadly classified as intentional or unintentional.

Now that I have reached the end this section, I am able to:

Course objective	Strongly agree	Somewhat agree	Neutral	Somewhat disagree	Strongly agree
Describe the components of a research report					
Discuss ethical, legal, and cultural and considerations in writing a research report					
Describe different forms of plagiarism					

SECTION 2: DISSEMINATING THE REPORT TO ACADEMIC AUDIENCES

By the end of this section, learners will be able to:

- Discuss the methods for selecting a suitable peer-reviewed journal for publication
- Discuss the ethical considerations of authorship
- Critically evaluate the structure and contents of a peer-reviewed article

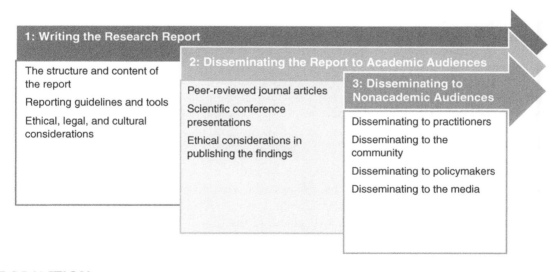

INTRODUCTION

There are standard formats and platforms for disseminating research findings to academic or research audiences, the most common being peer-reviewed journals, scientific conferences, dissertation and thesis reports, and research or scholarly newsletters.

Peer-Reviewed Journal Articles

Publishing the research study in a peer-reviewed journal is a common goal for researchers given the professional incentives associated with peer-reviewed publications, particularly in terms of career advancement and employment opportunities. The peer-review and publication process can be challenging, especially for students and novice researchers who have not experienced these procedures. Table 5.5 outlines the steps from developing a manuscript for publication to receiving the editorial board's final decision on the manuscript.

TABLE 5.5. **Steps in Developing and Submitting a Manuscript to a Peer-Reviewed Journal**

Step 1: Plan the manuscript

- Decide on the authorship and order of authorship.
- Compose a "working" title for the article.
- Select a suitable journal based on the focus, methods, intended audience, type of publication, quality of the journal.

Step 2: Develop the outline

- Review the journal's guidelines.
- Develop headings and subheadings based on the required structure (e.g., AIM(RaD)C), with bullet points outlining major discussion points.
- Prepare visuals or graphics from the data to support the narrative.

Step 3: Draft the manuscript

- Update the literature review if necessary
- Write the first draft following the structure of the outline
- Proofread the draft, taking note of spelling, grammar, and format
- Compile all sections if multiple authors are involved

Step 4: Allow time for all authors to provide internal review, feedback, and revisions

- Circulate the manuscript to all authors for internal review and feedback.
- Make revisions and recirculate manuscript to all authors as needed.
- Format the article and references based on the journal's guidelines.

Step 5: Submit the manuscript

- Review the journal's submission guidelines.
- Submit the manuscript and supplementary documents (e.g., title page, tables, figures).

Step 6: Act on editor and reviewers' decision

- Acceptance: review the proofs and provide feedback if needed.
- Revise and resubmit: read reviewers' comments, revise, and resubmit the revised manuscript along with a response to reviewers on how feedback was addressed.
- Rejection: revise (if given feedback) and submit to another journal.

Step 1: Plan the Manuscript

Deciding on Authorship

Discussing authorship, authorship order, and the expected contribution of each author prior to writing the manuscript enables an appropriate division of labor and prevents authorship disputes. The following are common authorship considerations when planning a manuscript: who to include as an author and on what basis, the authorship sequence and roles, and how many authors to include. While there is typically no limit on the number of authors, a number of journals specify the maximum number of authors to include on a single publication (American Journal of Public Health, n.d.). Authorship is associated with professional credits or prestige, but it also comes with responsibility and accountability. The International Committee of Medical Journal Editors (2019) define the following four criteria to qualify for authorship:

- *"Substantial contributions to the conception or design of the work; or the acquisition, analysis, or interpretation of data for the work; AND*

- *Drafting the work or revising it critically for important intellectual content; AND*
- *Final approval of the version to be published; AND*
- *Agreement to be accountable for all aspects of the work in ensuring that questions related to the accuracy or integrity of any part of the work are appropriately investigated and resolved."*

It is important to understand, frankly discuss, and carefully deliberate the authorship criteria and sequence based on each person's relative intellectual contribution to the research study and the manuscript. Many journals require a description of the specific contribution of each author to the study and the manuscript. The following is an example of the authors' contribution section from a published article by Desta et al. (2019, p. 9):

"KT, designed the study method, coordinated data collection, analyzed the data, and wrote the manuscript, JD, assisted the data collection and edition of the data write up. DK, facilitated the data collection for the TB treatment outcome and edited the manuscript. All authors have read and approved the manuscript" (Desta et al., 2019, p. 9).

The lead author is the individual who made the greatest intellectual contribution to the research and manuscript while the corresponding author is responsible for communicating with the journal throughout the submission, peer review, and publication process. The lead author is often but not always the corresponding author. The lead author position is highly coveted given its value in academic and professional circles. While the lead author is usually the first author listed on a manuscript, the significance of the authorship order varies by discipline. Regardless of the order, authorship implies the highest level of responsibility for the research and its conclusions. Individuals who do not meet the authorship criteria but made substantive contributions to the research project are recognized in the acknowledgements section. Examples of nonauthor contributions include funding, general administrative support, supervision of the research staff, and technical editing or proofreading. Below is an example of an acknowledgements section from one of our articles:

"The authors received travel funding from the Roberson Fund for African Studies, University of Louisville Graduate Student Council, and various donors through the University of Louisville School of Public Health and Information Sciences. We also acknowledge our partners at Kwame Nkrumah University of Science and Technology [KNUST] School of Public Health, KNUST Department of Theoretical and Applied Biology, KNUST Rotaract Club, as well as the community leadership and residents for their support during data collection, analysis, and dissemination." (Muvuka & Harris, 2019, p. 6)

There are several forms of unethical authorship practices, the most common being guest authorship, gift authorship, honorary authorship, and ghost authorship (Desai, 2012). Guest, gift, and honorary authorship involve listing as author an individual who does not meet the authorship criteria. More specifically, guest authorship involves listing an individual who did not make a substantive contribution to the research or the manuscript in an effort to boost the odds of publication given their influence in the field or publication record. Gift authorship involves including as author an individual who does not qualify for authorship based on friendship or the expectation of reciprocation (Gasparyan et al., 2013). Honorary authorship is when an individual who does not qualify is listed as an author given their position, seniority, or form of support that does not merit authorship (e.g., funding). Conversely, ghost authorship involves omitting an individual from the authorship list despite their major contribution to the research and eligibility for authorship (Desai, 2012). Another unethical authorship practice is citing one's own published work in subsequent manuscripts out of context of the current research being reported, to increase one's citation metrics (Sengupta and Honovar, 2017). In their guidance to publishers, the Committee on Publication Ethics (2018) has identified several red flags that can potentially indicate authorship issues including the following:

- The language quality in the manuscript does not match the cover letter
- Unspecified role in the acknowledgements section
- Questionable roles of contributors
- Unfeasibly long or short author list
- Similarity check that shows the work is from a thesis or dissertation, but the original author is not included either in the author list or in the acknowledgements
- Authorship changes during the revision stage without prior notification
- The manuscript is drafted or revised by individuals who are not listed as authors

Authors and researchers are ethically obligated to avoid such unethical or fraudulent authorship practices and to maintain professional integrity. They must proactively review and apply the ethical guidance for authors provided by journals or published by credible sources such as the Committee on Publication Ethics or the International Committee of Medical Journal Editors.

Developing the Working Title of the Article

The title of an article is critical for drawing attention to the study. The title is usually the first level of screening in a literature search, which informs a researcher's decision to review the abstract. Researchers typically start with a working title that is revised over the course of the research and writing process. Kumar (2013) describes a good title as one that gives a full yet concise and specific indication of the work reported since the goal is to create the first impression that will lead the reader to the full article. The title of a scientific article may contain punctuations and other characters such as quotation marks, question marks, and a colon. However, characters and punctuations should be used with caution since they may limit the article's discoverability in some databases.

Selecting a Suitable Journal for the Article

The proliferation of reputable journals in public health and related fields has expanded authors' options but challenged the identification of a suitable journal in which to publish. Investing time to identify potential journals early in the process increases the likelihood of success in finding a suitable journal (Sharman, 2015). There are several tools to facilitate journal selection, including the literature review, searchable databases, and online journal selection or matching. The literature review conducted early in the research process (Module 1) is a good starting point because the electronic databases and the reference lists of cited articles can also be searched for a list of relevant journals. Many publishers provide journal selection or matching tools to facilitate the search for a suitable journal. For instance, Wiley's Journal Finder Beta returns a list of potential journals based on the manuscript's title and abstract. Similarly, Elsevier's JournalFinder recommends potential journals based on the manuscript's title, abstract, key words, and field of research. Journal searches on these platforms returns the names of the journals along with information on their Impact Factor (IF), acceptance rate, and peer review timeline. JANE (Journal, Author Name Estimator) is a common online bibliographic journal selection tool that covers journals, authors, and articles indexed in PubMed/MEDLINE. It uses the title, abstract, key word searches, and additional parameters (e.g., open access, language, and publication type) to return a narrow or specific list of potential journals with their article influence (AI) score.

When selecting a suitable journal, the following key parameters should be evaluated in relation to the manuscript: overview of the journal, the journal's aims and scope, types of articles published, publication cost, selected author guidelines (e.g., word limit), and the journal's citation metrics. Additional parameters to be considered include acceptance rates, anticipated time to decision or publication, and the extent to which the journal is indexed in various databases. Authors can create a document containing a short list of relevant journals with their key parameters. For instance, an online search of the title "*The Importance of Trust in Partnerships Between Funders and Community-Based Organizations*" in JANE returned 35 journals, with *Milbank Quarterly, American Journal of Public Health* (AJPH), and *American Journal of Preventive Behaviors* having the highest AI scores. In addition, JANE provided a list of authors who had published articles with similar titles. Upon reviewing the search results, the *Evaluation and Program Planning* journal was the most appropriate considering the field, scope, and intent of the manuscript (Box 5.1).

BOX 5.1 Searching for a Suitable Journal for Publication

Title: The Importance of Trust in Partnerships Between Funders and Community-Based Organizations

Authors: Harris, M. J., Elmore, S., Osezua, V.

Synopsis: This qualitative study investigated the factors that influenced the relationship between a funder and a community-based organization. Trust was the overarching sentiment expressed by all participants. They revealed multiple dimensions of trust, including trust in each other, in the process, and in the outcomes even when they were different from what was expected. Community-based organizations want to trust, to have agency, and to do what they believe to be right without being micromanaged. Community-based organizations and funders should integrate cultural knowledge and reject community partnership approaches that reinforce dependency.

Key words: Community-based organizations, funders, partnerships, trust

The most appropriate journal identified for this article given its intent and placement in the field of public health was *Evaluation and Program Planning*

Citation metrics are widely utilized to indicate the quality and importance of a peer-reviewed journal. IF is an index that measures the number of times an average article published in a journal has been cited during a given period, usually a two- or five-year period. A journal with a high IF contains more frequently cited articles than one with a low IF. The IF should be interpreted with caution. It is a journal-level metric that does not reflect individual variations between articles and is usually influenced by a small number of highly cited articles (Haustein and Larivière, 2015; Seglen, 1997). Alternative quality measures have been developed to address the limitations of the IF. For instance, the AI indicates the relative importance or quality of a journal by measuring the average influence of each article in the journal. A mean AI Score higher than 1:00 indicates that each article in the journal has a higher-than-average influence while a score below 1:00 suggests that each article in the journal has below-average influence (Butler et al., 2017). Google Scholar produces its own metrics (i.e., Google Scholar Metrics) to assess the visibility and influence of recent articles by summarizing recent citations. Google Scholar's April 2022 metrics identified the *New England Journal of Medicine* and the *Lancet* as the top two publications in Health and Medical Sciences. Within the Public Health subcategory, the top two publications in April 2022 were the *International Journal of Environmental Research and Public Health* and the *AJPH* (Google Scholar, n.d.).

Selecting an appropriate journal involves careful deliberation and a trade-off between multiple parameters. For instance, while publishing in a top journal is coveted, acceptance rates are lower for such journals, and it may take longer to receive a decision due to the volume of manuscripts reviewed. Considering these factors, the top journal may not be the best option for a small and time-sensitive research project by a student or novice researcher. Depending on the previously listed parameters, this process could take the researcher a few attempts to find a suitable journal. At the minimum, the aim and scope of the journal should match the focus or subject area of the manuscript. We recommend that authors identify at least three priority journals in order of preference. In the event the manuscript is rejected by the first journal, it can be submitted to the next journal on the list.

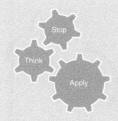

Identifying a Suitable Journal for the Manuscript

Imagine you have completed a research study on your topic of interest, and it is time to come up with an informative yet catchy title for your manuscript. Write down the title of your manuscript and conduct searches in JournalFinder, Journal Finder-Beta, and JANE, using the same information and see what these searches produce. Select one article from each platform's search result and review the abstracts. How similar or different were the titles and abstracts to your topic? Try changing the title, repeat the searches, and see what happens. What did you discover? Which journal would you select for your manuscript and why?

Online subscription and Open Access journals have significantly increased in the last 30 years, out-pacing traditional print versions. While subscription journals charge access fees to individual readers or institutions, Open Access journals and articles are accessible at no cost to the readers due to various funding models. One funding model for Open Access publishing involves charging the authors an Article Processing Fee (APC) once the article is accepted for publication. Another model does not charge authors an APC since the costs are covered by the journal's various funding sources (Springer, 2020). Open Access journals increase access to peer reviewed publications among diverse and global audiences, increase the visibility and citation of the articles, and expand opportunities for researchers to publish their work. There are two distinct categories of Open Access journals: (a) Gold open access makes the article permanently and freely accessible while enabling authors to maintain the copyright to the article with little to no restrictions on how the work can be used; and (b) Green open access or self-archiving enables the author to make a version (usually a preprint version) of their published article freely accessible after an embargo period determined by the publisher, with the publisher retaining the copyrights to the article (Laakso et al., 2011; Springer, 2020).

With the pressure for academics to publish and the popularity of Open Access journals requiring publication fees, there has been a proliferation of predatory journals and publishers who engage in a variety of deceptive, fraudulent, exploitive, or unethical publication practices for profits. Authors should be aware of these predatory journals. Examples of unethical practices by predatory journals include (a) charging high publication fees for guaranteed rapid publication without quality peer review, (b) aggressive solicitation using fake websites, contact information, or editorial staff, (c) requesting to publish manuscripts that have already been published elsewhere; and (d) publishing misleading impact scores. While some predatory journals have managed to infiltrate reputable databases, there are several safeguards against these journals. Beall's List of Predatory Journals and Publishers (https://beallslist.net) compiles a list of potential predatory journals and publishers. It also describes general criteria for detecting potential predatory journals but does not explain the reasons for including each journal or publisher on their list. We therefore recommend using this tool as a preliminary indication or red flag and engaging in an independent evaluation of the journal before making a definitive conclusion about its predatory nature. Additional safeguards against predatory journals include evaluating the journal's website and online presence and being cautious about direct requests for publications unless one has actively published in the journal or subscribed for email alerts from a reputable journal in their field. Shamseer et al. (2017) conducted a cross-sectional study to compare the characteristics of potential predatory biomedical journals listed on Beall's list to those of legitimate biomedical journals. They produced a list of common features of potential or suspected predatory journals, some of which are summarized in Box 5.2. Note that these features do not definitively indicate predatory journals but should raise red flags and stimulate further evaluation by the authors.

BOX 5.2 Features of Potential or Suspected Predatory Journals

- Poor writing mechanics (e.g., spelling and grammatical errors) on the website
- Distorted, blurred, or unauthorized versions of legitimate images
- Using language that targets authors (e.g., promising rapid publication)
- Missing description of the manuscript handling process
- Email submission of manuscripts rather than a website upload
- Absence of a retraction policy
- Missing information on whether and how journal content will be digitally preserved (e.g., no doi or ISSN)
- Very low article processing/publication charges (e.g., <$150 USD) compared to legitimate open access journals
- Missing information on copyright or retaining the copyright of published research while claiming to be open access
- Using nonprofessional and nonjournal affiliated email addresses (e.g., @http://gmail.com or @http://yahoo.com)

Shamseer et al. (2017)

Selecting the Type of Article

Before writing the manuscript, it is important to review the types of articles published by the desired journal (Table 5.6) to determine whether it fits into any of the accepted categories or how to frame the manuscript so that it fits into one of the categories. Each journal has its own submission guidelines including the types of articles, the word limit for each type of article, the required structure or format, as well as the required style manual for the references. The types of articles accepted by a journal are variable and range from brief reports to longer reports of original research or reviews. It is possible to submits an article for review under one category and receive an offer to resubmit it as an alternative category after the editorial or peer review. This may happen if the manuscript is of interest to the journal but does not meet the requirements for the category in which it was submitted. Revising and resubmitting the manuscript into the alternative format can increase the likelihood of acceptance. Conversely, the authors can respectfully decline this offer and submit their manuscript to another journal. For example, Harris et al. (2007) submitted a manuscript in response to a call for papers for a special edition of the journal following Hurricane Katrina. The authors accepted an alternative format request by the editor and the article was later published (Harris et al., 2009) and included in a compilation of articles edited by Virginia Brennan (2009) entitled "Disasters and Public Health: Hurricanes Katrina, Rita, and Wilma." Similarly, Muvuka et al. (2020) initially submitted an article entitled "Health Literacy in African American Communities: Barriers and Strategies" as a narrative review to *Health Literacy Research and Practice*, which was later resubmitted and published as a perspective article given the dearth of literature on the topic at the time of publication.

TABLE 5.6. Types and Characteristics of Journal Articles

Type of article	Characteristics
Book review	Provides a summary and critique of a published scholarly book
Case reports/clinical case study	Reports unique or pertinent phenomena in medical practice such as a previously unknown, rare, or emerging condition, treatment, or intervention
Editorial	Short articles written by invited authors or by the journal's editors to summarize or introduce the content of a specific issue of the journal
Essay	Analytical, historical, or theoretical pieces on a topic of interest to the journal or authors
Evaluation Report	Presents findings from program or policy evaluations commissioned by organizations or funders
Government Report	Reports on processes and outcomes of large government-funded programs
Methods	Describes new or expanded methodological approaches or procedures with the potential to advance research
Original Research	Covers empirical quantitative, qualitative, or mixed methods research studies. It often requires the AIM(RaD)C structure, comprising a structured abstract, introduction, methods, results, discussion, and conclusions. It may include restrictions on the number of tables, figures, and references
Perspective or Commentary	Presents the author's critical and evidence-based views or opinions related to pertinent issues in an analytical essay format
Review article	A critical synthesis and analysis of the literature on a specific topic that is usually formulated around a specific question. It can be a narrative review, review of best practice evidence, systematic review, meta-analysis, meta-synthesis, scoping review, or rapid review (see Module 1)
Short letter/Brief report	Brief reports of empirical data from original research that is often time sensitive or of special interest to the field
Theoretical	Presents a new theory or model or proposes new ways of applying or exploring existing theories
Updates	Short topical updates of the evidence-base

Step 2: Develop the Outline

Once the potential journal has been selected, the researcher ensures that the manuscript adheres to its specifications as it is being developed. It is often difficult to get started with writing a manuscript, however, a detailed outline for the manuscript is a good starting point. This outline enables the team to ensure that the manuscript covers all required sections, adheres to the recommended structure, and follows a logical sequence. In addition, breaking down key sections of the manuscript facilitates the division of tasks for multi-author manuscripts. Original research, evaluation, and review articles generally follow the AIM(RaD)C format (Table 5.7) while other types of articles follow various formats specified by the journals. As such, the outline of a research manuscript should be structured around the general AIM(RaD)C format or its variation as specified by the target journal. To keep the author(s) on track, the outline should contain the following key elements in bulleted form using a numbering scheme of choice for different levels of headings (e.g., I, A, 1, a,):

- The title of the article
- A list of all authors in the agreed upon sequence

- The target journal
- The total word limit
- The AIM(RaD)C headings and subheadings (where needed) with respective word limits and internal deadlines for each section
- Bulleted phrases concisely presenting key information or ideas to develop under each section or subsection
- The references

The outline may also list the visuals to be included in the manuscript. Kliewer (2005) provides detailed guidance on developing an outline for a manuscript in preparation for publication.

Step 3: Draft the Manuscript

Once the outline is complete, the manuscript can be drafted based on the outline and publication guidelines. While researchers will generally want to publish their work as soon as it is completed, there is often a substantial time lapse between the completion of the manuscript and when the original literature review was conducted. Considering our rapidly evolving field, there may be more recent publications that will be important to include in the introduction and discussion sections of the manuscript. Hence, updating the literature is important at this stage. Table 5.7 describes the general components of a research article (see Modules 2 and 3 for study-design specific guidelines and content).

TABLE 5.7. Major Components of a Research Manuscript for Publication

Section	Contents
Title	Provide a concise, informative, and engaging title highlighting the topic, study design, sample or population, and setting (if appropriate).
Authors	List the authors of the report, their credentials, and affiliations, and in some cases, their specific contributions to the project and/or manuscript
Abstract	Provide a brief overview of the entire study in 150–500 words, depending on the journal. The abstract is often followed by a list of relevant key words that are used to index and retrieve the article from databases.
Introduction	Describe the background and context of the issue using evidence from the literature review. This section justifies the need for the study, the research questions, the hypothesis, and the selection of methods to answer these questions. The first paragraph clearly articulates the research problem and provides sufficient contextual or background information on the problem. The next paragraphs discusses the issue in the context of the literature, highlighting debates, conflicts, or gaps in the literature. The last paragraph highlights the need for the study, specifies the purpose of the study, and clearly articulates the research question or hypothesis.
Methods	Describe the methods used to answer the research question and/or test the hypothesis. The methods specifically include the following information: the study setting, study design, philosophical, theoretical, or conceptual frameworks, sampling and recruitment procedures, the time frame, variables and their definitions, ethical considerations (e.g., protection of human subjects, IRB/ethics approval), data collection, analysis, and interpretation procedures, strategies for ensuring the validity or trustworthiness of the findings.

TABLE 5.7. (Continued)

Section	Contents
Results	Present the findings of the study as a result of the data collection and analysis. The first paragraph describes the sample using descriptive statistics in textual and visual forms. The next paragraphs describe the results of the analysis in response to the research questions or hypothesis, using text, statistics, tables, graphs, and figures or images. The data should be summarized and condensed as much as possible, featuring the most important findings of the study.
Discussion	Interpret the findings within the context of the literature. The discussion is an opportunity to tell the story of the research findings. It should be a critical interpretation of the research findings. Paragraph 1 reiterates the purpose of the study and discusses how it was met by responding to the research question or hypothesis. The next paragraphs compare and contrast the main findings of the study with findings from previous studies. They discuss any similarities and differences with existing literature and explain reasons for any differences. The next paragraph discusses the limitations of the study and how they influenced the interpretation of the findings, ending on a positive note that highlights confidence in the study. The last paragraph articulates implications of the findings on practice, policy, and future research (i.e., recommendations for future research).
Conclusion	Summarize the main study findings and the significance or contribution of the study to the literature and/or the field.
References	List the sources that were cited in the manuscript.
Acknowledgments	Acknowledge individuals or organizations that supported the project but do not meet the authorship criteria. This can include the funding agency, administrative staff, study participants (general mention only without names), gatekeepers, and other stakeholders. The authors should also specify any grants received for the research project.

Step 4: Internal Review, Feedback, and Revisions

Once the manuscript draft is written, it is compiled and proofread by the lead author, after which it is circulated to all coauthors for several rounds of review and feedback on its content and writing mechanics. The lead author makes all necessary revisions and formatting of the manuscript against the journal's guidelines. Prior to submission, the lead author should conduct a quality check to ensure that the manuscript is within the required word count, adheres to the journal's required formatting and citation style (e.g., APA, AMA), and that reference lists, figures, and tables are complete and properly labeled. All authors must have the opportunity to review and approve the final version of the manuscript before submission.

Step 5: Submit the Manuscript

Manuscript submission is an exciting milestone filled with anticipation. Most journals provide detailed submission guidelines, along with frequently asked questions, and contact information to ensure a smooth manuscript submission process. Submission guidelines vary but are not significantly different across journals. Many journals utilize online submission portals with tabs to enter author information and upload the manuscript and support documents. Examples of support documents include a cover letter addressed to the editor-in-chief, an acknowledgment file, and conflict of interest forms signed by each author (Table 5.8). The authors should adhere to the specific submission guidelines published by the journal to avoid an early rejection of the manuscript. A common submission guideline requires removing the names of the authors, their institutional affiliations, and funders/sponsors from the manuscript to enable

TABLE 5.8. Sample Required Documents for Manuscript Submission

Submission Guidelines – The goal is to "sell" the paper to the journal!

1. A title page with the title of the manuscript, the authors' names (in the sequence of authorship) along with their affiliations, contact information, and mailing addresses

2. An abstract (usually structured) with the title of the manuscript at the top and the key words at the end of the document

3. A blinded manuscript file that contains the following:
   - Page numbers
   - Numbered lines (not required by some journals)
   - 1.5 or double spacing with a 12-point font size (verify journal guidelines)
   - Table and figures at the end of the manuscript or uploaded as separate files

4. A concise cover letter (about 150 words) addressed to the Editor-in-Chief or editor with the following information:
   - A description of the title and specific type of manuscript (e.g., original research)
   - A statement that the manuscript has not been concurrently submitted elsewhere or is not currently under consideration or review by another journal
   - The novel nature, contribution, and public health importance of the current work
   - A sentence summarizing the findings of the paper and main idea that can be used for promotion purposes
   - The fit of the article with the journal's aims and scope, and readership
   - Confirmation of the approval of the manuscript by all authors
   - Name and signature of the corresponding author

5. Acknowledgements and contributions page as a separate document (some require placing theses sections after the references in the main manuscript document)

6. Conflict of interest and disclosure forms completed and signed by each author. These forms are often provided by the journal

7. Names and contact information of potential peer reviewers (not required by all journals)

---

an objective and blinded peer review process. For journals with a blinded peer review process, any documents identifying the authors, their organizations, and the sponsors, such as the title page and acknowledgements, are submitted as separate documents from the manuscript. Failing to properly blind the manuscript is a common reason for early rejection soon after submission (American Journal of Public Health, n.d.). Once the manuscript is submitted through the appropriate submission portal, the corresponding author or all authors receive a confirmation of submission from the journal. Most submission portals enable the corresponding author to track the status of the manuscript from submission until the final decision.

Step 6: Act on Editors' and Reviewers' Decisions

Acceptance rates and the times from submission to final publication decisions vary across journals. Journals may issue a decision in as little as four weeks of submission; however, it can take a year or more for a manuscript to be published, especially when taking into account several rounds of revisions and resubmissions. Authors should keep this in mind when developing project timelines or when presenting time-sensitive information in their manuscripts. In some cases, it takes time for the editors to identify subject matter experts or appropriate peer reviewers for the manuscript, in which case it can take even longer for the review process to be completed. Over time, journals have developed more efficient peer review mechanisms to shorten the times from submission to final decision. Some journals communicate average peer review and publication timelines on their websites.

Receiving a much-anticipated letter from the editor that is not an acceptance of the submitted manuscript is disappointing, let alone a rejection that requires the author to submit to an alternative journal. Several factors influence the acceptance or rejection of a manuscript. The manuscript is more likely to be published if it meets the following conditions:

- The manuscript aligns with the aims and scope of the journal.
- The manuscript is underpinned by a strong theoretical framework.
- The manuscript presents new knowledge with significant implications for practice, policy, or future research.
- The methodology is rigorous and/or novel.
- The manuscript adheres to the journal's formatting guidelines.

Similarly, there are several reasons for rejecting a manuscript. A well designed and carefully conducted research study will have addressed and avoided most of these potential flaws. The following factors increase the likelihood of a rejection for publication:

- The title does not communicate the focus of the manuscript.
- The study lacks novelty and innovation.
- The literature does not support the research methodology and discussion.
- There are inconsistencies across the manuscript in terms of purpose and content.
- There are major methodological flaws (e.g., poor study design, limited power).
- The manuscript overstates the findings.
- Conclusions are not supported by the results and methods.
- The abstract is poorly written; it contains erroneous content that does not reflect the research or is missing important information.
- The visuals are not adequately supported by the text or legends.
- The manuscript does not align with the journal's aims and scope.
- The manuscript does not adhere to the journal's formatting guidelines.
- The manuscript does not match the quality of similar articles published in the journal.

While not quite an acceptance or rejection, a decision to revise and resubmit the manuscript by a given deadline is in fact good news. This decision does not guarantee an acceptance after revision but enhances the likelihood of an acceptance. For revise and resubmit decisions, the reviewers indicate whether the manuscript requires minor or major revisions before being resubmitted. The reviewers' comments are often helpful in improving the quality of the manuscripts because they enable the authors to answer important questions and correct any major or minor flaws in the manuscript. Sullivan et al. (2019) and Springer (n.d.) provide helpful guidance when the editor's letter outlines a list of recommended revisions. If authors decide to revise and resubmit the manuscript, they must make the necessary revisions into the manuscript and attach a separate letter describing how they addressed each reviewer's comment. Some reviewers provide line-by-line revision suggestions, while others provide overarching comments regarding the manuscript. Table 5.9 depicts a sample response to reviewers.

It is important to issue a professional and polite response to reviewers' comments whether or not the authors agree with them. As much as possible, the authors should make the recommended changes if deemed reasonable after careful deliberation. In some instances, the authors are only able to partially address reviewers' comments, in which case they must provide an explanation or justification for the feedback they are unable to address. It may not be possible to add elements that were not included in the original conceptualization of the research study. For example, it may not be feasible for authors to address a reviewer's request for additional data, analysis, or theoretical framework. There are times that the recommended changes for major revisions are not feasible, forcing authors to make a difficult decision of either revising the manuscript to the extent possible and resubmitting to the same journal or abandoning the process with the current journal and submitting to a different journal. Should the authors decide to revise and resubmit, the revised manuscript and support documents must be resubmitted within the allotted timeframe unless the authors request an extension prior to the deadline.

TABLE 5.9. **Sample Response to the Reviewers' Comments**

Reviewers' comments	Response to reviewers	Reference lines
Please delete "and frequently reformed" in the background section.	We deleted "and frequently reformed" in the background section as suggested.	Line 3
You write: "In Florida, a video on"—and later "In North Carolina,"—delete "In Florida" and "—and later "In North Carolina,"" unless you explain how the state is salient to the point.	We removed the geographical information due to its lack of direct relevance.	Lines 77, 127, 149
You write: ". . . . ." Are these phenomena of culture or of health?	We re-worded the sentence for clarity and added an additional sentence elaborating the relationship between health and culture.	Lines 85–90

THE PEER-REVIEW PROCESS OF A JOURNAL ARTICLE

Peer review is a multi-phase process (Figure 5.4) conducted by a team of reviewers whose combined assessments inform the editor's decision to accept or reject a manuscript. Peer review is not limited to journal articles; it also applies to conference abstracts, books, and other types of research reports. It is important to understand what peer review entails as a researcher, author, and potential reviewer. Researchers, authors, and some public health practitioners are often invited to be peer reviewers for scientific journals, conference abstracts, books, and other reports based on their experience, expertise, and publication history. While it is an honor to receive a peer review request, it also comes with the responsibility of being critical, objective, and ethical in reviewing a submission that could potentially be published.

FIGURE 5.4. *The peer-reviewed publication process.*

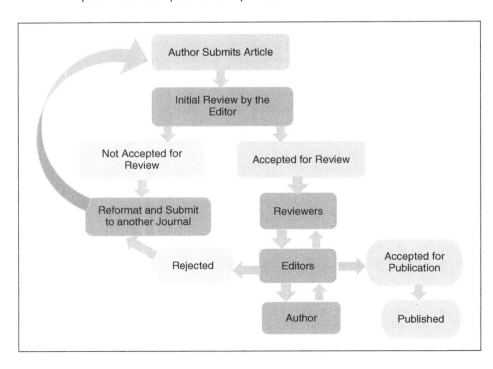

Once submitted, an article undergoes an initial review by the editor to ensure its suitability considering the aims and scope of the journal. The article is either rejected or accepted for review, in which case it is forwarded to peer reviewers who submit their assessments and recommended publication decisions to the editor. The editor evaluates the reviewers' assessments and communicates the final decision to the authors. Reviewers are often requested by the editor to submit their critical review of the manuscript or abstract within two to four weeks of accepting the request to review. Publishers communicate peer review expectations and provide reviewers with general but not prescriptive guidelines for the critical evaluation of the manuscript's scientific merits. In terms of expectations, the Committee on Publication Ethics Guidelines require that reviewers commit to the following (COPE Council, 2017):

- Reading the manuscript and reporting on it independently
- Maintaining confidentiality with respect to the content
- Remaining unbiased and reporting any conflicts of interest to the editor
- Reporting any suspected ethical violations in the manuscript

Some journals provide very specific guidelines, rubrics, or checklists to structure the review. For example, the *AJPH* adopted the Consolidated Standards of Reporting Trials (CONSORT), the Transparent Reporting of Evaluation with Nonrandomized Designs (TREND) and endorsed the Preferred Reporting Items for Systematic Reviews and Meta-Analyses (PRISMA) described in Section 1 of this module (McLeroy et al., 2012). The reviewer must first familiarize themselves with the review guidelines and tools prior to reviewing the manuscript.

Reviewing a manuscript requires several rounds of critical reading. The initial or preliminary round enables the reviewer to form general impressions of the merits of the manuscript and its potential for acceptance or rejection. During this first round, the reviewer takes into consideration the topic and its background, the research question, hypothesis, relevance, structure, and, more importantly, any obvious methodological flaws. The second reading is often more intense, purposeful, and critical. During the second round, the reviewer carefully rereads the article section by section, takes notes of the strengths and limitations of each section, and provides constructive feedback for addressing the limitations. The reviewer particularly spends time on the methodology, results, discussion, and conclusion sections. The reviewer can engage in additional rounds of review to provide additional feedback on less major yet important flaws.

Once the review is completed, the reviewer consolidates the notes and drafts a formal report of their review. While the structure of the peer review report varies across journals, most reviews will include (a) an overall impression of the reviewed manuscript, including its significance, strengths, quality, completeness, and any major flaws; (b) a summary of major weaknesses or limitations identified in each section; and (c) a summary of the minor weaknesses or limitations in each section. Journals also provide an option for reviewers to submit two reports: one for the authors of the manuscript and another confidential report that is submitted only to the editor (COPE Council, 2017). The latter contains any identified conflicts of interest, ethical misconduct, or concerns about the manuscript besides what is communicated directly to the authors. The authors receive one of three outcomes of the review: (a) reject, (b) revise and resubmit, or (c) accept. After an acceptance, authors are given an opportunity to make minor edits suggested by the editorial team and to approve the final version of the manuscript to be published.

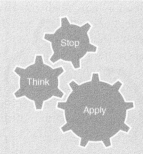

Evaluating a Published Systematic Review Using PRISMA

In groups of four, conduct a search of a *systematic review* article on your topic of interest using PubMed, Google Scholar or other search tools. The title will generally include the term *systematic review*. Evaluate the article using the PRISMA checklist (http://www.prisma-statement.org). Complete the checklist and write a summary statement summarizing your findings. Discuss and compare your findings within your group.

SCIENTIFIC CONFERENCE PRESENTATIONS

In addition to peer-reviewed journals, a scientific or research conference is another common dissemination platform that convenes academics, researchers, practitioners, and other stakeholders in the field. For most conferences, the abstracts or conference papers undergo a shorter peer-review process than that of journal articles. A conference call for abstracts is disseminated several months prior to a conference, requesting researchers and practitioners to submit abstracts or conference papers relevant to the conference theme. The structure of the abstract for a conference presentation is similar to that of a peer-reviewed article. Box 5.3 presents an example of an abstract submitted for a conference.

> **BOX 5.3** Sample Abstract for a Conference Presentation
>
> Abstract
>
> Title: Safe Water and Access to Sanitation in a Rural Community Adjacent to a Gold Mine
>
> Authors: _____
>
> **Introduction:** Having safe and accessible water is important for public health. Mining has negative effects on the quality of water sources in adjacent communities and a lack of development initiatives by multimillion-dollar enterprises leaves communities without basic infrastructure. The purpose of this study was to assess water quality and sanitation practices in a community adjacent to a gold mine.
>
> **Methods:** This cross-sectional study was conducted using the World Health Organization/United Nations Children's Fund "Core Questions on Drinking-Water and Sanitation for Household Surveys." Nonprobability sampling identified 30 residents who were administered the survey. Data were analyzed using SPSS®.
>
> **Results:** The sample was predominantly female, average age 53.9 years; 70% were employed. The majority were traders or farmers. Over half of the respondents drank preprocessed and prepackaged water, and 83% said it was "good." Most (86%) had piped water on their premises for household use, but 55% said it was "bad." Eighty-five percent had access to a flush toilet. Children's stools were disposed of in a toilet (28%) or in the garbage (14%). In cross-tabulations, the study found that water was more likely to be found on the premises when there were children in the household.
>
> **Conclusion:** Overall access to safe drinking water and adequate sanitation practice in this community was poor, undermining the health of the community. Multimillion-dollar companies must be more responsive to the needs of communities from which they benefit.
>
> Word count 232 (the word count does not include the title and the authors)

Authors are typically asked to select their preferred presentation format (e.g., oral, poster, roundtable) during the submission process. However, the final decision regarding the presentation format is largely based on the reviewers' recommendations. *Oral presentations* are formal moderated sessions, with speakers presenting individually or as part of a panel focused on a common theme. Conferences vary in the number and duration of sessions offered. Depending on the number of panelists, speakers may be given 10–20 minutes for their presentations and additional time for question-and-answer. A *roundtable presentation* is a smaller and less formal session where the presenter and small groups of participants sit around a table to discuss the presentation, then participants rotate to other tables featuring different but related presentations. A *poster presentation* allows a researcher to present their study in an engaging visual format that provides sufficient information for the reader to have a full understanding of the research project even without interacting with the presenter. A research poster includes the introduction/background, methods, results, discussion, conclusion, acknowledgements, and references (Figure 5.5). The presenting author is expected to remain by their poster during the designated session and actively interact with their audience.

Once submitted, the abstract or conference paper is blinded and assigned to peer reviewers who evaluate it based on review guidelines or checklists with a basic set of evaluation criteria (Box 5.4). The higher the scores across the reviewers, the more likely the submission is to be selected for presentation. Peer reviewers provide recommendations on the presentation format based on the topic, content, and overall score of the abstract. Oral presentations are generally more competitive than other presentation formats, and authors' preferences for oral presentations may not always be honored due to the limited number of oral sessions. Authors may be assigned alternative formats (e.g., poster or

FIGURE 5.5 *Example of a research poster presented at a scientific conference.*

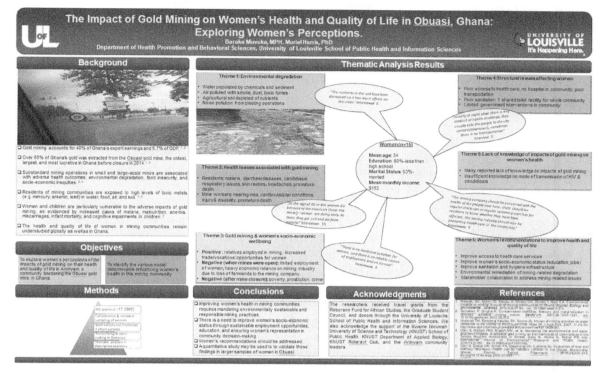

BOX 5.4 Sample Peer-Review Criteria for Conference Abstracts

1. **Topic prominence:** The topic is relevant, important, and significance to public health.
2. **Presentation objectives:** The "learning objectives" are clear, realistic, and measurable.
3. **Purpose:** The purpose or study objective is clear. The hypothesis or research questions are clearly articulated.
4. **Method:** The methods used in the study were clearly described and scientifically sound.
5. **Practice impact:** Evidence of the potential impacts on practice and policy is provided, and it supports and improves the science of public health practice (cites appropriate methods, data, and measurable conclusions).
6. **Academic impact:** The topic is significant to public health academia and imparts scholarship to advance academia's mission to improve education and policies for practitioners, researchers, and educators.
7. **Originality:** Originality/novelty and innovation are demonstrated.
8. **Tone:** A working knowledge of operations (e.g., development, challenges, infrastructure) is indicated toward improving public health education, training, or services.
9. **Structure:** The abstract adhered to submission guidelines.
10. **Overall:** The abstract is well-written, concise, and effectively outlines and communicates scope, context, and rationale.

---

roundtable) per the reviews' recommendations, unless they explicitly indicated only one specific preference in their abstract submission (e.g., oral presentation only).

Conference abstracts are often embargoed to prevent presentations in other forums or publication in a peer-reviewed journal until after the conference for which it was accepted. This ensures that the work presented at the conference is novel. Abstracts may be disqualified for several reasons including ethical violations such as promoting commercial interests, incomplete submission, nonadherence to the guidelines, or late submission. Once accepted, the peer reviewed abstracts are compiled into conference proceedings that can be accessed by conference participants.

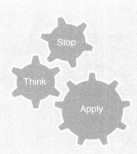

Evaluating and Revising an Abstract

Read the following abstract and provide an overall rating for the abstract using the peer-review criteria in Box 5.4. Rate the abstract on a scale of 1(lowest) to 5 (highest) for each of the 10 criteria. Sum up the final score across all 10 criteria and provide your final assessment:

Reject = 1–15; **Fair** = 16–30; **Good** = 31–44; and **Excellent** = 45–50

The body of the abstract (excluding the title) cannot be more than **250 words**. Revise the abstract for acceptance as an oral presentation at an international public health research conference, assuming that only **Excellent** scores lead to an oral presentation.

Title: Advocating for Effective Mining Policies: A Study of Health Effects of Gold Mining in a Rural Sub-Saharan Community

Background: While gold mining is vital to socioeconomic growth and development, it has been associated with adverse health and social impacts for vulnerable populations working in or living near the mines. Gold ore processing includes manual or machine assisted crushing, washing, and mercury amalgamation. Gold processing uses hazardous chemicals with known adverse environmental effects, including cyanide, sulfuric acid, mercury, lead, and diesel fuel.

Methods: This study assessed the effects of the mining environment on the health of individuals using a photo-elicitation process and short health and sociodemographic surveys in English or the local language. Participants photographed social and environmental factors they perceived affected their health and provided descriptions of their photographs. Descriptive statistics were calculated, and thematic analysis was conducted. Findings were disseminated to community leaders.

Results: Twenty-eight community members (79% male) participated. All had occupational or environmental exposure to the mines. The most common health problems reported were infectious diseases (26%), skin problems (19%), chronic diseases (19%), respiratory diseases (10%), and physical injury (9%). Photo-elicitation identified skin rashes, fumes emitted by mining equipment, polluted streams, cracked buildings, deforestation, and limited access to farmlands.

Conclusion: While acknowledging employment-related opportunities associated with gold mining, participants also delineated mining threats believed to adversely affect their health. The interdependency that exists between the mining company and the community is problematic because it is rooted in a context that prioritizes economic gain over health outcomes. Community leadership is cognizant of ecological destruction but point to the power differential between the mining company and the community as a barrier to successful advocacy for community centered mining policies and practices. Progress toward sustainable development goals require formal and intentional working relationships between multiple stakeholders including the community, mining company, and the government.

Key words: Advocacy, gold mining, photo-elicitation, environmental contaminants, health effects, social factors

ETHICAL CONSIDERATIONS IN PUBLISHING THE FINDINGS

Disseminating evidence to improve public health is a moral and ethical responsibility of public health researchers as it addresses the ethical values of reciprocity and solidarity (Langat et al., 2011). The failure to address ethical considerations in publishing research findings creates community mistrust in research and in the public health system, harms participants and communities, and results in professional consequences for the research team and their institution. Sengupta and Honavar (2017) identified the following six ethical considerations related to the publication of research findings, all of which have been integrated throughout the current and previous modules:

- Approval and consent
- Data accuracy, manipulation, falsification, and fabrication of the research and its conclusions
- Plagiarism and self-plagiarism
- Submission fraud
- Ethics of authorship
- Conflict of Interest

In addition, scholars have also stressed the importance and value of reporting all types of results, whether significant, nonsignificant, or inconclusive (Bhaskar, 2017). Many authors and journals were historically not interested in publishing studies that reported negative, null, or inconclusive results. However, as the scientific community recognizes the importance of publishing such results, authors, journals, and conferences have increasingly embraced even nonsignificant and inconclusive results.

SUMMARY

There are standard formats for disseminating the research findings to academic audiences, the most common being peer-reviewed journals and scientific conferences.

Authorship can be a contentious issue when working in teams. Discussing the authorship order and roles prior to writing a manuscript enables a division of labor and prevents conflicts. The lead author is the individual who made the greatest intellectual contribution to the work and the manuscript while the corresponding author communicates with the journal throughout the publication process.

Selecting an appropriate journal involves careful consideration of the journal's scope, purpose, types of articles accepted, cost, author guidelines, acceptance rates, and IF. Each journal has its own submission guidelines and types of articles. Peer-reviewed journal articles presenting original research generally follow the AIM(RaD)C format comprising the following: Abstract, Introduction, Methods, Results, Discussion and Conclusion.

The peer review of a manuscript is conducted by a team of reviewers who inform the editor's decision to reject, revise and resubmit, or accept the manuscript. The "revise and resubmit" decision requires revisions by the authors and a detailed response describing how they addressed each reviewer's comment.

The peer review process also occurs when an abstract is submitted for review prior to a conference, although it is often of shorter duration. The conference presentation format (e.g., oral, roundtable, or poster) depends on the author's preferences and reviewers' decisions.

Authors must engage in ethical dissemination practices, including avoiding plagiarism, unethical authorship practices, and data manipulation.

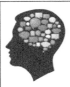

Now that I have reached the end this section, I am able to:

Course objective	Strongly agree	Somewhat agree	Neutral	Somewhat disagree	Strongly agree
Discuss the methods for selecting a suitable peer-reviewed journal for publication					
Discuss the ethical considerations of authorship and publication					
Critically evaluate the structure and contents of a peer-reviewed article					

SECTION 3: DISSEMINATING THE REPORT TO NONACADEMIC AUDIENCES

By the end of the section, the learner will be able to:

- Explain the importance of disseminating findings to nonacademic audiences
- Identify nonacademic audiences for the research study
- Utilize appropriate dissemination channels for the target audience

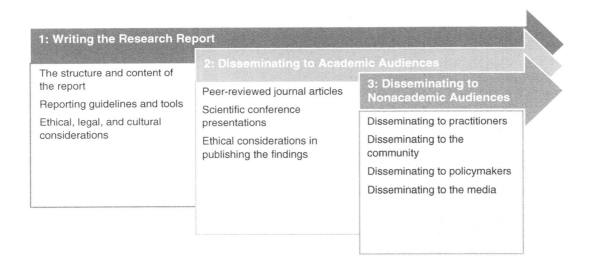

INTRODUCTION

Disseminating the research results to nonacademic/nonresearch audiences is not commonly practiced among researchers yet is crucial for increasing the visibility of the findings and bridging the gaps between theory, research, practice, and policy. Studies in samples of public health researchers in the United States ($N = 266$) and the United Kingdom ($N = 485$) found that while the majority of public health researchers acknowledged the importance of disseminating findings to nonresearch audiences, only one-third of the respondents produced research summaries for nonresearch audiences (Brownson et al., 2013; Tabak et al., 2014; Wilson et al., 2010). The most common dissemination methods used by the researchers in the UK study were academic journals (98%), conference presentations (96%), and reports to funders, while the least common methods were face-to-face meetings (40%), newsletters (39%), media interviews (32%), policy briefs (17%), and emails (18%) for nonresearch audiences (Wilson et al., 2010).

Targeting academic or research audiences alone has limited impact in stimulating and creating sustainable social changes. Contemporary public health issues are complex and sophisticated, requiring multi-level, transdisciplinary, and multisectoral action and policy for sustainable change. The changes in our public health and social landscape, along with the technological advancements have generated growing attention on knowledge translation (i.e., from research to action) and nontraditional dissemination methods for effective knowledge translation. To maximize the impacts of the research findings, researchers should strategically disseminate their findings to audiences with the capacity to act on them. This wide, purposeful, and targeted dissemination is both an ethical obligation and a form of professional accountability. In addition, it fosters trust and working relationships with various stakeholders. This section presents various traditional and novel dissemination tools that can be used to reach nonacademic/nonresearch audiences.

DISSEMINATING THE FINDINGS TO PRACTITIONERS

Some of the academic methods discussed in the previous section can reach public health practitioners. For instance, scientific conferences often convene researchers, academics, and public health professionals. Some practitioners also consult peer-reviewed journals, which they access through their organizational subscriptions. However, these academic dissemination methods are not suitable and accessible to all practitioners. For instance, in a study among practitioners ($N = 904$) in state public health departments in the United States (Harris et al., 2014), only 46% of the staff reported using academic journals (mostly open-access journals) to acquire research evidence. The most common practitioner-reported barriers in accessing these journals included time constraints and lack of access. Those who did not consult academic journals accessed research evidence primarily through seminars or workshops (65%), e-mail alerts (57%), and newsletters (33%) (Harris et al., 2014). Public health professionals or practitioners therefore benefit from more targeted and practical dissemination methods including workshops, trainings, seminars/webinars, and short courses (Brownson et al., 2018).

Most professional certifications require a minimum number of continuing education credits during a specific period, which practitioners can earn by attending workshops, trainings, short courses, or conferences. Researchers should actively seek opportunities and accept invitations to contribute to such practical platforms that benefit professionals and enhance knowledge translation. Some examples from the authors' experiences include, developing a health literacy training module for the public health workforce in a state, presenting dissertation findings on maternal mortality review committees in an obstetrics and gynecology grand rounds and at a conference organized by a professional organization for public health practitioners, and developing a short course on community engagement in public health practice. Such opportunities can be identified by reaching out to professional associations, local health departments, local institutions/organizations, or offices of public health practice or community-engagement that operate within many universities and research institutions.

DISSEMINATING THE FINDINGS TO COMMUNITIES OR THE GENERAL PUBLIC

Researchers have been criticized for engaging in what is commonly described as "helicopter research" or "fly-in, fly-out" research, where they fly into the community to collect data and fly out once data collection is complete, without feeding back the results to the community nor implementing any concrete actions that directly benefit the community. This practice is unethical and considered a violation of the principles of respect for persons, beneficence, and justice because it takes advantage of the participants yet deprives them of the potential benefits of the study, with mostly the researcher and organization ripping the benefits. In addition, helicopter research creates mistrust of researchers among community members, thus hampering future research efforts. While sharing the research findings with community members is a fundamental feature of community-based participatory research (CBPR), it should not be limited to CBPR. Rather, it should be viewed as an ethical and professional obligation to the community in any type of research. The research findings should be disseminated to community members who are affected by the issue, who can benefit from the findings, who need to act on the issue, and who collaborated with the researchers. For community-engaged research or research studies with an advisory council, the community stakeholders should spearhead the planning and coordination of the community dissemination of the research findings given their familiarity with the local context and communication preferences. The community-level dissemination of the research findings has several benefits including the following:

- Fosters interaction and dialogue between community members and researchers, providing the community an opportunity to ask questions and to provide immediate feedback on the findings (McDavitt et al., 2016)
- Builds and maintains trust between the community and the researchers
- Creates opportunities for future collaborative partnerships
- Mobilizes/stimulates community action or knowledge translation
- Enables the development of locally relevant and culturally appropriate interventions (McDavitt et al., 2016)

While communities can be geographically linked, communities can transcend geographical or physical boundaries because they involve a group of individuals who share something in common such as characteristics, location, beliefs, values, interests, behaviors, or experiences. Communities may or may not have a physical presence (a building), indicating the importance of utilizing a combination of in-person, in-print, and online/electronic dissemination channels (Box 5.5).

In Person

A traditional and common method for disseminating research findings in geographic communities and in communities is in person, with a physical presence. In-person community dissemination methods include community meetings, forums, interactive presentations, workshops, seminars, and trainings. For effective dissemination, the researchers should access the community through the local gatekeepers who were identified earlier in the research process. In addition to assisting with entry into the community during recruitment and data collection, these gatekeepers can also assist with contacting and convening the community members for dissemination purposes.

BOX 5.5 Community Dissemination Tools

In person
- Community outreach/campaigns
- Community meetings/townhalls
- Seminars, workshops, trainings
- Community forums/dialogue
- Community presentations

In print
- Posters and flyers
- Brochures and pamphlets
- Factsheets
- Community research briefs
- Community policy briefs
- Community reports
- Newsletters
- Other print media (e.g., newspapers, magazines)

Digital/Online
- Websites
- Podcasts
- Blogs
- Social Media
- Digital/electronic media (e.g., TV, radio, press releases)
- Emails and listservs

The researcher who chooses the in-person dissemination format should be prepared to conduct multiple visits to the community and several meetings with different subgroups, often starting with the gatekeepers or the community leadership itself. For instance, we conducted collaborative and independent studies on the impacts of gold mining activities on community health and on women's health in a small mining community in Ghana. After data collection and analysis, the research team presented the findings to the community council/leadership and engaged in a productive dialogue discussing concrete actions to address the issue. In addition, we submitted a copy of the report to the community leadership for broader dissemination. This has created a long-term relationship between the community and the researchers. For example, the principal investigator (Dr. Muriel Harris) and a team of public health students conducted a follow-up visit to this community, where they implemented an intervention to improve water quality as part of a long-term project.

In Print

Similar to in-person dissemination, print materials such as community research briefs and other health communication materials (e.g., flyers, brochures, posters) have been traditionally employed to disseminate the research findings to communities. Print materials have a wider reach than in-person dissemination methods because their distribution does not necessitate the presence of the researcher or research team.

Community research and policy briefs are particularly important community dissemination and advocacy tools since they present the main research findings in an actionable and nontechnical language. Some peer-reviewed journals and institutions, particularly those geared toward CBPR, require authors to submit community research briefs or community policy briefs in addition to their manuscripts. A *community brief or community research brief* is a short (one to two pages) summary of the research report, written in nontechnical language for community members and other nonresearch stakeholders. This brief is organized in bulleted form with simple headings and subheadings. It takes into account health literacy considerations to render it accessible to a lay audience. The NYU Center for the Study of Asian American Health (n.d.) publishes community briefs containing the following information:

- Title
- Authors and affiliations
- What is the problem?
- What is the purpose of the study?
- What is the intervention?
- What are the findings?
- Who should care the most?
- How does this study advance scientific research?
- Sources

A *community policy brief* is similar to a community research brief, but with emphasis on policy recommendations to address the issues identified in the study. The *Progress in Community Health Partnerships: Research, Education, and Action* (n.d.), a peer-reviewed journal dedicated to CBPR, requires authors to submit community policy briefs as part of manuscript submissions. These community policy briefs contain the following information:

- Title
- Authors and affiliations
- What is the problem?
- What are the findings?
- Who should care most?
- Recommendations for action

Print materials should be developed with inputs from members of the community or at the minimum, should be pretested in a sample of community members to assess their local and cultural relevance and comprehensibility prior to being widely disseminated.

Online

Advances in technology have expanded opportunities to disseminate interactive messages to larger and more diverse audiences even more rapidly than traditional dissemination methods. Among the online or electronic dissemination channels summarized in Box 5.5, social media is increasingly being utilized by researchers to establish connections with their stakeholders.

Social Media

Social media comprises a variety of interactive platforms including social networking sites (e.g., Facebook, Twitter, Instagram, Snapshot), microblogging (e.g., Twitter), media sharing (e.g., YouTube, TikTok), bookmarking (e.g., Pinterest), and social news sites that researchers can leverage to disseminate their findings (Bensley and Brookins-Fisher, 2019). While users vary by platforms, social media can reach the general public, practitioners, academics/researchers, and policymakers, all at the same time. Social media platforms offer unique benefits that cannot be achieved with traditional dissemination tools such as the rapid and interactive dissemination of research findings to large and diverse audiences, an opportunity to monitor responses or reactions to the research findings, and direct interactions with the readers. By reaching diverse audiences such as the general public, practitioners, policymakers, and academics/researchers, social media can create widespread awareness, stimulate advocacy, mobilize collective action, and facilitate knowledge translation.

Researchers, peer-reviewed journals, and other publishers are increasingly recognizing the value and potential impact of social media on knowledge dissemination and translation, as evidenced by their active social media presence, posts, hashtags, and audio-visual abstracts drawing attention to pertinent research findings or publications (Tunnecliff et al., 2015; Van Eperen and Marincola, 2011). Social media use by publishers and researchers has been associated with increased downloads and citations of peer-reviewed articles (Allen et al., 2013; Eysenbach, 2011). Despite these benefits, there are several pitfalls or challenges with using social media, including the proliferation of false information or misinterpretation of research findings. Reports have demonstrated that false information spreads more rapidly than credible information (Dijkstra et al., 2018), partly because they are more appealing, accessible, sensational, and novel, unlike traditional research articles that are not easily accessible, engaging, or comprehensible to the general public. Researchers must learn to strategically and effectively utilize social media platforms to disseminate their research findings to those affected by the issues and those with the capacity to act on the findings. Researchers should apply principles of health communications pertaining to segmenting the audience, understanding their social media behaviors and preferences, and developing targeted and accessible messages.

Health Literacy Considerations

Health literacy is an important consideration when disseminating health and public health information to the community or general public. Health literacy refers to the "degree to which an individual has the capacity to obtain, communicate, process, and understand basic health information and services to make appropriate health decisions" (Institute of Medicine Committee on Health Literacy, 2004, p. 2). Health literacy encompasses health numeracy, visual literacy, and eHealth literacy, among others, all of which should be taken into account when disseminating the research findings. Health numeracy is a component of health literacy that refers to an individual's capacity to access, process, interpret, and apply numerical, quantitative, and graphical health information to make effective health decisions (Golbeck et al., 2005). Visual literacy refers to an individual's ability to understand, interpret, and apply visual information such as images, graphs, and diagrams to make decisions about their health. Finally, eHealth literacy involves the capacity to use various electronic or digital technologies to search, access, understand, evaluate, and apply health information to make effective health decisions (Bautista, 2015).

While written communication alone cannot sufficiently address health literacy barriers, applying plain language or clear communication guidelines (Box 5.6) is one way of reaching individuals with lower health literacy. This includes ensuring that materials are produced at an appropriate reading level and that the words, images, and numbers used are understandable, engaging, and culturally appropriate. With respect to reading levels, the general recommendation in the United States is to write public information at or below the sixth grade reading level. However, lower reading levels should be considered in settings and populations with lower literacy and education levels since

> **BOX 5.6** **Basic Tips for Communicating with Individuals with Low Health Literacy**
>
> - Use simple, familiar, and culturally appropriate graphics and images.
> - Use short sentences and paragraphs.
> - Use common or familiar words, but be careful with slang.
> - Use concrete rather than abstract language.
> - Organize information in logical order, placing the most important information at the beginning.
> - Avoid jargon or explain technical terms. Consult the US CDC's "Everyday Words for Public Health Communication" website.
> - Use a combination of simple numbers, visuals (e.g., icon arrays), words, and illustrations/examples to represent numbers and their meanings (Pleasant et al., 2016).
> - Be precise with the numbers or do the math for the audience rather than providing complex measures that require further calculations.
> - Use familiar terms and use the same terms consistently.
> - Write in active voice..
> - Present actionable ("how to" or "what to do") information outlining practical steps.
> - Incorporate examples, case studies, illustrations, or real-life stories from community champions and opinion leaders.
> - Break down large chunks of texts using bullets, headings, and numberings.
> - Use a conversational tone (e.g., you).

these are predictors of low health literacy. In addition to tailored written communications, researchers can better reach individuals with lower health literacy through more interactive in-person and online/digital platforms discussed earlier.

Figure 5.6 illustrates an alternative strategy for presenting numerical information to individuals with lower health numeracy. The graphics were created using findings from a research study by Mugo et al. (2014) on the effects of HIV Pre-Exposure Prophylaxis (PrEP) on pregnancy incidence and outcomes.

FIGURE 5.6. *Example of an icon array summarizing findings from a study on HIV preexposure prophylaxis and pregnancy outcomes by Mugo et al. (2014). Images created by Iconarray.com. Risk Science Center and Center for Bioethics and Social Sciences in Medicine, University of Michigan.*

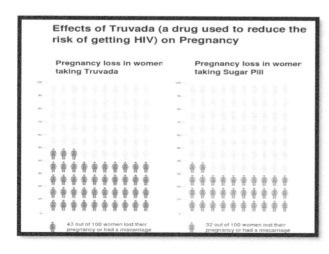
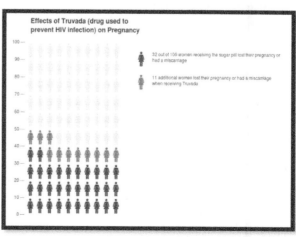

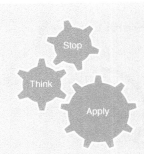

Disseminating Findings to your Priority Population

Think of a public health topic you are interested in researching and discuss how you would reach the community that is affected by the issue by responding to the following prompts:

1. What is the issue or research problem?
2. Who is primarily affected by the research problem you have selected?
3. Which specific dissemination methods would be best to reach your community? Why?

DISSEMINATING THE FINDINGS TO POLICYMAKERS

Policymakers and their constituents are a critical target audience for policy-relevant research findings given their capacity to influence and act on policies. Frieden's (2010) health impact pyramid and the socioecological model both demonstrate that policies have the greatest potential population-level impact because they rely less on individual efforts or voluntary behavior change, are more sustainable, and influence other levels of the socioecological model (e.g., individual, interpersonal, organizational, community levels). Researchers should therefore clearly articulate the policy implications of their research studies, alongside the practice and future research implications. The policy implications can be communicated to policymakers directly (e.g., in-person meetings, phone, or email) or indirectly (e.g., policy briefs, the media, social media).

Meeting with Policymakers

Making direct contact with policymakers and their staff members through in-person meetings, phone calls, or emails are effective methods for increasing the visibility of the issue among policymakers and influencing policy decisions. While often challenged by the limited availability of policymakers, in-person meetings provide an interactive platform for dialogue with policymakers and help in establishing trusting relationships with policymakers and staff. Note that staff members play a central role in gathering information for policymakers and are often influential in shaping their policy priorities and decision-making.

Developing Policy Briefs

A policy brief is one of several tools that can be used in disseminating the research findings to policymakers and their constituents, in addition to in-person meetings, emails, or phone calls. It is a concise narrative that outlines the evidence on a priority issue and provides evidence-based policy recommendations to address it, with the end goal of informing policy change or action. Targeted toward individuals with the capacity to influence policy change—including policymakers and constituents at local, state/regional, and national levels—the brief is mostly used for advocacy purposes rather than lobbying. Advocacy involves raising awareness among policymakers and the general public on a social or public health issue to stimulate or mobilize action without endorsing support or opposition for a specific piece of legislation. On the other hand, lobbying attempts to influence a policymaker's position (i.e., support or opposition) on a specific piece of legislation. While legal in many settings, lobbying is restricted to certain types of organizations and may conflict with many academic or research organizations' policies.

There are different types and formats of policy briefs, varying in emphasis. An *issue brief* provides detailed background information on the nature, magnitude, and contributing factors of the problem to raise awareness on the importance of the issue and the need for policy changes. A *policy analysis brief* presents a detailed analysis of one or more policies based on some specified criteria (e.g., impact, feasibility, cost) to inform policy recommendations (University

> **BOX 5.7** Tips for In-Person Meetings with Policymakers
>
> **Before the meeting**
>
> - Identify the appropriate policymakers based on their jurisdiction, background, voting history, interests, and position on the issue.
> - Invite two to three research team members, peers, or stakeholders to attend the meeting (designate roles such as spokesperson, data provider, storyteller).
> - Request a meeting by mail, email, fax, or phone. Introduce the team, the reason for the meeting, and your availability.
> - Follow-up on the initial request and schedule the appointment.
> - Prepare and rehearse talking points, providing an overview of the issue, your key findings, the research implications, and the recommended actions.
> - Prepare an information packet with a summary of your research and additional resources on the issue (e.g., one-page research summary, factsheets, policy brief).
> - Anticipate questions and prepare your responses.
>
> **During the meeting**
>
> - Introduce the team, organization, why you are interested on the issue, its relevance and importance to the constituents, and your expertise on the issue.
> - Tell a story using both empirical data and local anecdotal stories or illustrations.
>
> **Highlight your recommended actions and the supporting evidence**
>
> - Be concise and direct: deliver your message for three to five minutes and leave ample time for question-and-answer.
> - Answer questions clearly, concisely, politely, and professionally.
> - Offer to be a resource in your area of expertise for the policymaker and the staff.
> - Provide the information packet you prepared along with your contact information.
> - Thank the policymakers and the staff for their time.
>
> **After the meeting**
>
> - Follow up with a brief thank-you letter, attaching additional information as promised or requested during the meeting.
> - Check in regularly with the staff and policymaker and invite them to relevant events.
>
> *Sources:* American Public Health Association. (n.d.). Tips for making a visit to your policymaker. Retrieved June 1, 2020 from https://www.apha.org/-/media/files/pdf/advocacy/policymaker_visit_tips.ashx. Advocacy and Communications Solutions. (2015). Key tips for meeting with policymakers. Retrieved June 25, 2020 from https://www.advocacyandcommunication.org/wp-content/themes/acs/docs/resources/policy_maker_engagement_December_2015/ACS_Key_Tips_Policymaker_Meeting_Tips_.pdf

of Iowa Injury Prevention Research Center, 2017). This type of policy brief often ends with a recommendation of the best policy options based on the analysis. An *advocacy brief* provides an evidence-based argument for a specific course of action, thus includes strong policy recommendations to address the issue. A detailed policy brief generally contains the following sections (University of North Carolina at Chapel Hill, n.d.):

1. **Title:** Create a catchy heading that captures the reader's attention to the issue and communicates the content of the policy brief
2. **Executive summary:** Provide a short (one to two paragraphs) overview of the issue and the recommended/proposed policy
3. **Background:** Provide an evidence-based description of the nature and magnitude of the issue to justify its significance: What is the issue? Who is affected? How many? When? Where? Why does it exist?

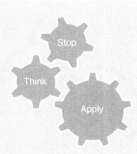

Identifying and Contacting a Local Policymaker

Think of a public health topic you are interested in researching and identify your elected local official. Conduct your research on the elected official you have selected and provide the following information:

1. Elected official's name and title/position:
2. Contact information and office address:
3. Does their history or background indicate an interest in public health?
4. Based on your research on the elected official's history, do you think this official would be interested in your research findings? Why or why not?
5. Discuss how you would contact the elected official and generally describe the kind of information you would like to share with them.

4. **Policy alternatives:** Discuss policy options to address the issue based on the best available evidence from the literature review and your research findings. This can include an evidence-based and objective analysis of each policy option based on the following criteria: intended and potential unintended effects, legality, population benefits, implementation costs, equity, administrative feasibility, political feasibility, acceptability, potential implementation barriers and mitigation strategies (Bardach and Patashnik, 2012; Bovbjerg et al., 2013; Bowen et al., 2009; Weiner, 2005). Shorter policy briefs omit this section and feature only the policy recommendation.

5. **Policy recommendation:** Propose the best policy solution(s) based on the objective analysis of the policy options in the previous step, including the concrete steps for implementing your policy recommendations. Alternatively, provide recommendations for addressing the limitations of the policy options that were analyzed.

6. **Sources/references:** Provide the resources used in developing the policy brief and additional resources with information on the issue or the policy.

7. **Appendices**: If needed, attach additional materials to support the policy recommendations (e.g., an asset map, a completed policy analysis matrix)

Policy briefs are succinct, varying in length from one to eight pages, depending on the type of brief and the audience. They can be presented in a plain text format or designed with images, headings and sub-headings, and other visual cues (textboxes, graphics, graphs) to highlight the key messages and draw the reader's attention (Figure 5.7).

The following are additional tips to keep in mind when developing a policy brief:

- Be concise: keep it short and simple.
- Focus on a single issue.
- Avoid jargon or technical terms.
- Use professional (not academic) or plain language depending on the audience.
- Provide actionable and applicable information: use active voice and action words.
- Incorporate simple and relevant graphics or visuals.
- Emphasize the proposed policy recommendations.
- Incorporate evidence from the literature and the research study to justify the problem and support the policy recommendations.

FIGURE 5.7. *Sample 2-page policy brief (note: the reference page has been omitted from the example).*

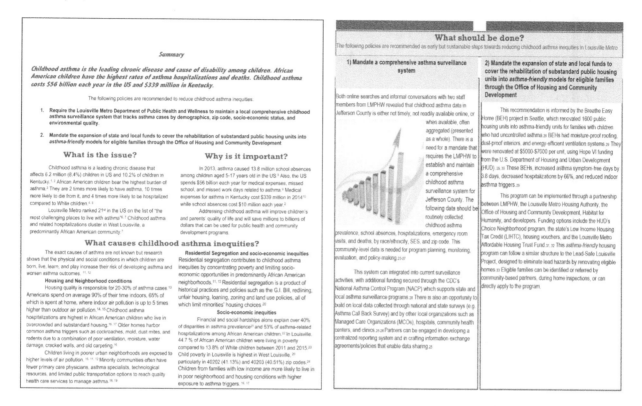

DISSEMINATING THE FINDINGS TO THE MEDIA

The news media is a powerful tool for disseminating public health messages and research findings given its wide coverage, diverse audience, and central role in shaping public debates and opinions. It is a primary source of information for many and has the capacity to reach both academic and nonacademic audiences. As previously mentioned, policies are the primary tool for creating sustainable changes in the social and physical conditions that bring about health issues. By creating awareness and increasing the visibility of public health issues, the media can mobilize the general public, opinion leaders, practitioners, and policymakers to take transformative actions at individual, community, institutional, and policy levels.

There are several media outlets that researchers can use depending on their target audience including: print media (e.g., newspapers, magazines), television, radio, digital media, and social media. Advances in technology have particularly expanded opportunities to disseminate interactive messages to larger and more diverse audiences even more rapidly. Unfortunately, this has also contributed to an "infodemic" or rapid proliferation of incorrect or false information that can hamper effective public health responses. As such, researchers should be more proactive and intentional in establishing positive media relations that enable an effective exchange of credible information between the producers of such information and the consumers or end-users of this information. There are a variety of media tools that researchers can leverage when working with media outlets including: press or news releases, op-eds, and media interviews.

Press or News Releases

Press or news releases are short (one to two pages) special announcements that are issued by organizations to disseminate important messages about special events or activities, projects (including research projects), or positions on important health and social issues. Press or news releases often serve as sources for news stories by local media outlets. A press release (Figure 5.8) generally contains the following elements (Bensley and Brookins-Fisher, 2019):

- Location and release date
- Contact information: contact person, email, phone, website for further questions or information
- Headline: a catchy title that communicates the focus of the press or news release
- Body: contains the key message (who, what, when, where), starting with the most important information and moving toward less important information (i.e., inverted pyramid); includes pertinent quotes from a spokesperson or an expert
- Boilerplate: closing statement with essential information about the organization or agency.

Op-Eds

An *op-ed* derived its name from its traditional location, which was opposite to an editorial page of a newspaper (Bensley and Brookins-Fisher, 2019). It is a short (one-column/approximately 800 words) persuasive argument or

FIGURE 5.8. *Sample press release from the Centers for Disease Control and Prevention. Centers for Disease Control and Prevention. (2020). CDC Marks the End of the 2018 Ebola Outbreak in Eastern Democratic Republic of the Congo. Retrieved July 1, 2020, from https://www.cdc.gov/media/releases/2020/p0625-cdc-marks-end-2018-ebola-outbreak.html.*

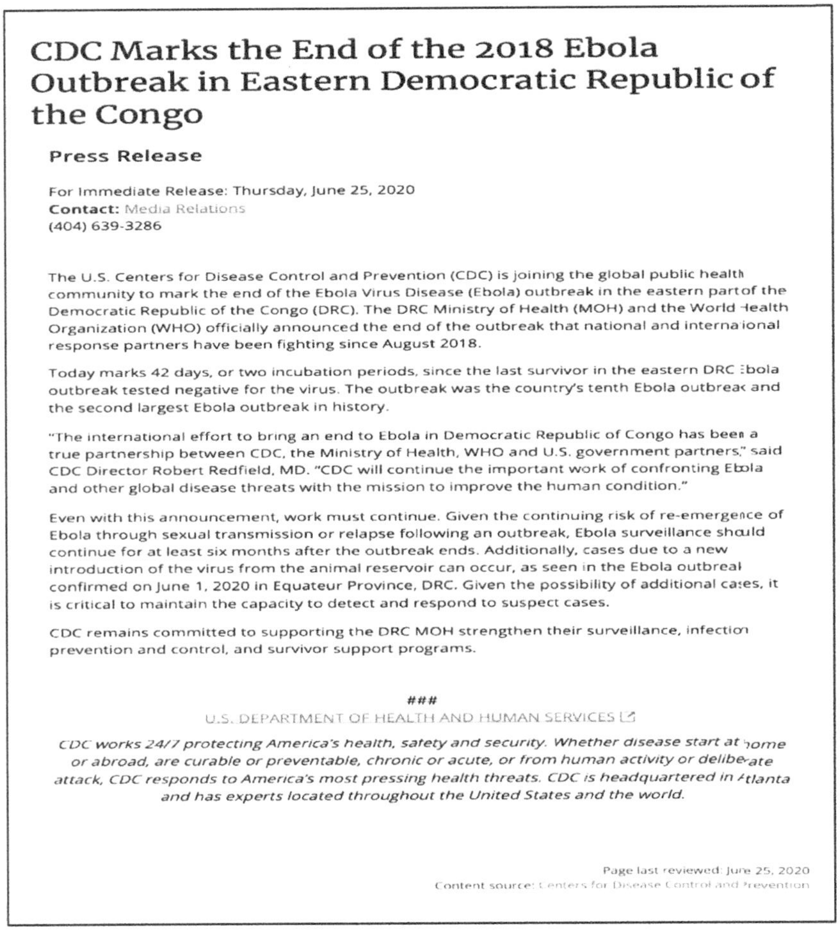

CDC Marks the End of the 2018 Ebola Outbreak in Eastern Democratic Republic of the Congo

Press Release

For Immediate Release: Thursday, June 25, 2020
Contact: Media Relations
(404) 639-3286

The U.S. Centers for Disease Control and Prevention (CDC) is joining the global public health community to mark the end of the Ebola Virus Disease (Ebola) outbreak in the eastern part of the Democratic Republic of the Congo (DRC). The DRC Ministry of Health (MOH) and the World Health Organization (WHO) officially announced the end of the outbreak that national and international response partners have been fighting since August 2018.

Today marks 42 days, or two incubation periods, since the last survivor in the eastern DRC Ebola outbreak tested negative for the virus. The outbreak was the country's tenth Ebola outbreak and the second largest Ebola outbreak in history.

"The international effort to bring an end to Ebola in Democratic Republic of Congo has been a true partnership between CDC, the Ministry of Health, WHO and U.S. government partners," said CDC Director Robert Redfield, MD. "CDC will continue the important work of confronting Ebola and other global disease threats with the mission to improve the human condition."

Even with this announcement, work must continue. Given the continuing risk of re-emergence of Ebola through sexual transmission or relapse following an outbreak, Ebola surveillance should continue for at least six months after the outbreak ends. Additionally, cases due to a new introduction of the virus from the animal reservoir can occur, as seen in the Ebola outbreak confirmed on June 1, 2020 in Equateur Province, DRC. Given the possibility of additional cases, it is critical to maintain the capacity to detect and respond to suspect cases.

CDC remains committed to supporting the DRC MOH strengthen their surveillance, infection prevention and control, and survivor support programs.

###
U.S. DEPARTMENT OF HEALTH AND HUMAN SERVICES

CDC works 24/7 protecting America's health, safety and security. Whether disease start at home or abroad, are curable or preventable, chronic or acute, or from human activity or deliberate attack, CDC responds to America's most pressing health threats. CDC is headquartered in Atlanta and has experts located throughout the United States and the world.

Page last reviewed: June 25, 2020
Content source: Centers for Disease Control and Prevention

informed opinion on a relevant issue. Unlike an editorial, which is written by an editorial staff or publisher, an op-ed is written by an individual who is not affiliated with the newspaper or magazine and has authority on the given topic based on expertise or experience. An op-ed should not express unsubstantiated or uninformed opinions, rather, the arguments made should be supported by strong evidence from one's research study and from the literature review. The OpED Project (n.d.), a useful resource for developing skills in writing an OpED, proposes the following basic structure of an OpED:

- Lead/opening statement: Start with a compelling statement that captures the reader's attention. It can be built around a groundbreaking research finding, a powerful anecdotal story, a recent event, or an anniversary of a historical event.
- Thesis: Clearly articulate the main argument of the op-ed.
- Body: Develop the main argument using supporting evidence from various sources including empirical research, scholarly products, experts, professional or personal experience.
- "To be sure" paragraph: Anticipate, address, or acknowledge any counterarguments or critiques.
- Conclusion/kicker: Provide a call to action or propose solutions to the issue and conclude by re-iterating the lead.

Media Interviews

Media outlets often reach out to academics, researchers, and other professionals with interview requests for news stories on topics of interest to their audiences. The misinterpretation of research findings by the media can be partly attributed to ineffective information exchanges and relationships between researchers and media personnel. Many researchers, academics, and other experts decline media interview requests for diverse reasons including their unavailability, limited training on media relations, failure to recognize the media as an important dissemination channel, prioritization of incentivized platforms (e.g., scientific journals), perceptions of media as agenda-driven or politically biased, or organizational restrictions related to the media. With limited resources and assistance from subject matter experts or researchers, media personnel are sometimes left to interpret and translate complex health and public health research information for their audiences. This story highlights the importance of developing effective working relationships with the media to disseminate and translate public health research.

Prior to engaging in any media activities, researchers should familiarize themselves with their organization or institution's policies related to media relations. Many organizations have designated media/public relations/communications personnel who coordinate any communications between the organization and the media. These individuals can provide more information about the policies as well as technical assistance with developing media products (Brownson et al., 2018). Media interviews can be administered on various platforms including print media (e.g., newspaper), radio, television, and videoconferencing. They can be individual or group interviews. Since media outlets and personnel operate with tight deadlines or time constraints, it is important to provide a prompt and respectful response (i.e., acceptance or decline) to an interview request after considering the following key questions:

- Is the interview with this media outlet permitted by my organization's policies? What are the organization's procedures for accepting a media interview request?
- Is the media outlet trusted and utilized by my target audience?
- What are my objectives for the interview?
- How will this interview benefit my target audience, me, and my organization?
- Am I comfortable and prepared to participate in the interview?
- Am I available for this interview?
- Which aspect of my research can I share?

Box 5.8 provides some basic tips for preparing and participating in a media interview.

BOX 5.8 Preparing and Participating in a Media Interview

Pre-interview
- Gather information about the interview format, focus/subject, interviewer, other interviewees, and duration.
- Review previous interviews by the same interviewer or media outlet.
- Review your work and develop talking points summarizing key findings (include relevant statistical information or specific details that are easily forgotten).
- Select three to five takeaway messages for your audience (American Pyschological Association, 2004).
- Anticipate questions and prepare your responses. Some may provide the main questions or subject areas in advance, others may ask for a summary of your research, from which they derive the questions.
- Identify co-panelists, their backgrounds, and areas of expertise.

Actual interview
- Refrain from using jargon or technical terms, if used, explain the terms.
- Break down complex statistics into simple numbers or proportions.
- Elaborate your responses but be brief.
- Do not disclose confidential or sensitive information (American Pyschological Association, 2004).
- Be transparent or honest when the question is beyond the scope of your study or your area of expertise.

Post interview
- Thank the interviewer and co-panelists.
- For print interviews, request to review the final story (if possible) prior to publication to ensure its accuracy. Note that this may not be possible given their time constraints. If not possible, highlight the importance of maintaining an accurate representation of your research findings (American Pyschological Association, 2004).

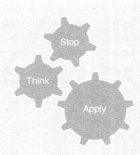

Identifying Local Media Outlets for Dissemination Purposes

Think of a public health topic you are interested in exploring through your research and identify the potential target audiences for your results. List the top three local media outlets (e.g., newspapers, radio, and/or television) that you would be interested in sharing your results with. Discuss why you have selected these media outlets.

 SUMMARY

Disseminating the research results beyond the academic/research audience is crucial for bridging the gaps between theory, research, practice, and policy. Nonacademic audiences include the community, practitioners, policymakers, and media personnel.

> Public health professionals or practitioners benefit from more targeted dissemination methods including workshops, trainings, seminars/webinars, and short courses given their accessibility, practicality, and the continuing education credits acquired from participating in such sessions.
>
> The research findings should be disseminated to community members who are affected by the issue, who can benefit from the findings, who need to act on the issue, and who collaborated with the researchers, using a combination of in-person, in print, and online/electronic dissemination channels. Health literacy is an important consideration when communicating with communities. Applying plain language or clear communication guidelines, is one way of reaching individuals with lower health literacy. In the United States, health information should be presented at or below the sixth grade reading level.
>
> Policymakers and their constituents are a critical target audience for policy-relevant research findings given their capacity to influence and act on policies. The study's policy implications and recommendations can be communicated to policymakers using direct (e.g., in-person meetings, phone, or email) or indirect methods (e.g., policy briefs, the media, and social media).
>
> The media is a powerful tool for disseminating public health messages and research findings given its wide coverage, diverse audience, and central role in shaping public debates and opinions. There are several media outlets that researchers can use depending on their target audience including: print media (e.g., newspapers, magazines), television, radio, and digital media, and social media. To prevent and combat the rapid proliferation of incorrect information, researchers should be more proactive and intentional in establishing media relations that enable an effective exchange of credible information between producers and consumers.

Now that I have reached the end this section, I am able to:

Course objective	Strongly agree	Somewhat agree	Neutral	Somewhat disagree	Strongly agree
Explain the importance of disseminating findings to nonacademic audiences					
Identify nonacademic audiences for the research study					
Identify appropriate dissemination channels for the target audience					

REFERENCES

Achkar, J. M., & Macklin, R. (2009). Ethical considerations about reporting research results with potential for further stigmatization of undocumented immigrants. *Clinical Infectious Diseases*, 48(9), 1250–1253. http://dx.doi.org/10.1086/597587

Allen, H. G., Stanton, T. R., Di Pietro, F., & Moseley, G. L. (2013). Social media release increases dissemination of original articles in the clinical pain sciences. *PLoS One*, 8(7), e68914. http://dx.doi.org/10.1371/journal.pone.0068914

American Journal of Public Health. (n.d.). Frequently asked questions. https://ajph.aphapublications.org/page/SubmissionFAQs

American Pyschological Association. (2004). How to work with the media. https://www.apa.org/pubs/authors/working-with-media

Bardach, E., & Patashnik, E. M. (2012). *A practical guide for policy analysis: The eightfold path to more effective problem solving*. CQ press. https://www.ethz.ch/content/dam/ethz/special-interest/gess/cis/international-relations-dam/Teaching/cornerstone/Bardach.pdf

Bautista, J. R. (2015). From solving a health problem to achieving quality of life: Redefining eHealth literacy. *Journal of Literacy and Technology*, 16(2), 33–54.

Bensley, R. J., & Brookins-Fisher, J. (2019). *Community and public health education methods: A practical guide* (4th ed.). Jones & Bartlett lvLearning.

Bhaskar, S. B. (2017). Concealing research outcomes: Missing data, negative results and missed publications. *Indian Journal of Anaesthesia*, 61(6), 453–455. http://dx.doi.org/10.4103/ija_361_17

Bovbjerg, R.B., Eyster, L., Ormond, B.A., Anderson, T., and Richardson, E. (2013). Opportunities for community health workers in the era of health reform. The Urban Institute. http://www.urban.org/sites/default/files/publication/32551/413071-Opportunities-for-Community-Health-Workers-in-the-Era-of-Health-Reform.PDF

Bowen, D. J., Kreuter, M., Spring, B., Cofta-Woerpel, L., Linnan, L., Weiner, D., . . . Fernandez, M. (2009). How we design feasibility studies. *American Journal of Preventive Medicine*, *36*(5), 452–457. http://dx.doi.org/10.1016/j.amepre.2009.02.002

Brennan, V. M. (2009). *Natural disasters and public health: Hurricanes Katrina, Rita, and Wilma.* Johns Hopkins University Press.

Brownson, R. C., Eyler, A. A., Harris, J. K., Moore, J. B., & Tabak, R. G. (2018). Getting the word out: New approaches for disseminating public health science. *Journal of Public Health Management and Practice*, *24*(2), 102–111. http://dx.doi.org/10.1097/phh.0000000000000673

Brownson, R. C., Jacobs, J. A., Tabak, R. G., Hoehner, C. M., & Stamatakis, K. A. (2013). Designing for dissemination among public health researchers: Findings from a national survey in the United States. *American Journal of Public Health*, *103*(9), 1693–1699. http://dx.doi.org/10.2105/AJPH.2012.301165

Butler, J., Sebastian, A., Kaye, I., Wagner, S., Morrissey, P., Schroeder, G., , & Vaccaro, A. (2017). Understanding traditional research impact metrics. *Clinical Spine Surgery*, *30*(4), 164–166. http://dx.doi.org/10.1097/BSD.0000000000000530

Centers for Disease Control and Prevention. (2019). Reducing stigma. https://www.cdc.gov/coronavirus/2019-ncov/daily-life-coping/reducing-stigma.html

Chilisa, B. (2012). *Indigenous research methodologies. SAGE.* Publications

Committee on Publication Ethics. (2018). How to recognize potential authorship problems. https://publicationethics.org/files/Recognise_Potential_Authorship_Problems.pdf

Cook, D. A., & Bordage, G. (2016). Twelve tips on writing abstracts and titles: How to get people to use and cite our work. *Medical Teacher*, *38*(11), 1100–1104.

COPE Council. (2017). Ethical guidelines for peer reviewers. https://publicationethics.org/files/Ethical_Guidelines_For_Peer_Reviewers_2.pdf

Desai, C. (2012). Authorship issues. *Indian Journal of Pharmacology*, *44*(4), 433–434. http://dx.doi.org/10.4103/0253-7613.99294

Desta, K. T., Kessely, D. B., & Daboi, J. (2019). Evaluation of the performance of the National Tuberculosis Program of Liberia during the 2014-2015 Ebola outbreak. *BMC Public Health*, *19*(1221)), 1–10. http://dx.doi.org/10.1186/s12889-019-7574-7

Dijkstra, S., Kok, G., Ledford, J. G., Sandalova, E., & Stevelink, R. (2018). Possibilities and pitfalls of social Media for translational medicine. *Frontiers in Medicine*, *5*(345), 1–6. http://dx.doi.org/10.3389/fmed.2018.00345

Duquia, R. P., Bastos, J. L., Bonamigo, R. R., González-Chica, D. A., & Martínez-Mesa, J. (2014). Presenting data in tables and charts. *Anais Brasileiros de Dermatologia*, *89*(2), 280–285. http://dx.doi.org/10.1590/abd1806-4841.20143388

Efron, S. E., & Ravid, R. (2019). *Writing the literature review: A practical guide.* Guildford Press.

EQUATOR Network. (n.d.). Library for health research reporting. https://www.equator-network.org/library/

Eysenbach, G. (2011). Can tweets predict citations? Metrics of social impact based on twitter and correlation with traditional metrics of scientific impact. *Journal of Medical Internet Research*, *13*(4), e123. http://dx.doi.org/10.2196/jmir.2012

Fah, T. S., & Aziz, A. F. A. (2006). How to present research data? *Malaysian Family Physician*, *1*(2–3), 82–85. https://www.ncbi.nlm.nih.gov/pmc/articles/PMC4453119/pdf/MFP-01-82.pdf

Frieden, T. R. (2010). A framework for public health action: The health impact pyramid. *American Journal of Public Health*, *100*(4), 590–595. http://dx.doi.org/10.2105/AJPH.2009.185652

Gagnier, J. J., Kienle, G., Altman, D. G., Moher, D., Sox, H., Riley, D., & CARE Group. (2013). The CARE Guidelines: Consensus-based Clinical Case Reporting Guideline Development. *Global Advances in Health and Medicine*, *2*(5), 38–43. http://dx.doi.org/10.7453/gahmj.2013.008

Gasparyan, A. Y., Ayvazyan, L., & Kitas, G. D. (2013). Authorship problems in scholarly journals: Considerations for authors, peer reviewers and editors. *Rheumatology International*, *33*(2), 277–284. http://dx.doi.org/10.1007/s00296-012-2582-2

Golbeck, A. L., Ahlers-Schmidt, C. R., Paschal, A. M., & Dismuke, S. E. (2005). A definition and operational framework for health numeracy. *American Journal of Preventive Medicine*, *29*(4), 375–376. http://dx.doi.org/10.1016/j.amepre.2005.06.012

Google Scholar. (n.d.). Top publications: Health and medical sciences-Public health. https://scholar.google.com/citations?view_op=top_venues&hl=en&vq=med_publichealth

Harris, J. K., Allen, P., Jacob, R. R., Elliott, L., & Brownson, R. C. (2014). Information-seeking among chronic disease prevention staff in state health departments: Use of academic journals. *Preventing Chronic Disease*, *11*, E138. http://dx.doi.org/10.5888/pcd11.140201

Harris, M., Powell, M., & Stamp, E. (2009). Re-establishing a home after Katrina: A long and winding road. In V. M. Brennan (Ed.), *Disasters and public health: Hurricanes Katrina, Rita, and Wilma.* Johns Hopkins.

Harris, M. J., Powell, M. H., & Stampely, E. (2007). Re-establishing a home after Katrina: A long and winding road. *Journal of Health Care for the Poor and Underserved*, *18*(2), 492–495. http://dx.doi.org/10.1353/hpu.2007.0032

Haustein, S., & Larivière, V. (2015). The use of bibliometrics for assessing research: Possibilities, limitations and adverse effects. In I. Welpe, J. Wollersheim, S. Ringelhan, & M. Osterloh (Eds.), *Incentives and performance.* Cham: Springer. http://dx.doi.org/10.1007/978-3-319-09785-5_8

Husereau, D., Drummond, M., Augustovski, F., de Bekker-Grob, E., Briggs, A. H., Carswell, C., . . . CHEERS 2022 ISPOR Good Research Practices Task Force. (2022). Consolidated Health Economic Evaluation Reporting Standards 2022 (CHEERS 2022) Statement: Updated Reporting Guidance for Health Economic Evaluations. *Value in Health*, *25*(1), 3–9. http://dx.doi.org/10.1016/j.jval.2021.11.1351

In, J., & Lee, S. (2017). Statistical data presentation. *Korean Journal of Anesthesiology*, *70*(3), 267–276. http://dx.doi.org/10.4097/kjae.2017.70.3.267

Institute of Medicine Committee on Health Literacy. (2004). *Health literacy: A prescription to end confusion.* National Academies Press. http://dx.doi.org/10.17226/10883

International Committee of Medical Journal Editors. (2019). Defining the role of authors and contributors. http://www.icmje.org/recommendations/browse/roles-and-responsibilities/defining-the-role-of-authors-and-contributors.html

iThenticate. (2013). Research Ethics: Decoding plagiarism and attribution-Types of plagiarism in research. http://www.ithenticate.com/resources/infographics/types-of-plagiarism-research

Kliewer, M. A. (2005). Writing it up: A step-by-step guide to publication for beginning investigators. *American Journal of Roentgenology*, *185*(3), 591–596. http://dx.doi.org/10.2214/ajr.185.3.01850591

Kumar, M. J. (2013). Making your research discoverable: Title plays the winning trick. *IETE Technical Review*, *30*(5), 361–363. http://dx.doi.org/10.4103/0256-4602.123113

Kumar, P. M., Priya, N. S., Musalaiah, S., & Nagasree, M. (2014). Knowing and avoiding plagiarism during scientific writing. *Annals of Medical and Health Sciences Research*, *4*(3), S193–S198. http://dx.doi.org/10.4103/2141-9248.141957

Laakso, M., Welling, P., Bukvova, H., Nyman, L., Bjork, B., & Hedlund, T. (2011). The development of open access journal publishing from 1993-2009. *PLoS One*, *6*(6), e20961. http://dx.doi.org/10.1371/journal.pome.0020961

Langat, P., Pisartchik, D., Silva, D., Bernard, C., Olsen, K., Smith, M., Sahni, S., & Upshur, R. (2011). Is there a duty to share? Ethics of sharing research data in the context of public health emergencies. *Public Health Ethics*, *4*(1), 4–11. https://doi.org/10.1093/phe/phr005

McDavitt, B., Bogart, L. M., Mutchler, M. G., Wagner, G. J., Green, H. D., Jr., Lawrence, S. J., . . . Nogg, K. A. (2016). Dissemination as dialogue: Building trust and sharing research findings through community engagement. *Preventing Chronic Disease*, *13*, E38. http://dx.doi.org/10.5888/pcd13.150473

McLeroy, K. R., Northridge, M. E., Balcazar, H., Greenberg, M., & Landers, S. J. (2012). Reporting guidelines and the American Journal of Public Health's adoption of preferred reporting items for systematic reviews and meta-analyses. *American Journal of Public Health*, *102*(5), 780–784. http://dx.doi.org/10.2105/AJPH.2011.300630

Moher, D., Liberati, A., Tetzlaff, J., Altman, D. G., & PRISMA Group. (2009). Preferred reporting items for systematic reviews and meta-analyses: The PRISMA statement. *PLoS Medicine*, *6*(7), e1000097. http://dx.doi.org/10.1371/journal.pmed.1000097

Mugo, N. R., Hong, T., Celum, C., Donnell, D., Bukusi, E. A., John-Stewart, G., . . . Baeten, J. M. (2014). Pregnancy incidence and outcomes among women receiving preexposure prophylaxis for HIV prevention: A randomized clinical trial. *JAMA*, *312*(4), 362–371. http://dx.doi.org/10.1001/jama.2014.8735

Muvuka, B., Combs, R. M., Ayangeakaa, S. D., Ali, N. M., Wendel, M. L., & Jackson, T. (2020). Health Literacy in African-American Communities: Barriers and Strategies. *Health Literacy Research and Practice*, *4*(3), e138–e143. https://doi.org/10.3928/24748307-20200617-01

Muvuka, B., & Harris, M. J. (2019). A rapid assessment of the impacts of gold mining on Women's health and quality of life in Ashanti region, Ghana. *Journal of Public Health Issues and Practices*, *2*, 138), 1–9. http://dx.doi.org/10.33790/jphip1100138

NYU Center for the Study of Asian American Health. (n.d.). Community Briefs. https://med.nyu.edu/asian-health/resources/community-briefs

O'Brien, B. C., Harris, I. B., Beckman, T. J., Reed, D. A., & Cook, D. A. (2014). Standards for reporting qualitative research: A synthesis of recommendations. *Academic Medicine*, *89*(9), 1245–1251. http://dx.doi.org/10.1097/ACM.0000000000000388

O'Cathain, A., Murphy, E., & Nicholl, J. (2008). The quality of mixed methods studies in health services research. *Journal of Health Services Research & Policy*, *13*(2), 92–98. http://dx.doi.org/10.1258/jhsrp.2007.007074

Omar, E. M. (2014). How to publish a scientific manuscript in a high impact journal. *Advances in Digestive Medicine*, *1*(4), 105–109. http://dx.doi.org/10.1016/j.aidm.2014.07.004

Page, M. J., McKenzie, J. E., Bossuyt, P. M., Boutron, I., Hoffmann, T. C., Mulrow, C. D., . . . Moher, D. (2021). The PRISMA 2020 statement: an updated guideline for reporting systematic reviews. *BMJ*, *372*, n71. http://dx.doi.org/10.1136/bmj.n71

Pleasant, A., Rooney, M., O'Leary, C., Myers, L., & Rudd, R. (2016). Strategies to enhance numeracy skills. *NAM Perspectives*, 1–6. http://dx.doi.org/10.31478/201605b

Pollock, M., Fernandes, R. M., Pieper, D., Tricco, A. C., Gates, M., Gates, A., & Hartling, L. (2019). Preferred reporting items for overviews of reviews (PRIOR): A protocol for development of a reporting guideline for overview of reviews of health care interventions. *Systematic Reviews*, *8*(335), 2–9. http://dx.doi.org/10.1186/s13643-019-1252-9

Progress in Community Health Partnerships: Research, Education, and Action. (n.d.). Author Guidelines. https://www.press.jhu.edu/journals/progress-community-health-partnerships-research-education-and-action/author-guidelines

Schulz, K. F., Altman, D. G., & Moher, D. (2010). CONSORT 2010 statement: Updated guidelines for reporting parallel group randomized trials. *Annals of Internal Medicine*, *152*(11), 726–732. http://dx.doi.org/10.7326/0003-4819-152-11-201006010-00232

Seglen, P. O. (1997). Why the impact factor of journals should not be used for evaluating research. *BMJ*, *314*(7079), 498–502. http://dx.doi.org/10.1136/bmj.314.7079.497

Sengupta, S., & Honavar, S. G. (2017). Publication ethics. *Indian Journal of Ophthalmology*, *65*(6), 429–432. http://dx.doi.org/10.4103/ijo.IJO_483_17

Shamseer, L., Moher, D., Maduekwe, O., Turner, L., Barbour, V., Burch, R., . . . Shea, B. J. (2017). Potential predatory and legitimate biomedical journals: Can you tell the difference? *A cross-sectional comparison. BMC Medicine*, *15*(1), 28. http://dx.doi.org/10.1186/s12916-017-0785-9

Sharman, A. (2015). Where to publish. *Annals of the Royal College of Surgeons of England*, *97*(5), 329–332. http://dx.doi.org/10.1308/rcsann.2015.0003

Springer. (2020). Open Access. https://www.springer.com/gp/authors-editors/authorandreviewertutorials/open-access

Springer. (n.d.). Revising and responding. https://www.springer.com/gp/authors-editors/authorandreviewertutorials/submitting-to-a-journal-and-peer-review/revising-and-responding/10285584

Steven, A., Garritty, C., Hersi, M., and Moher, D. (2018). Developing PRISMA-RR, a reporting guideline for rapid reviews of primary studies (Protocol). https://www.equator-network.org/wp-content/uploads/2018/02/PRISMA-RR-protocol.pdf

Stroup, D., Smith, C. K., & Truman, B. I. (2017). Reporting the methods used in public health research and practice. *Journal of Public Health and Emergency*, *1*, 89. http://dx.doi.org/10.21037/jphe.2017.12.01

Sullivan, G. M. (2012). Writing education studies for publication. *Journal of Graduate Medical Education*, *4*(2), 133–137. http://dx.doi.org/10.4300/JGME-D-12-00044.1

Sullivan, G. M., Simpson, D., Yarris, L. M., & Artino Jr., A. R. (2019). Writing author response letters that get editors to "yes". *Journal of Graduate Medical Education*, *11*(2), 119–123. http://dx.doi.org/10.4300/JGME-D-19-00161.1

Tabak, R. G., Stamatakis, K. A., Jacobs, J. A., & Brownson, R. C. (2014). What predicts dissemination efforts among public health researchers in the United States? *Public Health Reports*, *129*(4), 361–368. http://dx.doi.org/10.1177/003335491412900411

The OpEd Project. (n.d.). Op-ed Writing: Tips and Tricks. https://www.theopedproject.org/oped-basics/#structure

The University of Iowa Injury Prevention Research Center. (2017). Writing & disseminating policy briefs: A communications guide for injury and violence researchers and practitioners. https://iprc.public-health.uiowa.edu/wp-content/uploads/2018/03/Writing-and-Disseminating-Policy-Briefs.pdf

Tong, A., Sainsbury, P., & Craig, J. (2007). Consolidated criteria for reporting qualitative research (COREQ): A 32-item checklist for interviews and focus groups. *International Journal for Quality in Health Care*, *19*(6), 349–357. http://dx.doi.org/10.1093/intqhc/mzm042

Tricco, A. C., Lillie, E., Zarin, W., O'Brien, K. K., Colquhoun, H., Levac, D., . . . Straus, S. E. (2018). PRISMA Extension for Scoping Reviews (PRISMA-ScR): Checklist and Explanation. *Annals of Internal Medicine, 169*(7), 467–473. http://dx.doi.org/10.7326/M18-0850

Tunnecliff, J., Ilic, D., Morgan, P., Keating, J., Gaida, J. E., Clearihan, L., . . . Maloney, S. (2015). The acceptability among health researchers and clinicians of social media to translate research evidence to clinical practice: Mixed-methods survey and interview study. *Journal of Medical Internet Research, 17*(5), e119. http://dx.doi.org/10.2196/jmir.4347

University of Cambridge. (n.d.). Authorship and intellectual property. https://osc.cam.ac.uk/copyright-issues/authorship-and-intellectual-property

University of North Carolina at Chapel Hill. (n.d.). Policy briefs. https://writingcenter.unc.edu/tips-and-tools/policy-briefs

US Centers for Disease Prevent and Control. (2020). CDC marks the end of the 2018 Ebola outbreak in Eastern Democratic Republic of the Congo. https://www.cdc.gov/media/releases/2020/p0625-cdc-marks-end-2018-ebola-outbreak.html

US Copyright Office. (n.d.). Chapter 1: Subject matter and scope of copyright. https://www.copyright.gov/title17/92chap1.html#107

Van Eperen, L., & Marincola, F. M. (2011). How scientists use social media to communicate their research. *Journal of Translational Medicine, 9*, 199–199. http://dx.doi.org/10.1186/1479-5876-9-199

von Elm, E., Altman, D. G., Egger, M., Pocock, S. J., Gøtzsche, P. C., & Vandenbroucke, J. P., and STROBE Initiative (2014). The Strengthening the Reporting of Observational Studies in Epidemiology (STROBE) Statement: guidelines for reporting observational studies. *International Journal of Surgery, 12*(12), 1495–1499.

Weiner, J. (2005). Health policy analysis checklist. http://ocw.jhsph.edu/courses/IntroHealthPolicy/PDFs/Bardach_Outline_IHP_7b.pdf

Wilson, P. M., Petticrew, M., Calnan, M. W., & Nazareth, I. (2010). Does dissemination extend beyond publication: A survey of a cross section of public funded research in the UK. *Implementation Science, 5*, 61–61. http://dx.doi.org/10.1186/1748-5908-5-61

World Intellectual Property Organization. (n.d.). What is intellectual property? https://www.wipo.int/copyright/en

INDEX

Page numbers in *italics* refer to figures and page numbers in **bold** refer to tables.

5 C approach, 49

A

Aarons, D., 18
ABLENESS, 6
accuracy, 109, 205
Achkar, J. M., 305
action research, 9, 234
active learning, **15**
Adichie, Chimamanda Ngozi, 10
adverse events, 18
Africa, 16, 100, 187
African Americans, 232, 240, 272, 283, 287–288
age, 5, 6, 10, 81, 199
agency, 100
AI *see* article influence
AIM(RaD)C format, 118, 214, 297, 315, 316, 325
Ali, N. M., 199
Alzheimer's Foundation of America, 32
AMA *see* American Medical Association
American Medical Association (AMA), 126, 303
American Psychological Association (APA), 88, 126, 303
American Public Health Association, 165
American Statistical Association, 109
Americans with Disabilities Act (ADA), 106
analysis of covariance (ANCOVA), 110
analysis of variance (ANOVA), 111, 114, 230
analytical studies, 60–61
analytic memos, 211
ANCOVA *see* analysis of covariance
ANOVA *see* analysis of variance
annotated bibliography, 21
APA *see* American Psychological Association
APF *see* article processing fee
article influence (AI), 312–313
article processing fee (APF), 313
arts-based approaches, 8, **9**
ATLAS.ti, 29, **211**
attrition, **64**, **80**, 83
audio recordings, 29, 197, 202, 206, 207
audiovisual documents, 203
audit trials, 206
authenticity, 58, 204, 205
authorship, 310–312
auto-ethnography, 156
autonomy, 16, 28, 100
auto-plagiarism, 307
axiology, 151

B

back-translation, 99
Bandura, A., 71
bar graphs, 111, *114*, 300
Baxter, P., 155
behavior, 4, 5, 27, 91, **194**, 267, 291
  researcher's, 201–202
  theory of planned, 70
behavioral research, 91
Behavioral Risk Factor System Survey (BRFSS), 280, 283, 285, **286**, **287**, 288
beliefs, 5, 7, 155, 213, 224
  cultural, 90, 236, 265, 273, 279
bell (Gaussian) curve, 111, *112*
Belmont Report, 13, 14, 19, 183
beneficence, 57, 58, 183, 241
Bernard, H. R., 189
Bhuyan, M. R., 250
biases, 63, 79, 97, 103, 116, 117
bimodal distribution, 111
biomedical research, 13, 16, 17
biosketch, 127, 128
bivariate analysis, 113–114
Black men, 13, 14
Blaney, C. L., 91
blinding, 61
blood pressure, 110
Boateng, G. O., 92
Boaz, A., 6
Boolean operators, 40–41
Booth, A., 34
bracketing, 158, 178
brainstorming, 23, 24, 167, 176
Braun, V., 208, 211
breast cancer research, 32
BRFSS *see* Behavioral Risk Factor System Survey
Brinkmann, S., 194
Brislin, R. W., 207–208
BRUSO model, 92
budget, 128–130
Burris, M. A., 159

C

Camacho, S., 250
Canada, 155
Caribbean countries, 18
Caribbean Public Health Agency (CARPHA), 18
Carrico, C., 196
case–control studies, **8**, 59
case studies, 8, **9**, 154–155
  data sources for, 155
  mixed methods research, 264–291
  purpose statement, 175
  research questions, 177
  types of, 155

Integrated Research Methods In Public Health, First Edition. Muriel Jean Harris and Baraka Muvuka.
© 2023 John Wiley & Sons, Inc. Published 2023 by John Wiley & Sons, Inc.
Companion website: www.wiley.com/go/harris/integratedresearchmethods

CBPR *see* community-based participatory research
CDC *see* Centers for Disease Control and Prevention
cell phones *see* mobile phones
census data, 83
Centers for Disease Control and Prevention (CDC), 70, 259, 305
cervical cancer, 249–250
CFR *see* US Code of Federal Regulations
Charmaz, K., 157, 209
chart method, 48
child health, 4
   see also children
children, 4, 13, 57, 250, 281
Chilisa, B., 10, 28, 74, 100, 232, 305
China, 159
chi-square test, 111, 113
CINAHL (Cumulative Index of Nursing and Allied Health Literature), **43**
CIOMS *see* Council for International Organizations of Medical Sciences
citations, 47, 312–313
Clandinin, D. J., 158
Clarke, V., 208, 211
clinical trials, 5–6, 60, 61
clusters, 84
CMap, 7
Cochrane library, **43**
code book, 63
code–recode strategy, 206
coding, 29, 209–210
Coding Analysis Toolkit (CAT), **212**
cognitive process, 92, *93*
cognitive skills, 47, 52
cohort studies, **8**, 59
Collaborative Institutional Training Initiatives (CITI), 17
collective action, **15**, 159
collective cultures, 4
collective ethics philosophy, 100
Collins, C. S., 178
Collins, K. M. T., 262
Combs, J. P., 258
Committee on Publication Ethics, 307, 311–312, 321
common-sense reasoning, 56
communicable diseases, 4
community-based participatory research (CBPR), 5, 9–10, 14–16, 58, 123, 165, 327, 329
community engagement 5, 9–10, 14–16, 58, 100, 123, 249
community policy briefs, 329
community research briefs, 329
community transformation, 10, 28
computers, 104
concentration camps, 13
concept mapping, 48, 74–75, 167, 249
conceptual framework, 11–13, 22, 24, 27
   mixed methods research, 248–251
   qualitative research, 178–180
   quantitative research, 74–76
conciseness, 51
confidentiality, 14, 102, 109, 141, 199, 207
confirmability, 30, 206
conflict of interest 325
Connelly, F. M., 158
consent, 5, 6
   form, 101–102, 140–142, 185–187
   see also informed consent
consistency, 29
CONSORT (Consolidating Standards of Reporting Trials), 123, 321
constant comparative method, 209, 210, 261, 284
constant comparison approach, 29, 157
constructivism, 8, 28, 51, 225

control groups, 26, 61, 63, 83
convergent designs, 229–230, **238**, **239**, 243, 260–261
Cooper, L. A., 104
copyright laws, 304–305
Corbin, J. M., 157, 170, 174
COREQ (Consolidated Criteria for Reporting Qualitative Research), 214, 302
Cornell method, 47
correlation coefficient, 60
correlational studies, 59–60, **77**
correlations, 59–60, **77**, 113, *114*
COSMIN checklist, 88
COSMIN database, 78
Council for International Organizations of Medical Sciences (CIOMS), 13, 18
cover letters, 108
COVID-19, 74, 106, 165, 305–306
creative relationship framework, 57, 65
credibility, 29–30, 204, 205
Creighton, G., 161
Crenshaw, K., 72
Creswell, J. D., 10, 28, 228
Creswell, J. W., 10, 28, 155, 224, 225–226, 228, 232–233, 236–240, 248, 251, 253, 260
critical race theory, 3
critical realism perspective, 225
critical research, 8
critical theory, 3, 9
critical thinking, 3
Cronbach's alpha (α), 96
cross-cultural research, 4–5, 10, 17, 19, 104, 105
cross-cultural validity, 96
cross-sectional studies, **8**, 59, 110
CRPD *see* United Nations Convention on the Rights of Persons with Disabilities
cultural appropriateness, 169, 176
cultural awareness, 4, 19
cultural beliefs, 90, 236, 265, 273, 279
cultural connectedness, 104, 120
cultural desire, 4, 19
cultural dexterity, 4, 19
cultural differences, 57
cultural phenomena, 155–156
cultural responsiveness, 58, 67, 68, 90, 119, 241, 254
cultural sensitivity, 4, 5, 19
cultural skills, 58
cultural values, 58, 67, 241, 254
culture, 4–5, 16, 58, 65
curriculum vitae (CV), 127
customs, 5, 58, 65

D

data,
   categorical, 110
   coding, 29, 209–210
   fabrication, 18
   falsification, 18
   integrity of, 109–110
   interval, 92, 110, 111
   nominal, 110
   ordinal, 110
   phishing of, 18
   primary 62, **63**, 89
   qualitizing, 253, 261, 262
   quantitizing, 237, 253, 261–262
   ratio, 92, 110, 111
   recoding, 63
   repositories, 62
   saturation, 188, 198

secondary, 62, **63**
  transformation, 261–262
  visualization, 63
  see also data analysis; databases; data collection; data management
data analysis, 22, 28–29, 110
  mixed methods research, 239–241, 258
  qualitative research, 208–211, **212**, 218
  quantitative research, 62–63
  software, 29, 206, 211, **212**
  surveys, 109–118
  validity, 117–118
databases, 40–41, **43–44**, 78, 270
data collection, 28–29
  adequate engagement in, 205
  methods, 24
  mixed methods research, 253–258
  qualitative research, 24, 192–205
  quantitative research, 24, 78–79
  surveys, 88, 94, 103–106, 120
data management **182**, 206–208, 210–211
debriefing, 156
deception, 156
Declaration of Helsinki, 13
Dedoose, 29, 206, 210, **211**
deductive process, 153, 178
deidentification, 207
De Leeuw, E. D., 105
dementia-related research, 32
Demir, S. B., 230
democratic participation, **15**
Democratic Republic of Congo (DRC), 154, 170
Demographic and Health Surveys program, 106
demographic profiles, 83, 291
dependability, 205–206
descriptive analysis, 111, **112**
descriptive studies, 58–60, **77**, 154
Desta, K. T., 311
DeVellis, R. F., 92, 253
deviant cases, 29
diabetes, 32, 38, 81, 168, 173, 232, 280–281
diagrams, 12
diets, 281
  see also healthy eating
digital documents, 203
digitization, 206–207
Dillman, D. A., 105
dimension reduction, 115
direct costs, 128
disabilities, 57, 58, 106
  emotional, 57
  predisposing factors, 71
disadvantaged groups, 5, 14, 67, 184
discriminant analysis, 115
dissertations, 38, **298**
document review, 203–204, 218, 257–258, 271
documents, 203
  see also document review
Donabedian, A., 179
drama, 8
DRC *see* Democratic Republic of Congo

E

Ebola epidemic, 74
ecological studies, **8**
economic policies, 71–72
education, 71
educational attainment, 111, *113*
Edwards, C., 93, 103
Egleston, B. L., 95

eHealth literacy, 330
electronic files, 206
elimination of mother-to-child transmission of HIV (EMTCT)
  program, 172
Elsevier's Journal Finder, 312
Embase, **43**
embedded review, 21
emergencies, 18
emergency preparedness, 81
emotional ability, 10
emotional disability, 57
emotional health, 4
employment, 72
empowerment, 3, 9, 10
EMTC *see* elimination of mother-to-child transmission of HIV
  (EMTCT) program
EndNote, 47
environment, 4
environmental hazards, 71
environmental reevaluation, 91
epidemiology study designs, **8**
epistemology, 151
equality, **15**
Equator (Enhancing the QUality and Transparency Of health Research)
  network, 302
equity, 4, 9
  health, 3, 85, 291
ERIC (Education Resources Information Centre), **44**
errors,
  sampling, **80**, 83, 104, 255
  type 1, **64**, **81**, 83
  type 2, **64**, **81**, 83
ethical codes, 183
ethical considerations, 13–19
  ethnographic studies, 156
  mixed methods research, 241, 242, 262
  photovoice, 161
  qualitative research, 183–184
  quantitative research, 57–58
  research report, 118–119, 305–306
  research topic, 168
  surveys, 109–110, 120
Ethical Guidelines for Statistical Practice, 109
ethical review board (ERB), 13
ethics committees, 13–18, 131, 183
ethics review and approval process, 16–18
ethics review boards, 13–17, 19, 57
ethics training, 17
ethnicity, 6, 110
ethnic research, 6–7, 10
ethnography, 8, **9**, 155–156, 175, 177, 209
European Commission, 6, 121
Euro-Western research, 6
evaluation design, *236*, 268–269, 282
evaluation reports, **298**
experience, 8
experimental research designs, 26, 61, 81
explanatory sequential design, 232–233, **238**, **239**, 240
explanatory studies, **77**
exploratory sequential design, 231, **233**, **238**, **239**, 240
exploratory studies, 59, **77**, 154

F

factor analysis, 96, 115
family, 72
feasibility, 168–169
federally qualified health center (FQHC), 229, 236, 265, 268–270, 272
feedback, 147, 205, 317
feminism, 3

feminist theory, 3
field notes, 205
Fisher's exact test, 113
Flesch-Kincaid Grade Level Test, 97
"fly-in, fly-out" research, 327
Flyvbjerg, B., 154, 155
focused codes, 210
focus groups, 29, 198–200, 256–257
foundations, 32
FQHC *see* federally qualified health center
Freire, Paulo, 10
Frieden, T. R., 335
Frongillo, E. A., 92
funding, 18, 31–33, 121–122, 131

G

Galama, T. J., 72
gatekeepers, 189–190, 202
gender, 5, 6, 110, 111
generalizability, 57, 63, 65, 79
Gennaro, S., 268
Geographic Information Systems (GIS), 106, 225, 234, *235*, 250, 255, 271, 284–285, 287
geographic residence, 10
gestures, 5
Ghana, 100, 154, 160, 250
GIS *see* Geographic Information Systems
Glaser, B. G., 156–157, 174, 208
Global Health (database), **44**
gold mining, 154, 160–161, 195
gonorrhea, 14
Google Scholar, 313
Google Translate, 99
graffiti, 8
GRAMMS (Good Reporting of a Mixed Methods), 302
Grant, M. J., 34
Grant, R. W., 191
grants, 31–32, 121–131
 award process, 131
 review, 130–131
 writing the application, 121–130
gray literature, 44
Green, J., 225, 226
Grewal, A., 43
grounded theory method (GTM), 12–13, 154, 156–158, 170, 226
 classic, 157
 constructivist, 157
 fundamental concepts, 157
 purpose statement, 175
 research questions, 177
 Straussian, 157
 theoretical saturation, 188
group work, 145–146
GTM *see* grounded theory method
Guatemala, 14
Guba, E. G., 205, 218
Guest, G., 226
Guidelines and Policies for the Conduct of Research in the Intramural Research, 131
Guttman scale, 92

H

Hagan Collier technique, 283
Hagiwara, N., 231
Hart, T. C., 49
Hawthorne Effect, **64**, 79, **80**, 201, 257

Hays, D. G., 213, 214
health,
 definition, 70
 equity, 3, 85, 291
 literacy, 330–331
 numeracy, 330
 as a right, 4
 social determinants of, 9, 70
 see also health belief model; health care; health impact pyramid; health insurance
Health and the General Social Survey, 88
health belief model, 70, 165
health care, 4, 71, 90–92, 266–268, 279
health impact pyramid, 335
health insurance, 199
health-related outcomes, 27, 71, 72, 81
health-related research, 6
health-seeking, 71
healthy eating, 280, 285–290
healthy environments, 281
healthy living, 4, 285
 see also healthy eating; physical activity
heart disease, 32, 71, 81, 280–281
"helicopter research", 327
Hendricks, T. C. C., 121
Herrmann, A., 165
history, **64**, **80**
HIV/AIDS, 14, 74, 154, 167, 172, 249, 306, 331
Hlongwa, P., 14
holy trinity approach, 213
honesty, 109
household surveys, 106
housing, 72
Huang, G. D., 5
Hulton, L. A., 179
human fetuses, 13
human papillomavirus (HPV), 250
human rights, 13, 14
Human Subjects Protection, 13–19, 127
HyperRESEARCH, **212**
hypotheses, 12, 23, 60–61, 82–83
 alternative, 23, 82–83
 null, 23, 82–83

I

ICPSR *see* Inter-University Consortium for Political and Social Science Research
IF *see* impact factor
illicit drug use, 103, 155
iMindMap, 75
immigrants, 90, 188, 250, 266
immigration policy, 267–268
impact factor (IF), 312–313
IMRADC format, 299
incentives, 105, 191–192
inclusion, **15**
income, 72
indigenous communities, 100
indigenous culture, 6–7
indigenous people, 6–7, 28
indigenous research, 6–7, 10, 28, 57, 74
indirect costs, 128
inductive process, 153, 157, 178
inferential statistics, 63, 111
information saturation, 45
 see also data saturation
informed consent, 16, 140–142, 185–187
 continuous, 186

in emergencies, 18
in mixed methods research, 241
parental permission, 185
person's capacity to give, 16, 57–58
in qualitative research, 184–187
in quantitative research, 100, *101*, 106
signed, 184–185
waiver of, 184–185
see also consent
institutional review board (IRB), 13–14, 19, 100, 127, 131, 141, 156, 188, 189, 232–233
instrumentation, **64**, **80**
integrity,
of data and methods, 109–110
personal, **15**
intellectual property, 304–305
International Ethical Guidelines for Biomedical Research Involving Human Subjects, 13
International Guidelines for Ethical Review of Epidemiological Studies, 13
international postdoctoral scholars (IDPs), 250
international research studies, 17
internet surveys, 104–105, 255
see also web-based surveys
interpretivist research, 8
interrater reliability, 96, 206, 284
Inter-University Consortium for Political and Social Science Research (ICPSR), 62
intervention studies, **8**, 61, **77**
interviews, 8, **9**, 192–198
conducting, 197–198
data from, 29
developing a guide, 195–197
face-to-face, 105–106, **107**
individual, 26, 199, 226, 249, 255–256
media 337–338
recording, 29, 197
semistructured, 192, 193, 195, 256
structured, 192, 193, 256
types of questions in, 193–195
unstructured, 192–193, 195, 256
investigational therapy, 18
Ipsos, 105
IRB Regulation for the Review of Research, 100, 139
IRB *see* institutional review board
I-we relationship, 6

J

Jack, S., 155
JANE (Journal, Author Name Estimator), 312
Johns Hopkins University, 43
Johnson, A. G., 58
Johnson, R. B., 238
Johnson-Thornton, R. L., 279
journal articles, **298**, 309–321
authorship issues, 310–312
choosing the title, 312
developing the outline, 315–316
drafting the manuscript, 316, **317**
peer-review process, 320–321
planning the manuscript, 310–314
reviewing, 318–319, **320**
selection of a journal, 312–314
selecting the type of, 314, **315**
submitting, 317–318
justice, 57, 58, 183, 184, 241
see also social justice

K

Kendal's tau, 113
key words, 40
Klykken, F. H., 186
Knowledge Panel, 105
Korinek, K., 268
Krieger, N., 72
Krusal-Wallis test, 114
Kuder-Richardson-20 test (KR-20), 96
Kumar, R., 11, 74, 248, 312
Kvale, S., 194, 195

L

Lahman, Maria, 16
language, 5, 6, 8, 99–100, 184, 186, 207–208
barriers, 266–267, 274, 279
Latkin, C. A., 93, 103
letter of intent (LOI), 32–33, 123–125
letters of support, 127–128
Likert scale, 81, 91–92, 96, 97
Likert-type scale, 78, 110
Lincoln, Y. S., 205, 218
linear regression model, 115
literature review, 21–22, 34–52, 90, 126
critical and analytical reading, 47, 52
defining the topic, 40
distinguished from other types of reviews, 21–22
integrative, 68, 70, 245
in mixed methods research, 245–246, *247*, 249, 265
planning stage, 39–45
preliminary, 166, 171
in qualitative research, 170–171
in quantitative research, 68–70
questions, 40, 46
search statements, 40–42, 45, 52
selection criteria, 44–45
synthesis of the findings, 49
three-stage process, 38–51
types, 34, **35–38**
utility of, 21, *22*
see also literature review report
literature review report, 48–52, 70
length, 50
sections of, 50
literature search, 45–47
logic statements, 12
logistic regression model, 115
LOI *see* letter of intent
longitudinal studies, 59
Love, P., 6
low-income populations, 71
Luquis, R. R., 4, 19

M

Macklin, R., 305
mail surveys, 88, 104, 105, **107**
maleficence, 57, 58
see also nonmaleficence
Mann–Whitney U test, 111
mapping method *see* concept mapping
marginalized people, 5, 10, 74, 159, 249
marketability, 73
marriage, 72
maternal death surveillance and response (MDSR), 154, 170
maternal health, 4
maternity services, 179
maturation, **64**, **80**, 117

Mauriën, K., 249
MAXQDA, **211**
Maxwell, J. A., 179
McGorry, S., 99
MDSR *see* maternal death surveillance and response
MEAL approach, 49
media, 164, 335–338
   campaigns, 285, 287
   interviews, 337–338
   see also social media
Medicaid, 267–268
medical records, 203
Medical Research Council, 121
medical research protocols, 13
Melgar-Quinonez, H. R., 92
member checking, 30, 205, 237, 241
memorandum of understanding (MOU), 127–128
Mendeley, 47
mental health, 4
Merriam, S. B., 152, 154, 201, 202, 203, 209
Mertens, D. M., 233, *234*, 264
meta-analysis, **36**, *46*
meta-synthesis, 34, **36**
Microsoft Excel, 29, 110, 270, 271
Microsoft Vision, 75
Microsoft Word, 97, 206, 209, 210, 271
migration, 10, 250
   see also immigrants; immigration policy
misconduct, 18
mixed methods research, 11, 26, 28, 223–291
   case studies, 264–291
   complex designs 233–234
   conceptual framework, 248–251
   convergent designs, 229–230, **238**, **239**, 243, 260–261
   cultural responsiveness, 241
   data analysis, 239–241, 258
   data collection, 253–258
   ethical considerations, 241, 242, 262
   informed consent, 241
   literature review, 245–246, *247*, 249, 265
   philosophical underpinning, 225–226
   planning process, 243–244
   problem statement, 246–247, 265
   reporting the findings, 260–261
   research question, 248
   sampling, 251–253
   sequential designs, 231–232, **238**, **239**, 240
   strengths and weaknesses, 226, **227**
   theoretical frameworks, 226–241
   validity in, 237–238, 242
mobile phones, 105–106, 173
Morse, J., 227
mortality, 71, 74, 170, 281
MOU *see* memorandum of understanding
multiple levels of influence, **27**
multiple realities, 151, 157
multiple regression models, 115
multivariate analysis, 110, 115
mutual respect, **14**, 57, 241
Muvuka, B., 154, 155

narrative inquiry, 8, **9**
narrative profiles, 262
narrative research, 158–159, 175, 177
narrative review *see* traditional review
National Academy of Sciences, 2
National Education Association, 4
National Institute of Diabetes and Digestive and Kidney Diseases, 131
National Institute of Minority Health, 131
National Institutes of Health (NIH), 6, 31, 103, 118, 121, 123, *124*, 130, 131
National Survey on Drug Use, 88
Nazi Germany, 13, 183
NCDs *see* noncommunicable diseases
needs assessment, 27, 123, 126, 236, 250
neighborhoods, 72, 281–291
Neilands, T. B., 92
neonates, 13
Nepal, 105
neutrality, 30
newsletters, 165
NIH *see* National Institutes of Health
noncommunicable diseases (NCDs), 4, 167–168, 280, 281, **286**
nonequivalent group designs, 61
nonmaleficence, 183
   see also maleficence
nonparametric tests, 111–113
nonparticipation, 83, 183, 201, 257
notations, 237
note-taking methods, 47–48, 52
Nuremberg Code, 183
Nuremburg Trials, 13
NVivo, 29, **211**, 230, 284

obesity, 280–281
objective truth, 7
observational studies, 61, *235*
observations, 201–202, 257, 271
O'Leary, Z., 203
ontology, 151
Onwuegbuzie, A. J., 238, 258, 262
Oparah, J. C., 10
op-eds, 337
Open Access journals, 313
operators, 40–41
oral storytelling, 158
otherness, 6, 10
outline method, 47
overciting, 51
overweight, 280–281

Palinkas, L. A., 26
Papers (software), 47
parametric tests, 111–112
paraphrasing, 307
parental permission, 185
parentheses, 40, 41
Parkinson's disease, 119
participant assent, 143
participatory research, 9–10, 225
   qualitative, 159–161
   see also community-based participatory research (CBPR)
patient-centred care (PCC), 267
Patient Education Materials Assessment Tool, 259
Patton, M. Q., 29, 193
PCA *see* principal component analysis
PCC *see* patient-centred-care
Pearson's correlation, 111, 113, 230
peer-review, 44, 56, 57, 205, 206, 320–321
   see also peer-review journals
peer-review journals, 308–321, 327
Perez, M. A., 4, 19

permissions, 5, 185, 202
personal documents, 203, 258
personal experience, 164
phenomenology, **9**, 158, 175, 208
   hermeneutic, 158
   transcendental, 158
philosophical worldviews, 28
photo-elicitation, 159–160
photographs, 8, 159–160
photovoice, 8, **9**, 159–161
physical ability, 10
physical activity, 81, 94, 280–285, 287, 289
physical harm, 14
physical materials, 203, 258
PI *see* principal investigator
pie charts, 111, *113*, 300
pilot testing,
   distinguished from pretesting, 197
   interviews, 196–197
   survey instruments, 88, 89, 98, 104, 120
Pismek, N. 230
plagiarism, 48, 51, 69, 306–307
Plano Clark, V. L., 224–226, 228, 232–234, 236–240, 248, 251, 253, 260
PNC *see* prenatal care
policies, 267–268
   developing briefs, 332–335
   economic, 71–72
   immigration, 267–268
   social, 71–72
   see also policymakers
policymakers, 332–335
poor, the, 14
   see also socioeconomic status (SES)
population level data, 87
positionality, 153, 156, 169, 180
positivism, 3, 7–8, 28, 151, 225
postcolonial discourse, 3
postpositivism, 3, 7–8, 56–57, 66, 70, 225
power, 5, 8, 10, 58
   see also empowerment
pragmatism, 10–11, 28, 151, 225, 264
predatory journals, 313–314
predisposing factors, 71
preliminary readings, 166
prenatal care (PNC) 229, 236, 255, 257, 259, 264–280
   barriers to early entry, 274, 279
   best practices in, 268
   recommendations for, 278, 280
prenotifications, 88, 105
Prescott, F. J., 196
press releases, 336
pretesting, 89, 120, 196–197, 256
PRIMSA framework, 250
principal component analysis (PCA), 115
principal investigator (PI), 4, 58, 68, 130
PRISMA (Preferred Reporting Items for Systematic reviews and Meta-Analysis), 46, 47, 302, 321
prisoners, 13, 57
privacy, 14, 161
privacy statement, 141
privilege, 58
Privilege, Power and Difference, 58
problem statement,
   mixed methods research, 246–247, 265
   qualitative research, 172–174, 180
   quantitative research, 72–74, 126
process coding, 209
professional experience, 164
project managers, 130

project timeline, 126, **127**
Protection of Human Subjects (US), 13
PsycINFO, **44**
psychological harm, 14
psychometric testing, 96, 98
public documents, 203, 258
public health, definition, 4
PubMed, **43**
purpose statement, 174–175
p-value, 82, 300

Q

QDA Miner, **212**
qualitative codebooks, 210
qualitative codes, 261
qualitative-quantitative approach, 225
qualitative research, 3, 11–12, 28–29, 149–218
   attributes of, 151–153
   conceptual framework, 163–170, 178–179
   data collection, 24, 192–205
   data management, 206–208
   disseminating the findings, 212–213
   ethical considerations, 183–184
   literature review, 170–171
   overview of approaches, **9**
   philosophical underpinnings, 151
   process, 161, *162*
   purpose of the study, 174–175
   recruitment and selection process, 190–192
   reporting the findings, 212–217
   research area, 164–165
   research designs, 154–161
   research problem, 171–174
   research proposal, 181–182
   research questions, 23, 73–74, 175–177
   research topic, 165–170
   theoretical framework, 178–179
   theory in, 12–13
   validity and reliability, 29–30
qualitative researchers, 152–153
qualitizing, 253, 261, 262
quality of care, 179
Qualtrics, 87
quantitative research, 7, 11–12, 55–132
   data collection, 24, 78–79
   ethical considerations, 57–58
   philosophical underpinnings, 56–57
   planning for, 66–67
   primary methodologies, **8**
   reporting the findings, 116, 118, 120
   research designs, 58–62, **77**
   research questions, 23, 73–74, 76–77
   theoretical framework, 12, 70–72, 91
   validity, 29, 58, 61, 63–64, 116–118
quantitizing, 237, 253, 261–262
quasi-experimental research designs, 26, 61, 81
questions,
   in applied research, 3, 23
   in basic research, 3, 23
   closed-ended, 7, 78–79, 94, 193
   direct, 194–195
   focused, 23
   indirect, 194–195
   in interviews, 192–193
   in literature review, 40, 46, 47
   open-ended, 78–79, 94, 152, 154, 176, 193
   order of, 95
   sociodemographic, 194, 196
   in surveys, 93–95

Quirkos, **212**
quotation marks, 41, 42
quotations, 51
quoting, 307

R

race, 5, 6, 10
race theory, 3
racism, 70
Randolph, J., 40
random digit dial (RDD), 283
rapid assessments, 187, 237
rapid reviews, **38**
readability, 97
realism, 151
reality, 28, 151
reciprocity, 9, 57, 191, 241, 325
recruitment, 5–6, 10, 17, 189, 190–192
Redwood-Jones, Y. A., 161
reference management software 47
reflectivity process, 6, 250
reflexivity, 16, 152–153, 156, 158, 169, 176, 178, 180, 205, 206
RefWorks, 47
reliability, 96–98
Rennison, C. M., 49
replicability, 46
request for proposal (RFP), 121, 122, 130
research,
   applied, 3, 9
   basic, 3, 9
   conducting, 4
   cross-cultural, 4–5, 10, 19, 104, 105
   definition, 2–3, 19
   formal, 3
   fundamental concepts in, 2–20
   identifying assumptions about, 7
   intent of, 2–3
   multicultural, 10
   philosophical underpinnings, 7–11
   relational approach to, 6
   "scientific", 7
   systematic, 4
   transformative, 10, 28, 225
   translational, 6
   see also mixed methods research; participatory research; qualitative research; quantitative research; research findings; research problem; research proposal; research questions; research reports; research study design framework; research team
research ethics board (REB), 13
research ethics committee (REC), 13
research findings,
   disseminating, 22, 212–213, 326–339
   reporting, 30–31, 116, 118, 120, 212–217, 260–261, 296–326
   see also research report
research problem, 22, 171–174
   see also problem statement
research proposal, 181–182
research questions, 23, 33, 120
   distinguished from literature review questions, 40
   formulating, 24
   identifying, 22
   in mixed methods research, 248
   purpose of, 23
   in qualitative research, 23, 73–74, 175–177
   in quantitative research, 23, 73–74, 76–77
   and research design, 24, **25**, **77**
research reports,
   abstract, 299

acknowledgments section, 298
appendices, 302
body of, 299–301
dedications, 298
discussion section, 300–301
disseminating, 309–339
end matter, 301–302
ethical and cultural considerations, 118–119, 305–306, 325
executive summary, 299
front matter, 297–299
guidelines and tools, 302–304
introduction, 299
legal considerations, 304–305
literature review section, 299
methodology section, 299
qualitative, 213–218
reference section, 301
results/findings section, 300
structure, 30–31, 297–301
table of content, 299
title page, 298
types of, 298
writing, 296–309
research study design framework, 20–34
research team, 4, 23, 66–68, 167, 244–245
resources, 137–147
respect for persons principle, 57, 106, 183, 191, 241
respondent validation, 205
retrospective studies, 59
RFP *see* requests for proposal
rights, 4, 141
risks, 14, 16, 101, 140, 183
Rolstad, S., 96

S

SafeAssign, 307
sampling,
   chain referral, 188
   cluster, 84, 85, **252**
   convenience, 85–86, 187, **252**
   heterogenous, 188, **252**
   homogenous, 188, **252**
   maximum variation, 188
   in mixed methods research, 251–253
   nonprobability, 187
   probability, 187
   purposive, 85–86, 187, **252**
   in qualitative research, 187–188
   in quantitative research, 83–87
   quota, 85, 188
   random, 83, *84*, 86, 87, **252**
   size calculations, 87–88, 117, 120, 187–188, 251–253
   snowball, **86**, 188, **252**
   stratified, 83–84, **86**, **252**
   systematic, 84–85, **87**, **252**
   theoretical, 157, 188, **252**
Sandelowski, M., 262
Saxe, John Godfrey, 3
scaterrplots, 113
scientific conference presentations, 322–323
"scientific" research, 7
scientific reasoning, 56
scooping review, **37**
Scopus, **44**
SDGs *see* sustainable development goals
search engines, 40, 43, 44
search statements, 40–42, 45, 52
search terms, 40

security, 141
selection, **64**, **80**
self-determination, 28
self-plagiarism, 307, 308
self-reflection, 159, 169
self-reporting, 103, 117
SEM *see* Socioecological Model
semester-long activity, 146
sentence method, 48
SES *see* socioeconomic status
sexually transmitted infections, 14
sexual orientation, 6, 10
Shaffer, C. F., 266
SHOWeD acronym, 159
Sierra Leone, 74, 100
Silaigwana, B., 16
Silverman, D., 26
Singer, E., 105
Singh, A. A., 213, 214
Smith, K. R., 268
Smith, S., 158
snowballing, 43, 44
snowball sampling, **86**, 188, **252**
social behavioural educational research, 17
social change, 159
social constructivism, 8, 31
social desirability, 93, 103, 120
social exclusion, 70
social justice, 4, 8, 9, 10, 28, 74, 241, 249, 250
social media, 164, 287, 330
social oppression, 10, 28
social policies, 71–72
social studies classes, 230
social support, 81
Socioecological Model (SEM), 27, 265–267, 284, 332
socioecological systems perspective, 70, *71*
socioeconomic development, 71
socioeconomic disparities, 72
socioeconomic status (SES), 6, 10, 72
   see also low-income populations; poor, the
software,
   anti-plagiarism, 307–308
   concept mapping, 75
   data analysis, 29, 206, 211, **212**
   reference management, 47
   sample size calculations, 87
songs, 8
South Africa, 16
sovereignty, 28
Spearman's rank-order correlation, 111
Spearman's rho, 113
split-half technique, 96
SRQR *see* Standards for Reporting Qualitative Research
Stake, R. E. 154
stakeholder engagement, 5–7, 74
Standards for Reporting Qualitative Research (SRQR), 214
statistical analysis, 3, 109–115
statistical regression to the mean, **64**, **80**, 117
statistical significance, 82
statistical tests, **115**
stemming, 40
stigmatization, 305–306
Stockton, C. M., 178
Strauss, A. L., 156–157, 170, 174, 208
Strekalova, Y. A., 6
stress, 71, 158
STROBE (Strengthening the Reporting of Observational Studies in Epidemiology), 123, 302
study sites, 189–190, 199

style manuals, 301, **302–303**
Sudman, S., 92
Sugarman, J., 191
Sullivan, G. M. 299
survey fatigue, 95
survey instruments, 78
   already existing, 88, 120, 253
   designing, 89–98, 254
   pilot testing, 88, 89, 98, 104, 120
   readability, 97
   reliability, 96–98
   translating, 99–100
SurveyMonkey, 105, 255
surveys, 3, 7, 59, 60, 270
   advantages and disadvantages, **79**
   analyzing and interpreting data, 109–118
   comparison of primary and secondary data, 62, 63
   completion, 88, 105, 106, 108
   data collection, 88, 94, 103–106, 120
   design, 78–79
   distribution and delivery, 88, 104–108, 254–255
   ethical considerations, 109–110, 120
   household, 106
   incentives to participate, 105
   interview-mediated, 105–106
   population-based, 62
   prenotification of, 88, 105
   questions in, 93–95
   response rate, 104–106
   self-completion, 105
   semi-structured, 93–94
   structured, 93–94
   telephone, 88, 105, 106, 107
   training of interviewers, 103–104
   validity, 79, 80, 83, 93, 95–96, 103, 104, 120
   web-based, 88, 104–106, 107, 255
   see also survey fatigue; survey instruments
sustainable development goals (SDGs), 70
symbols, 40–41
synthesis, 49, 68
syphilis, 13, 14
systematic research, 4
systematic reviews, **35**, 44, *46*

tables, 111, 300
Taguette, **212**
Tashakkori, A., 225, 265
teachers, 230
teamwork, 91
technical reports, **298**
technological development, 71
Teddlie, C., 225, 264
telephone surveys, 88, 105, 106, **107**
term papers, **298**
terms of reference (ToR), 68, 245
test-retest reliability, 96
text messaging, 88, 105
thematic analysis, 208–209
thematic approach, 30–31, 70
thematic saturation, 188
theoretical framework, 11–13, *22*, 27
   in mixed methods research, 226–241
   in qualitative research, 178–180
   in quantitative research, 70–72, 91
theoretical saturation, 188
theory of planned behavior, 70
thesis, 38, **298**

Thorpe, C. T., 92
Thurstone scale, 92
thyroid cancer, 158
Tomasi, J., 261
topic selection, 23
ToR *see* terms of reference
Torrance, H., 241, 244
traditional (narrative) review, **35**, 38, 52
training, 17, 103–104
transcription, 29, 207
transferability, 30, 206
transformative research, 10, 28, 225
translation, 99–100, 144, 207–208
transparency, 46, 48, 119, 214
travel expenses, 130
TREND (Transparent Reporting of Evaluation with Nonrandomized Designs, 321
triangulation, 26, 65, 155, 205, 206, 226–228, 241
truncations, 40, **42**
trust, 9, 58, 75, 104
trustworthiness, 29, 205–206, 218
truth, 7
truthfulness, 30
t-tests, 111, 114
tuberculosis, 305
Turkey, 230
TurnitIn, 307
Tuskegee Study of Untreated Syphilis in Negro Male, 13, 14, 183

U

ubuntu, 57
United Nations Convention on the Rights of Persons with Disabilities (CRPD), 57
univariate analysis, 110
US Code of Federal Regulations (CFR), 13, 18
US Department of Health and Human Services, 13
US National Commission for the Protection of Human Subjects in Biomedical and Behavioral Research, 13

V

vaccine trials, 14
validity, 26, 29
    concurrent, 29, 95
    construct, 29, 95, **96**
    content, 29, 95, **96**
    criterion, 95, **96**
    cross-cultural, 96
    definition, 95
    external, 63, 79
    internal, 63, **64**, 79, **80**, 103
    mixed methods research, 237–238, 242
    predictive, 29, 95
    qualitative research, 29–30
    quantitative research, 29, 58, 61, 63–64, 79, **80**, 83, 116–118
    structural, 95
    surveys, 79, **80**, 83, **93**, 95–96, 103, 104, 120
    types of, 95
values, 58, 67, 151, 241, 254
van Kippersluis, H., 72
verification, 207
video recordings, 202, 206
Viergever, R. F., 121
violence, 4
virtual interviews, 200–201
visual literacy, 330
voluntary participation, 141
vulnerable populations, 14, 19, 58, 159, 165, 170, 184, 191

W

Wang, C., 159, 160
Wassenaar, D., 16
Watkins, D. C., 240
web-based surveys, 88, 104–106, **107**, 255
Web of Science (database), **44**
websites, 43
well-being, 70
WHO *see* World Health Organization
Wilcoxon signed-rank test, 111
wild cards, 40, **42**
Wiley's Journal Finder Beta, 312
Wilson, A. T., 264
Wolcott, H. F., 208
women, 10, 154, 159, 165, 199, 250
    and childbirth, 179
    immigrant, 90, 266–268
    pregnant, 13, 172
    prenatal care, 264–280
Woolf, S. H., 6
World Health Organization (WHO), 13, 70, 121, 281, 306
World Medical Association, 13
worldviews, 6, 9, 28, 29, 57

Y

Ye, C., 105
Yin, R. K., 154–155
Young, S., 92

Z

Zhang, Y., 250
zip codes, 255, *256*
Zotero, 47